Transplantation: A Companion to Specialist
Surgical Practice
Third Edition

Take a look at the other great titles in the Companion Series...

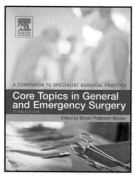
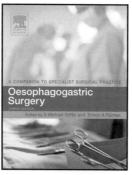
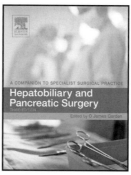
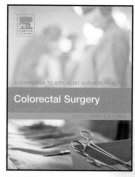
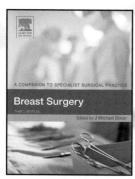
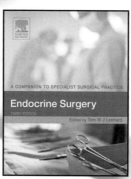
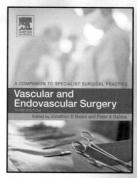
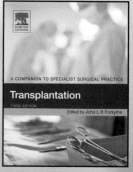
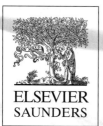

A Companion to Specialist Surgical Practice
Third Edition

Series Editors
O. James Garden
Simon Paterson-Brown

Transplantation: A Companion to Specialist Surgical Practice

Third Edition

Edited by
John L.R. Forsythe
Consultant Transplant Surgeon
Transplant Unit
Royal Infirmary of Edinburgh

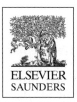

ELSEVIER
SAUNDERS

ELSEVIER
SAUNDERS

An imprint of Elsevier Limited

First edition 1997
Second edition 2001
Third edition 2005
© 2005, Elsevier Limited. All rights reserved.

ISBN 0 7020 2737 5

British Library Cataloguing in Publication Data
A catalogue record for this book is available from the British Library

Library of Congress Cataloging in Publication Data
A catalog record for this book is available from the Library of Congress

Notice
Medical knowledge is constantly changing. Standard safety precautions must be followed, but as new research and clinical experience broaden our knowledge, changes in treatment and drug therapy may become necessary or appropriate. Readers are advised to check the most current product information provided by the manufacturer of each drug to be administered to verify the recommended dose, the method and duration of administration, and contraindications. It is the responsibility of the practitioner, relying on experience and knowledge of the patient, to determine dosages and the best treatment for each individual patient. Neither the Publisher nor the editor assumes any liability for any injury and/or damage to persons or property arising from this publication.
The Publisher

Printed in The Netherlands
Last digit is the print number: 9 8 7 6 5 4 3 2 1

Commissioning Editor: Michael Houston
Project Development Manager: Sheila Black
Editorial Assistants: Kathryn Mason, Liz Brown
Project Manager: Cheryl Brant
Design Manager: Jayne Jones
Illustration Manager: Mick Ruddy
Illustrator: Martin Woodward
Marketing Managers: Gaynor Jones (UK), Ethel Cathers (USA)

Contents

Contributors

Murat Akyol MD FRCS
Consultant Transplant Surgeon
Royal Infirmary of Edinburgh;
Honorary Clinical Senior Lecturer
University of Edinburgh
Edinburgh, UK

Simon T. Ball MA PhD MRCP
Consultant Nephrologist
University Hospital
Birmingham, UK

John J. Casey MB ChB PhD FRCS
Consultant Transplant Surgeon
Royal Infirmary of Edinburgh
Edinburgh, UK

Stephen C. Clark BMedSci BM BS DM FRCS(CTh)
Consultant Cardiothoracic Surgeon
Freeman Hospital
Newcastle upon Tyne, UK

Margaret J. Dallman DPhil
Professor of Immunology
Imperial College London
London, UK

Philip A. Dyer PhD FRCPath
Consultant Clinical Scientist
Transplantation Laboratory
Manchester Royal Infirmary;
Honorary Reader in Transplantation
Science
University of Manchester
Manchester, UK

Olivier Farges MD PhD
Professor of Surgery
Hôpital Beaujon
Clichy, Paris, France

Robert S. Gaston MD
Professor of Medicine
Medical Director, Kidney and
Pancreas Transplantation
University of Alabama at
Birmingham
Birmingham, AL, USA

Keith P. Graetz MA MB BChir MRCS
Specialist Registrar
Nottingham City Hospital
Nottingham, UK

Asif Hasan FRCS(CTh)
Consultant Cardiothoracic Surgeon
Freeman Hospital
Newcastle upon Tyne, UK

Benjamin E. Hippen MD
Clinical Instructor of Medicine
University of Alabama at
Birmingham
Birmingham, AL, USA

Alison Langton BSc MPhil
Senior Clinical Scientist
Transplantation Laboratory
Manchester Royal Infirmary
Manchester, UK

Helen Liggett BSc MSc
Senior Clinical Scientist
Transplantation Laboratory
Manchester Royal Infirmary
Manchester, UK

Lorna P. Marson MD FRCS
Senior Lecturer in Transplant
Surgery
Transplant Unit
Royal Infirmary of Edinburgh
Edinburgh, UK

Rafael Matesanz MD PhD
President, Transplant Committee
Council of Europe;
Director, Spanish National
Transplant Organization
Madrid, Spain

Charles G. Newstead BSc MB BS MD MRCP FRCP
Consultant Renal Physician
Leeds Teaching Hospital Trust
Leeds, UK

Neil R. Parrott MD FRCS
Consultant Transplant Surgeon
Manchester Royal Infirmary
Manchester, UK

William D. Plant BSc MB MRCPI FRCP
Consultant Renal Physician
Cork University Hospital
Cork, Ireland

Keith M. Rigg MD FRCS
Consultant Surgeon
Nottingham City Hospital
Nottingham, UK

Christopher J. Rudge BSc MB BS FRCS
Medical Director
UK Transplant
Bristol, UK

A.M. James Shapiro MD PhD FRCS FRCSC
Director, Clinical Islet Transplant
Program
University of Alberta
Edmonton, Canada

Stephen J. Wigmore BSc MB BS MD FRCS(Ed) FRCS
Senior Lecturer and Wellcome
Fellow
University of Edinburgh;
Honorary Consultant Surgeon
Royal Infirmary of Edinburgh
Edinburgh, UK

Karen Wood BSc MSc
Senior Clinical Scientist
Transplantation Laboratory
Manchester Royal Infirmary
Manchester, UK

Judith Worthington BSc
Senior Clinical Scientist
Transplantation Laboratory
Manchester Royal Infirmary
Manchester, UK

Preface

The *Companion to Specialist Surgical Practice* series was designed to meet the needs of surgeons in higher training and the practising consultant who wish up-to-date and evidence-based information on the subspecialist areas relevant to their surgical practice. In trying to meet this aim, we have recognised that the series will never be as all-encompassing as many of the larger reference surgical textbooks. However, by their very size, it is rare that the latter are completely up to date at the time of publication. The first edition of this series was published in 1997, with the second following in 2001. In this third edition, we have been able to bring up to date the relevant specialist information that we and the individual volume editors consider important for the practising subspecialist surgeon. Where possible, all contributors have attempted to identify evidence-based references to support key recommendations within each chapter. These should all be interpreted with the help of the guidance summary 'Evidence-based practice in surgery', which follows this preface.

We are extremely grateful to all volume editors and to their contributors to this third edition. It is thanks to their enthusiasm and hard work that the relatively short time frame between each of the editions has been maintained, thereby providing to the reader the most accurate and up-to-date information possible. We were all immensely saddened by the sudden and tragic death of Professor John Farndon, who edited the first and second editions of the volumes *Breast Surgery* and *Endocrine Surgery*. While recognising that he was a unique and talented individual, we are pleased to welcome the additional editorial skills of Mike Dixon and Tom Lennard for this third edition.

We are also grateful for the support and encouragement of Elsevier Ltd and hope that our aim – of providing up-to-date and affordable surgical texts – has been met and that all readers, whether in training or in consultant practice, will find this third edition a valuable resource.

O. James Garden BSc, MB, ChB, MD, FRCS(Glasg), FRCS(Ed), FRCP(Ed)
Regius Professor of Clinical Surgery, Clinical and Surgical Sciences (Surgery), University of Edinburgh, and Honorary Consultant Surgeon, Royal Infirmary of Edinburgh

Simon Paterson-Brown MB, BS, MPhil, MS, FRCS(Ed), FRCS
Honorary Senior Lecturer, Clinical and Surgical Sciences (Surgery), University of Edinburgh, and Consultant General and Upper Gastrointestinal Surgeon, Royal Infirmary of Edinburgh

EVIDENCE-BASED PRACTICE IN SURGERY

The third edition of the *Companion to Specialist Surgical Practice* series has attempted to incorporate, where appropriate, **evidence-based practice in surgery**, which has been highlighted in the text and relevant references. A detailed chapter on evidence-based practice in surgery, written by Kathryn Rigby and Jonathan Michaels, has been included in the volume on *Core Topics in General and Emergency Surgery*, to which the reader is referred for further information on assessing levels of evidence. We are grateful to them for providing this summary for each volume.

Critical appraisal for developing evidence-based practice can be obtained from a number of sources, the most reliable being randomised controlled clinical trials, systematic literature reviews, meta-analyses and observational studies. For practical purposes three grades of evidence can be used, analogous to the levels of 'proof' required in a court of law:

1. **Beyond reasonable doubt** – such evidence is likely to have arisen from high-quality randomised controlled trials, systematic reviews, or high-quality synthesised evidence such as decision analysis, cost-effectiveness analysis or large observational data sets. The studies need to be directly applicable to the population of concern and have clear results. The grade is analogous to burden of proof within a crimimal court and may be thought of as corresponding to the usual standard of 'proof' within the medical literature (i.e. *P*<0.05).

2. **On the balance of probabilities** – in many cases a high-quality review of literature may fail to reach firm conclusions owing to conflicting or inconclusive results, trials of poor methodological quality or the lack of evidence in the population to which the guidelines apply. In such cases it may still be possible to make a statement as to the best treatment on the 'balance of probabilities'. This is analogous to the decision in a civil court where all the available evidence will be weighed up and the verdict will depend upon the balance of probabilities.

3. **Not proven** – insufficient evidence upon which to base a decision or contradictory evidence.

Depending on the information available three grades of recommendation can be used:

a. strong recommendation, which should be followed unless there are compelling reasons to act otherwise;

b. a recommendaton based on evidence of effectiveness, but where there may be other factors to take into account in decision-making, for example the user of the guidelines may be expected to take into account patient preferences, local facilities, local audit results or available resources;

c. a recommendation made where there is no adequate evidence as to the most effective practice, although there may be reasons for making a recommendation in order to minimise cost or reduce the chance of error through a locally agreed protocol.

The text and references that are considered to be associated with reasonable evidence are highlighted in this volume with a 'scalpel code', leaving the reader to reach his or her own conclusion.

Editor's note

Although part of a surgical series, this volume is not just for surgeons. It is for all those who play an important role in the transplant procedure. Thus it has been designed to interest nursing staff who care for organ failure patients, transplant coordinators, theatre staff, immunology laboratory staff, para-medical personnel, physicians and surgeons. Modern techniques in transplantation and new forms of immunosuppression, emphasised throughout this volume, have increased the complexity of clinical and ethical dilemmas that face the whole team caring for the transplant patient. Appropriate responses to such dilemmas are required to ensure the continued success of transplantation medicine.

John L.R. Forsythe MD FRCS(Ed) FRCS
Consultant Transplant Surgeon, Transplant Unit,
Royal Infirmary of Edinburgh

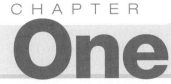

The ethics of transplantation

Stephen J. Wigmore and
William D. Plant

The medical profession has long subscribed to a body of ethical statements developed primarily for the benefit of the patient. As a member of this profession, a physician must recognise responsibility to patients first and foremost, as well as to society, to other health professionals, and to self.

American Medical Association[1]

Philosophy, n. A route of many roads leading from nowhere to nothing.

Ambrose Bierce[2]

INTRODUCTION

The sentiment of Ambrose Bierce may still retain adherents within the transplant community. This is unfortunate. Ethical and moral dilemmas pervade the practice of organ transplantation. This chapter advances the thesis that best practice in organ transplantation requires:

1. sensitivity to the ethical dimension within clinical situations;
2. fluency in the language of ethical discussion;
3. skill in the practical resolution of ethically complex scenarios.

These complement the parallel sensitivities, fluencies and skills in immunology, pharmacology, nursing, medicine, surgery and logistic organisation upon which successful transplant programmes are built. Perhaps we do not acknowledge the ethical issues as explicitly as the others.

The spectrum of ethical dilemmas is broad

How do we decide to whom we should allocate scarce resources such as liver allografts? Should we favour those with the greatest immediate need (such as victims of self-poisoning with paracetamol) or those with the greatest potential for long-term benefit (such as young patients with chronic cholestatic disease)? Should we perform living-donor allograft procedures when there is a high probability of early primary disease recurrence? How much information must we transmit to patients to be sure that we can establish truly informed consent to a transplant procedure? Is it ever right to financially reward organ donors? Is xenotransplantation morally acceptable?

These are some of the core paradigms repeatedly encountered in organ transplantation. In this chapter we seek to explore some of them in more detail, using reflection upon examples to illustrate the more general principles underlying the nature of particular ethical dilemmas. The examples are not real cases, but have been assembled to exhibit particular issues.

We do not feel that the explicit use of philosophical terms should be confined to the seminar room or to the bar-room discussion. Description facilitates discussion, and both of these facilitate understanding. If, as clinicians of conscience, good character and integrity, we can become more comfortable working through such a process then, perhaps, we will be more skilled in the practice of resolving ethical dilemmas.

These issues impact upon us in a number of ways – as healthcare professionals, as citizens and as individuals. The remarkable advances in transplantation over the last 30 years have presented ever more challenging scenarios at a bewildering pace. In performing 'new' procedures we have developed our technological capacity more rapidly than the philosophical, legal and cultural procedures with which to decide how best to resolve the ethical dilemmas that these present.

We live in a pluralist society in which individuals hold different, but reasonable, views on how ethical issues should be resolved. Traditional medical ethics focused almost exclusively upon the professional ethics of physicians and on the doctor–patient relationship. In contemporary times (and in parallel with the revolution in biotechnology) the term 'bioethics' has come to enjoy a broader usage. This retains traditional medical ethics at its core but also acknowledges interplay with the more general ethics of biology, science, sociology and culture.[3]

SYSTEMS AND PRINCIPLES IN MEDICAL ETHICS AND BIOETHICS

The ethical basis of Western medicine is characterised by a number of traditions,[3] which find expression in codes of practice and in the culture of healthcare workers. Prominent amongst these are the deontological (duty-based) and the utilitarian (consequence-based) traditions.

The deontological tradition[3] stresses the duties of practitioners and the rights of patients. Many codes[3] of practice, such as the Hippocratic Oath, the Declaration of Geneva and the General Medical Council Statements[4] on 'Duties and Responsibilities of Doctors' are of this tradition. There is a strand of rational, universalising deliberation within deontology that may, in some circumstances, seem uncompromising and excessively rigid. Clinicians 'ought' to act in particular ways because this is 'right', often irrespective of the consequences. Any act should be capable of being expressed as a universal law. The great strength of the deontological tradition is its stress on the autonomy of the patient and on the primacy of doctor–patient relationships. It asserts that individuals should always be viewed as **ends** in themselves, never as **means** to an end. Its weakness is in application. 'Absolute' principles that are contradictory may co-present in particular circumstances (e.g. 'never cause pain', 'always preserve life' – what if life-saving interventions cause pain?).

On the other hand the utilitarian tradition[3] aspires always to do that which leads to a 'good' or 'best' outcome. It is commonly paraphrased as 'Seek the greatest good of the greatest number'. If the 'right' action does not lead to the 'best' outcome then it should be reviewed or abandoned. The necessity for rationing of healthcare resources brings utilitarian analyses into particular prominence. On occasion, the individual may be the 'loser' in the greater scheme of things – a common criticism of this approach.

It is important to remember that utilitarian analysis can be applied to an individual case – what is in a patient's, as opposed to all patients' best interests (or will lead to the best outcomes)? Two strands may be identified – 'rule' utilitarianism and 'act' utilitarianism. 'Rule' utilitarianism weighs up the consequences of acting according to a **general moral rule** (e.g. that patients over 65 years with type II diabetes should never receive transplants as the long-term survival of this group is likely to be less than that of a younger non-diabetic group). 'Act' utilitarianism weighs up the consequences of **a particular act** (e.g. deciding not to proceed with living donation in a case where there is a high risk of recurrence of a primary disease in the recipient).

It is important to stress that these traditions are **not** opposite ways of viewing and acting upon ethical dilemmas. Most analyses will show that they tend to derive the same conclusions when 'working' moral issues are at stake.

Both traditions have a strong flavour of universalisability. However, as all ethical analyses ultimately focus on **particular** cases, the importance of **context** may well have been understated in the past. Some current intellectual traditions, notably existentialism, situation ethics and postmodernism[3] are less convinced of the existence of general laws/principles that can be applied to particular cases. Rather, they focus on how to solve specific problems as they arise and are open to the insights of other religious, racial, philosophical and cultural traditions. The principal criticism of these traditions is that moral relativism may easily drift into moral anarchy (although, of course, moral absolutism may similarly drift into moral fascism).

In real life, we recognise a spectrum between cases in which context and situation need to be the dominant consideration and those in which universally derived general principles can be applied. No one tradition or perspective is 'more correct' – they offer different perspectives to problem solving.

PRINCIPLES

A number of prima facie principles (commonly distilled to four) are widely accepted as forming the bedrock of medical ethics.[3,4] As we shall see, in individual cases there is often conflict between the simultaneous adherence to all of these. Depending on the context (and on whether a deontological or utilitarian approach is favoured), a 'least unsatisfactory' trade-off between principles must be negotiated or achieved. Skill in identifying and achieving the best balance is that which characterises best practice in dealing with moral dilemmas.

1. Beneficence: doing good[3,4]

A central tenet of medical ethics is the obligation to strive at all times to do good for the patient. Deontologists view this as a universal moral duty, utilitarians as achieving the universally desired best outcome. It is instructive to reflect upon the secondary obligations that follow from acceptance of this principle. Beneficence demands competence. Accreditation and continuing medical education are central to this, as are elements such as professional

development, clinical and basic research, and audit. Transplant programmes with clinical governance processes in place are expressing vigorous adherence to this principle. Communication skills are vital – weighing up possible outcomes is one thing, sharing them with the patient and negotiating choices quite another.

2. Non-maleficence: avoiding harm[3,4]

Since the days of Hippocrates, clinicians have endorsed the principle of 'Primum non nocere' ('First, do no harm'). All interventions, however well intentioned, may cause harm. Making sure that the balance between benefit and harm is appropriate is an important clinical judgement. In the past, professional decisions (i.e. that the balance achieved by a particular course of action was acceptable) often paid scant attention to the patients' perspectives of the balance. This might be called **paternalism** – classically according predominant weight to clinicians' judgement on the balance between beneficence and non-maleficence, with little weight given to patient autonomy.

The other end of the spectrum is where overwhelming emphasis is placed on respect for patient autonomy, with little reflection on professional judgement of beneficence/non-maleficence trade-offs. This is equally undesirable and might be called **consumerism**.

3. Respect for autonomy[3–5]

Individuals should be treated as ends, not as means. Respect for the dignity, integrity and authenticity of the person is a basic human right. Deriving from this principle are the important issues of consent and confidentiality. Patients with capacity to understand relevant information (explained in broad terms and with simple language), to consider its implications in terms of their own values, and come to a communicable decision, are deemed to have decision-making capacity. (The legal default is that conscious adults are assumed to have capacity unless evidence to the contrary can be advanced.) Some patients, because of transient or irreversible cognitive impairment, may not have this capacity. It is important to note that even a decision that seems irrational to the physician **must** be respected if the patient has decision-making capacity. The issue is more complex regarding children under 16 years.

Informed consent is central to the doctor–patient relationship. Its definition is difficult – in countries such as Australia and Canada there is a **legal** duty to provide patients with information that a **prudent or reasonable patient**, in that patient's particular circumstances, would wish to know in order to arrive at a decision. In the UK, the amount of information that a **reasonable doctor** would provide, in that patient's particular circumstances, is required.[6] (However, a court might decide that, in unusual circumstances, failure to disclose certain risks of procedures might be negligent, **even if this is accepted practice** as attested by a responsible body of medical opinion.) Information about certain possible risks may be retained under so-called **therapeutic privilege**, if it is honestly felt that this would needlessly harm the patient psychologically (justified by an 'act' utilitarian attitude with heavy emphasis on non-maleficence). This privilege cannot be invoked when informed consent to participation in a research study is being obtained – for obvious reasons. No overt or covert pressure to consent should exist. Many guidelines[7] exist to help deal with difficulties in obtaining consent.

Case history

A 23-year-old man has developed fulminant hepatic failure after taking an overdose of paracetamol following the breakdown of a long-term relationship. This is his first attempt at self-harm and after consultation with his family he is listed for urgent liver transplantation. A donor organ becomes available and the transplant is successful. During the recovery period the recipient expresses his dismay at having received a transplant. He states that he still wishes to die and refuses to take his immunosuppressive medication.

In this case it could be argued that transplantation in an individual who has expressed, by his actions, a wish to die, is a breach of his autonomy. In general terms, interventions made when patients do not have the capacity to offer consent should follow certain principles. Any advance directives should be consulted; persons with knowledge of the patient's previous views should be consulted for their insight into the possible choices that the patient might have made were he able to participate. Family cannot consent to any procedure on his behalf, unless there is a legal guardianship in existence. The decision as to how best to proceed should be taken by the doctor with overall responsibility for the case. Choices should be limited to those that are in the patient's best interests and that least limit the patient's future choices should he regain the capacity to consent. In this situation the clinicians have used the principle of beneficence to justify the act of transplantation, in the hope that the attempt at self-harm was, at best, accidental or, at worst, not intended to result in death. A utilitarian perspective might argue against transplantation in this situation, giving priority in the allocation of organs to individuals who have unequivocally expressed a desire to live. Alternatively, it could be argued that the circumstances precipitating this act of self-harm are transient or that the normal mental state of the individual may have been temporarily disturbed. This could respond to a change in circumstances or to treatment with appropriate counselling or medications. In this unusual scenario, the reiteration by the patient that he wishes to die and his refusal to continue with treatment necessary to keep the transplant functional, presents a complex matrix of interaction between differing principles. If he has regained the capacity to consent, then his autonomy must be respected. On the other hand, this should prompt a discussion as to the reasons why the original choice was made. Beneficence and non-maleficence may prompt the clinicians strongly to counsel him to continue with treatment. It should be pointed out (in the spirit of justice) that he has received a scarce resource and that a range of individuals have done their best to make the right choice for him. One might wish to use this as a pragmatic 'emotional lever' in the discussion – however, primacy must be given to his autonomy.

4. Justice: promoting fairness[3,4]

This is a very important principle in the ethics of transplantation, where demand far outstrips supply. In that context, the allocation of organs requires a rank-ordering system with some philosophical justification for the method chosen. There are many theories of justice, some deriving from the deontological and utilitarian traditions. If scarce resources are to be allocated, then how should this be done?

A 'rule' utilitarian approach might suggest that we always seek to maximise the overall welfare of the group or minimise the waste of resources. Many transplant services have allocation systems loosely built upon the premise that selecting and organising allocation around a limited number of criteria predictive of best outcome (such as HLA types) best serves this purpose.

This disadvantages some patients. Other systems operate very strict acceptance criteria for listing – again meeting some of the requirements for fairness, but not all. Discrimination on the basis of race, gender, age or 'social worth' obviously violates the principle of justice.

It is important to acknowledge that justice and fairness need to be applied broadly. These principles apply to the individual patient, but also to other patients whose circumstances may be influenced by events relating to that patient. Similarly, we need to be fair to other members of the transplant team and to the broader needs of society.

Implementation of the four principles: interactions

Although the four principles listed above are the central principles in medical ethics and bioethics, there are different interactions between different 'players' in their implementation. Issues relating to beneficence and non-maleficence lie very much in the domain of the clinician/doctor–patient relationship, with particular focus on individual patient events. Issues of respect for autonomy and justice interact much more widely, with greater roles for the law, social policy, politics and culture. In addition, these latter apply more readily to groups of patients rather than to individuals. Despite this, all four principles should be given due and equal consideration in case analyses.

A second trend is worthy of comment: autonomy and justice are themes enjoying considerably more attention now than in the past, when medical paternalism may have been a more culturally dominant phenomenon than in the present.

CADAVERIC ORGAN DONATION

There has been an increase in live-donor organ procurement in recent years. However, the majority of available organs still come from cadaveric donors – predominantly donors confirmed as dead by brainstem testing, but with non-heart-beating donor procurement programmes in place in a number of transplant centres. This resource base is shrinking. This, in combination with the ever-increasing rise in potential recipients, is a cause of considerable pressure on transplantation programmes. Various solutions to this problem have been advanced. All pose difficult ethical problems.

The cadaveric organ donor

Case history

A 25-year-old man suffers a serious head injury in the workplace. He lives in a stable relationship with his girlfriend of 6 years. He has an extensive, loving family. He does not carry a donor card. He requires emergency ventilation whilst investigation and treatment proceeds. He is found to have suffered irreversible brain damage and, although his heart is still beating, brainstem function tests confirm that he is dead.

This is the classic paradigm at the heart of the enterprise of organ transplantation.

1. SHOULD THIS MAN'S ORGANS BE USED FOR TRANSPLANTATION?

We have no idea as to this man's wishes. Up to 20% of the population are believed to carry organ donor cards, but these are found in fewer than 10% of potential donors when the moment of choice arises. This man has never discussed this situation with another person in so far as it can be established. He has not been added to a register of organ donors (the United Kingdom Transplant Organ Donor Register exceeded 11 million at the beginning of 2004). This currently leads to the application of the classic processes in cadaveric organ procurement.

One analysis would be to presume, in the absence of evidence to the contrary, that he consents to organ donation. If no advance directive exists, then enquiry needs to be made of his family as to whether or not they feel that he would have objected. If they are in agreement that his organs be removed then permission to do so may be given. This is, therefore, largely a pragmatic process. What is the status of his girlfriend? What if there is family disagreement? Although primarily utilitarian in intent, this approach exhibits a deontological commitment to autonomy and justice.

This action presumes consent **subject to family agreement**. A utilitarian argument might be that this approach does not facilitate maximum possible organ procurement. Indeed, in the UK up to 45% of families in a recent study are reported as declining to consent to organ retrieval. Different approaches have been advanced in face of this.

Some would argue that consent **should** be presumed unless the man himself has previously expressed an objection (i.e. has **opted out** of this presumption). Family agreement, although desirable, would not be necessary. An approach similar to this has been adopted in a number of European countries, and debate rages as to the impact this strategy makes on procurement. The societal logistics of this are complex – to what degree should the state ensure that individuals have had access to a process allowing him or her to 'opt out'? One strategy is to provide opportunities for **mandated choice**. This would present individuals with the opportunity to record their choice at times when selected documentation is being completed (e.g. application for driving licences). Pilot studies, however, suggest that this will not achieve total coverage of populations.

Opponents of an 'opt-out' strategy argue that it places a different (and perhaps lesser) emphasis on the principle of autonomy; that it treats individuals as means rather than ends; that it may be less fair to surviving relatives; and that (from a utilitarian standpoint) it may be counterproductive. Public opinion is notably fickle. An incident in which, for example, family objections or distress were dealt with insensitively could lead to adverse publicity, potentially compromising organ donation in general.

Ultimately this is a conflict between a deontological view that the individual's right to beneficence, non-maleficence and respect should not be accorded lesser weight than a utilitarian view that other patients have similar rights (manifest as their need for a transplant).

2. HOW SHOULD THE FURTHER MANAGEMENT OF THIS MAN PROCEED?

The patient is brainstem dead, a concept now widely accepted. It is argued that a certificate of death could be issued at the time of completion of brainstem function tests, rather than when the heart finally stops.[8] Most of the major religious traditions accept this concept.[9]

The primary obligation of those caring for this man is to administer treatment that is to **his** benefit. It could be argued that human rights include the right to dignity at the end of life, the right to die as one might wish, and to be remembered as an individual.

If the patient has consented to be an organ donor, then facilitating the expression of this altruistic act may be the last expression of autonomy and, as such, is beneficent. In circumstances where consent has been presumed, then the same principles apply.

However, it is inevitable that management of the patient's fluid balance and cardiovascular status will differ if he is being managed as a donor. There is a sense that this, in some ways, violates the primary obligation of treating him only to his benefit. However, **he is now dead**, and, as such, the issue of beneficence/non-maleficence does not apply in the same way. It is difficult to know what ethical principles apply to 'treatment' of the dead. Certainly, respect for the dignity of the recently deceased is appropriate and mandatory.

Case history continued

Having granted consent to the procedure of organ donation the family of the donor is informed about a clinical trial of a promising treatment that has the potential to improve the functional quality of organs destined to be used for transplantation. They are informed that involvement in this study will require the donor to be given a drug by injection before the organs are removed but will not involve any other variation from the normal protocol of organ retrieval. They are asked to give their consent to this procedure.

Objection to treatment administered to the donor for the potential benefit of the future recipient might be on the grounds that there is no conceivable benefit to the donor; that such treatment assumes consent that might have been withheld and that, on utilitarian grounds, adverse events accompanying such treatment might prejudice public opinion about organ donation. Alternative arguments might be that improved transplant outcomes following such treatment would increase the 'value' of the altruistic gift, increasing beneficence and, again on utilitarian grounds, might increase the availability of organs for transplant thus benefiting society as a whole. No clear ethical precedent exists to help resolve this question, but examples of optimising donor management already include administration of antibiotics, vasopressors and fluids to donors. These are generally accepted as part of normal management.

3. ARE THE ISSUES DIFFERENT IF (A) HE HAS NOT ALREADY BEEN PLACED ON A VENTILATOR OR (B) HIS HEART HAS STOPPED BEATING?

The first of these has been the subject of considerable discussion.[10,11] The stimulus to electively ventilate potential organ donors (particularly those with major intracerebral injury) who will suffer what would otherwise be a terminal respiratory arrest has been utilitarian – an attempt to correct the ongoing shortfall between the supply of donor organs and the demand for these. From the perspective of the potential donor, there are arguments against such a strategy, particularly if analysed within the deontological model. It would be difficult to argue that such an intervention would do any good to the potential donor, thereby violating the principle of beneficence.

It is a considerable upgrading of therapy compared with that mentioned above **if its only objective is to facilitate organ procurement**. If the patient had previously expressed a desire to be an organ donor, then one might contend that fulfilling his wish to participate in an altruistic act is beneficent. In practice, this would be an uncommon occurrence. Another unlikely (but possible) outcome might be that the patient might not, if ventilated at the point of respiratory arrest, subsequently develop brainstem death. Instead he might recover sufficient respiratory function to survive in a persistent vegetative state – a disastrous outcome clearly violating the principle of non-maleficence.

If the moment of intervention (to ventilate) occurs at or before the point of respiratory arrest then a different situation pertains, especially if the patient has not consented to **this particular intervention** (ventilation) for **this specific purpose** (facilitation of organ donation). The patient is **alive** at this point. Doctors may only treat a living patient from whom consent has not been obtained if it is to his or her benefit **and for no other purpose**. It is further

argued that relatives may not give consent in this circumstance, unless acting as properly designated health proxies or with power of attorney.

This argument, within a deontological analysis, suggests that none of the four principles (with the possible exception of fairness to potential organ recipients) are particularly adhered to with an elective ventilation programme, and that this practice may be unethical. A utilitarian analysis, on the other hand, would argue that many beneficial outcomes may follow. These might include improved health (or even life) for patients with organ failure, and happiness for the family that 'some good came from the situation'. It is further contended that the risk of **real** (as opposed to theoretical) harm to the patient is very low.

This issue is at a 'stand-off' in the UK at present, although clarification of the legal issues would be welcome. It also helps to consider the background to this problem in terms of justice and fairness. It is important that medical and nursing staff in intensive therapy units (ITUs) are comfortable with this concept and happy to participate if such an endeavour is deemed legal, ethical and desirable. Such staff may also wonder if using (scarce) resources in this way does not compromise the care of other patients requiring ITU care. This issue needs to 'sell' to an extensive constituency of stakeholders, and a simple 'rule' utilitarianism suggestion that 'We must maximise organ procurement, come what may' is probably not a sufficient justification.

The use of non-heart-beating donors is again driven by utilitarian considerations and may occur in two circumstances. First, consider a patient who is ventilated, but not brain-dead, with such severe injuries that a decision is taken to discontinue therapy. Within 60 minutes of the terminal cardio-respiratory arrest there is a window of opportunity to remove organs for use in donation. In this situation there is little difference from the general principles addressed above, because the patient is **dead**.[12] The speed of procurement may seem a little distasteful, but probably does not pose a substantive additional moral problem.

A second, more controversial, area is when a patient suffers sudden unexpected death (usually a witnessed out-of-hospital cardiac arrest). It may be possible to preserve kidneys for the purposes of transplantation (after establishing that resuscitation has been unsuccessful) if facilities are available to initiate in situ cooling of the kidneys by insertion of an intra-aortic balloon catheter. This will give an opportunity to discuss organ donation with the family.

The main ethical issues relate to the morality of initiating a procedure on a dead body without consent having been obtained, and before consultation with family members (which may be impractical within the necessary timeframe). Once the opportunity to consult with family members has occurred then the issues discussed previously apply.

The introduction of the Human Tissue Act 2004 resolves some of the ethical issues faced by non-heart-beating organ donation programmes. In this legislation, it is agreed that placement of the catheter maintains the possibility of donation (which would otherwise be lost) and is therefore lawful. These issues have been the subject of much commentary,[13,14] but a number of such programmes (which have usually been commissioned only after extensive discussion with local stakeholders, especially the coroner) have now been successfully established.

Allocation of cadaveric organs

CASE STUDY

A 45-year-old mother of three children has progressive hepatic failure due to primary biliary cirrhosis. She is on the waiting list for hepatic transplantation. Over the last several weeks a number of suitable organs have been procured, but on each occasion these have been given to patients presenting with fulminant hepatic failure. These have included a reformed alcoholic who has taken a paracetamol overdose and a prisoner (serving a life sentence for the sexual assault and murder of two schoolchildren) who had developed non-A non-B fulminant hepatitis.

Who 'owns' these organs? In whose gift is the decision as to allocation? No legal answer to this currently exists in the UK (or in many other states).[15] Indeed, it is not entirely clear if the notion of 'property' in a dead body (or part of a dead body) exists unless it has been subjected to 'a process or application of human skill' (including stuffing or embalming).[5] It is an issue in need of clarification.[16] However, there is a general presumption that the state has a responsibility for the allocation or disposal of the said organ(s), which it discharges by delegation to the appropriate agency or transplant team.[15]

The notion of **distributive justice** applies here. Some models are generally unacceptable on ethical, cultural or political grounds. These might include systematic discrimination on the grounds of race, gender, religion or political beliefs. To date, the notion that cadaveric donation and allocation can be made conditional (by the donor/donor's family) to attributes of the recipient is not an accepted premise. This was reaffirmed in the February 2000 report of an investigation (chaired by Chris Kelly, Permanent Secretary at the UK Department of Health) into an event where racist conditions had been attached to procurement of organs from a cadaveric donor. In this context, the principle of justice in a deontological analysis was felt to hold precedence over any utilitarian analysis.

Slightly less obviously, there may be a (natural human) tendency to see some individuals as having greater social 'worth' or 'merit' (the 'blameless' mother-of-three versus the self-harming paracetamol self-poisoner or the decidedly unappealing prisoner). We may like some patients more than others. Whereas these may be understandable sentiments, there is an obligation of impartiality, transparency and justice in making these decisions. Furthermore, the perceptions of the clinician could easily be construed as prejudices, reflecting his or her value systems rather than those of the profession or society as a whole.

Some extreme solutions have been advocated. Cahn[17] has suggested that if not everybody can have access to scarce resources, then nobody should! This values an extreme sense of equity, but is hardly appealing in any other fashion. Doyal[18] suggests randomisation – again appealing to an absolute model of equity. Systems involving attempts at welfare maximisation are more generally accepted. Stratifying likely outcomes by criteria such as human leucocyte antigen (HLA) matching in kidney transplantation is one such model. This is a form of 'rule' utilitarianism that meets some of the necessary criteria of justice, but not all. Some patients will be disadvantaged, perhaps because of their being of uncommon HLA types. Again, many of these models feature 'medical success' as the pre-eminent criterion for evaluating outcomes, placing less emphasis on broader improvements in the predicaments of patients' lives that might follow transplantation.

One approach that may improve equity at the margins is to apply the formal principle of justice of Aristotle (first promulgated in his *Nicomachean Ethics*). This suggests that 'equals' should be treated 'equally', but where 'inequality' exists, then 'unequal' treatment should occur to correct this imbalance. This is not as abstruse as it sounds!

In the case cited above, the patients with fulminant hepatic failure clearly had a more immediate and life-threatening need than the patient with chronic hepatic failure. Allocating an organ to them thus acts, in part, to redress the 'inequality' in the situation. This kind of decision-making will be very familiar in particular to those engaged in intra-thoracic and hepatic transplantation. Similarly, Aristotle's principle of justice is the basis of various points systems to 'tie-break' when an allocation based on HLA matching in kidney transplantation produces a number of (apparently) equally suitable recipients.

There is usually broad societal consensus that some kind of system that seeks to balance welfare maximisation with equity is acceptable, particularly if it is transparent and reactive to the identification of systematic imbalances. However, the individual patient may not share this view and may feel that his or her case is the 'most deserving'. This produces a dilemma for the clinician.

If there is a prima facie obligation to seek to achieve the best outcome for one's patient, how can one be supportive of an allocation system that does not place them 'top of the list'? From a deontological perspective one could argue that the patient's interests are best served by supporting a transparent (respecting autonomy by communication and information sharing) system with a commitment to justice (which applies equally to your patient as well as others).

Abandoning this position might lead to a free-for-all in which your patient's needs might have even less chance of being met. Notice the drift into a utilitarian analysis – reflecting again the way in which similar conclusions are reached by both traditions of ethical analysis.

How do we deal with those who have behaviour patterns that are self-harming? Should alcoholics receive liver transplants or smokers heart transplants? The principle of justice is again central. In terms of allocation, it may well be unfair to other patients who have not contributed to their own ill health. In reality, it is much more difficult! In truth much of the workload of many specialties is involved in the treatment of individuals whose disease is a direct or indirect consequence of their actions – consider peripheral vascular surgery and coronary heart disease. True moral dilemmas always present us with a variety of uncomfortable choices and usually leave us somewhat uncomfortable with the one we have chosen.

The context in which these decisions need to be made is so wide ranging that it is impossible to establish core rules. We do owe it to our patients, however, to be explicit when justifying why choices are made. The extreme of immediate clinical need (in which beneficence is likely to be the dominant relevant principle) is particularly challenging. Will the 'slightly less unwell' patients always get 'shoved back in the queue' when new emergencies present? In the imaginary case above, there is a fair likelihood that those sentiments may well be those of the patient with chronic hepatic disease.

Finally, we mention the theory of justice of John Rawls.[19] This suggests that a device that renders us impartial might enhance our reflection on justice. Modifying this slightly, let us advance the following for reflection by the reader. Imagine that you will be born into a society whose rules are not known to you. You will develop organ failure (of which organ, at what age and in what context you do not know). You do not know what will be your race, gender or position in society. You will hope that whatever system of allocation of organs exists will offer you the best chance of an early transplant, whoever you are. In such an analysis **what model of distributive justice in organ allocation would *you* favour?**

Identifying, accepting and prioritising candidate recipients

CASE STUDY

A 74-year-old female patient with end-stage renal failure has had two previous renal allografts. She is now back on dialysis and experiencing multiple difficulties with this. She has chronic obstructive airways disease (COAD), aortic stenosis and ischaemic heart disease. She has a very high titre of panel reactive antibodies. She is insistent that she be added to the waiting list for a further allograft. She asserts that she is prepared to accept a very high risk of intraoperative/postoperative complications, including death. She threatens to electively withdraw from dialysis unless her wish is granted.

This patient has a high risk of intraoperative problems and given her age and comorbid conditions she may well not survive very long even with a successful allograft. A 'commonsense' reaction (almost certainly with a utilitarian bias, and a focus on issues of justice) to this scenario might be to express incredulity if she were added to the waiting list again, and outrage if she were to receive a favourably matched cadaveric organ from a 20-year-old donor.

A traditional deontological approach, centred on the individual clinician's responsibility to an individual patient, might suggest that it is the duty of her physician to seek further transplantation on the grounds of beneficence. Certainly she has a poor prospect of longer-term survival with this, but that is also the case if she is to remain on dialysis. Even a short period with an allograft might give her a better quality of life. This case is on the borderline of clinical judgement with regard to non-maleficence. Certainly there is a high risk of harm with proceeding to transplantation, but it is possible that this will not be the case. Context is important here – the beneficence/non-maleficence scale is likely to be even more dramatically tipped against her if the organ transplant in question were a heart.

Although it is probable that denial of transplant could be justified on the grounds that non-maleficence should be accorded a higher weighting than beneficence (with a deontological or an 'act' utilitarian analysis), we might conclude that clinical uncertainty cancels these out. If the supply of organs were unlimited, then respect for autonomy (her determination, in the face of what would hopefully have been clear counselling as to risk, to proceed) might tip the balance towards agreeing to list her. Communication to establish that she truly is expressing informed consent would be critical here.

However, organs **are** in limited supply and the transplant programme does have a responsibility to justice. There is a need to be fair to this patient, but also to others. Both an 'act' utilitarian and a 'rule' utilitarian approach would argue that the potential organ would be best used for another patient. This might be one with greater potential to benefit, or who has not previously had a transplant (this woman has previously had two transplants) – equity is often as important as maximising utility. Furthermore, the transplant team has an obligation to be fair to its own members – it may be unjust to expect an anaesthetist to anaesthetise, or a surgeon to operate upon, a patient whom they expect may well die during, or shortly after, the procedure.

If this is the decision taken then it is important to acknowledge that the principle of justice has been given priority over the principles of beneficence, non-maleficence and respect for autonomy. What to do if the patient (as seems likely) disagrees or complains? In this circumstance it is important to be honest with the patient and explain the rationale for the decision. The patient should be offered recourse to another opinion and, if appropriate, to the mechanisms for making a complaint.

As the patient is highly immunologically sensitised (and might reasonably be listed for an age-matched organ) there exists the possibility of an 'easy option' – to list the patient in the expectation that she will not be offered a suitable kidney, or that discretion could be employed in rejecting any offers made. This is a most unethical route, difficult to justify by any means.

To deceive the patient in this way violates all respect for her autonomy. To abuse the transplant list in this way violates the principle of justice to other patients, to other colleagues and to the transparency necessary to exhibit that such rationing choices as are made are rational, consistent and honest. The obligation to these principles and to other patients demands this honesty, however uncomfortable may be the discussions engendered by the decision.

Would the situation be different if a live donor were available? Perhaps, but only insofar as the issue of justice to other potential recipients is removed. Should the surgeon remain convinced that the balance of principles still argues against transplantation then that decision should again be made and discussed. For the professional, judgement may well be difficult, but it is an obligation. Even if the patient demands the procedure (backing this up with threats of self-harm), the reluctant surgeon should abide by his or her decision.

In the past the principles of beneficence and non-maleficence were crudely subsumed into the cultural vice of paternalism. In the present the welcome increase in respect for autonomy should not slide into the equally unethical vice of consumerism. Healthcare workers must offer their considered best advice after balancing the relevant ethical principles. They cannot merely agree to patient demands, howsoever fervently expressed.

LIVE DONORS

Procurement of organs from live donors exposes them to a hazardous procedure. It can be argued that they derive no specific benefit other than the externality of having discharged an altruistic desire (and possibly, indirectly, the personal and material benefits that flow from the improvement in health status of a family member).[20] It is an almost unique situation – exposing one individual to potential harm for the benefit of another. Many surgeons and physicians remain less than enamoured of live donation. Some view it as a particularly difficult choice if there is a higher-than-standard risk of an adverse outcome in the recipient.

The level of risk to the donor is also important – donating a kidney is a widespread activity with extensive data on outcomes in large numbers of patients over a 30-year period.[21] Donating part of one's lung, liver, pancreas or small bowel could be viewed as a procedure with considerably more risk and uncertain long-term outcome.

Consent

CASE STUDY

A 45-year-old woman wishes to donate a kidney to her 68-year-old father. She has hypertension, which is well controlled by a single agent. She has no left ventricular hypertrophy (LVH) on echocardiography, no microalbuminuria, normal renal function and no other comorbidities. She is married with two teenage daughters. Her educational attainment was to age 16 in secondary school, she is dyslexic and has poor reading skills. She is of a retiring personality type and has not asked many questions other than along the lines of 'When can I give a kidney to my Dad? I don't care about the risk. I just want to get on with it …'.

In the UK, living donor transplantation is governed by the Human Organ Transplants Act, 1989. A number of guidelines are laid down. These include establishing that the asserted genetic relationship is likely, providing information for monitoring purposes, and prohibiting commercial transactions. It is important to ensure that there are no absolute contraindications to nephrectomy of a donor kidney. The British Transplantation Society,[22] among others, has issued guidelines on this. Although this lady has some comorbidity, it is not of a sufficient extent to exclude her as a candidate on purely medical grounds. However, there is inevitably some harm and risk inherent in a nephrectomy.

There is a common law principle that no individual can give consent to being killed or seriously injured. Live donation of a kidney is felt to be **relatively** safe (risk of death ~0.06%, with good long-term outcomes), so this does not apply. But what is an acceptable level of risk? And who should be the arbiter of this – the clinician, weighing beneficence and non-maleficence, or the patient expressing her autonomy?

The elements necessary to ensure that informed consent is present include the absence of coercion. It is important to explore with this woman her motivation to donate to ensure that there are no currently unidentified unacceptable pressures. These can be subtle or extreme, incorporating manipulation, bribery, family pressures and an internal desire to do (reluctantly) 'the right thing'. The surgeon needs to be satisfied that these issues have been fully explored before proceeding. One mechanism that may be helpful is the use of a 'donor advocate'.[23]

An example of subtle familial pressure that is encountered not infrequently is when a number of siblings are assessed as potential donors to another sibling. It may be that, for example, three out of four siblings are blood-group-incompatible with the potential recipient. This leaves one sibling as the sole potential donor, who may feel unable to stop the process, whatever misgivings he or she may have. A sense of obligation can be a very powerful pressure.

In this circumstance, it may be that the assessing team or the surgeon provides the potential donor with an opportunity to voice their anxiety and find 'a way out'. It may be that the potential donor seeks some kind of 'medical' reason to be 'let off the hook'. Is it ethical in this situation for the surgeon to manufacture a reason for excluding the potential donor that will allow them to 'save face' with the rest of the family? This is difficult. From a deontological viewpoint, lying can rarely be justified. From an 'act' utilitarian viewpoint, the surgeon may feel that non-maleficence (avoiding the need for the secretly unwilling potential donor to consent to donation) gives justification to the expression of a falsehood. Alternatively, looking at it from a different (but still 'act' utilitarian) perspective, one could argue that the moral hazard of the lie (it may eventually come to light with worse intrafamilial problems) may ultimately cause more difficulties.

It is well documented[23] that potential donors often have made a decision to donate at the earliest stage of the assessment process, often before they have had access to a full explanation of the potential outcomes. Revisiting this will minimise the potential that the patient has not understood the exact risks and benefits of the procedure. In the particular case outlined above, a potential donor with a high possibility of being very poorly informed seems to be behaving in this way.

If appropriate processes are in place, then there is every opportunity to ensure informed choice. Without it, nothing further should occur. In some patients (perhaps this one) extra attention to communication and information sharing will be necessary.

Moral hazards and the effect of future outcomes on current decisions

CASE STUDY

A 52-year-old woman offers to make a living donation of her kidney to her sister who is on haemodialysis. The potential recipient has a past medical history of metastatic teratoma that while it has responded well to chemotherapy has prevented her from being placed on the cadaveric renal transplant waiting list.

All sorts of ethical principles are in conflict in this case. Respect for the autonomy of the donor within the deontological tradition would suggest that the operation should go ahead. The immediate medical risk to the donor will not differ whatever the outcome for the recipient. If her sister had an illness with little or no risk of recurrence, then it is likely that this would be viewed as a straightforward case, presenting the standard ethical dilemmas of live donation. It is obviously a case that we would like to 'think over'. Why?

Initially, there is the issue of whether or not the immunosuppression entailed by the transplant operation greatly increases the recipient's likelihood of recurrence of malignancy – a typical 'informed consent' problem. However, more than just non-maleficence and respect for autonomy are at stake here. Justice may argue that this patient has a greater uncertainty as to post-transplant outcomes and, as such, should be given a 'lower' priority for cadaveric allocation. However, most patients do better with transplantation than with dialysis, and this is an unusual malignancy, the longer-term outcome of which is difficult to predict.

A central issue here is the possibility of early graft loss/recipient loss due to recurrence of malignancy in the recipient – a risk over and above the standard risk of graft rejection. This is inexplicably linked with the risk of potential harm or death in the recipient. Should this risk to the recipient modify our view as to the 'reasonableness' of the risk being run by the donor? From a utilitarian perspective, especially an 'act' utilitarian analysis, we should contemplate the impact that consequences will have on our decision.

Not to proceed avoids risk to the donor (non-maleficence). She may argue that whatever her sister's outcome, the level of risk to the donor is unchanged. The recipient might well be a patient in whom further cadaveric donation might be ruled out on the (utilitarian/justice) grounds that such kidneys would be better used for other patients, in whom the risk of early (patient) loss is less. In this context, now may be the only chance that this woman has for another kidney. Donation will then have a beneficial effect. Alternatively she could wait for some years – medical progress may make it possible for future transplantation without such risk of malignant disease recurrence.

If uncertain, the surgeon should seek a second opinion, but ultimately the decision hangs on whether or not one accepts the premise that the transplant outcome should modify the decision to remove a kidney from a well-informed individual expressing a strong desire to donate.

Conditional donation of organs (in a highly unusual context)

CASE STUDY

A woman is admitted as an emergency with a subarachnoid haemorrhage and is diagnosed as being brainstem dead. She was in the early stages of living donor assessment as a potential donor for her son, who has renal failure secondary to post-streptococcal glomerulonephritis. Her family are approached about organ donation and agree to the donation of her organs on the condition that one kidney is dedicated for the use of her son. The transplant coordinator and intensivist explain that it is not possible to make such guarantees but the family cannot understand why her decision to donate a kidney to her son made in life should be effectively invalid following her death and threaten to withdraw consent if this wish is not met.

Consent to cadaveric organ donation is taken to imply that such organs should be 'freely given'. This latter point excludes the imposition of conditions upon the donation of organs. The confusion of the family in the above case is easy to understand. Their relative was already preparing to donate a kidney to her son while alive and now that she has died this may no longer be possible because to do so would jeopardise ethical principles of equity of access and allocation. There is no doubt as to her 'advance intent'. As a consequence of an event involving conditional donation with a racist bias, a report recommended that **no conditions** should be attached to donation.[24] While the request of the family may seem to be reasonable, the 'case law' principle exists in this scenario. If the conditions placed by the family on organ donation are accepted there is a concern that this exceptional case might be used to justify conditional donation on other grounds such as gender, age, disease, race or religion. If the condition placed by the family is not met there is a risk that the donation of the other organs may not go ahead and the wider transplant recipient waiting lists might lose an opportunity. This case is, however, illustrative only – a 'pragmatic' resolution following widespread consultation (difficult at short notice) might well be the outcome in reality.

Remuneration of expenses and payment of organ donors

CASE STUDIES

The father of a physician working in the UK is resident in a non-EU state in the developing world. Civil war, social chaos and economic stagnation have afflicted this state. Renal replacement therapy facilities are practically non-existent. The father has advanced renal failure, but is wealthy. He and his family feel that transplantation is the only reasonable course of action available. There are no suitable family donors and he is prepared to pay another person to donate a kidney. His son seeks general advice from a transplant surgeon in the UK as to how his family can overcome their problem.

A man has been assessed as a living kidney donor for his brother. He has a well-paid job running a small building company and has considerable financial commitments in the form of a large mortgage and three children at independent school. He is reluctant to proceed with donation unless he receives reasonable reimbursement of his expenses including loss of income. The regional health authority has agreed to reimburse part of the potential loss of income but this would fall short of the amount required to meet his expenses. His brother states that he will make up the difference between his brother's loss and the health authority reimbursement.

There is a generally held view that there is a substantial moral difference between the sale of an organ and voluntary donation. Much of this revolves around the notion that bodily integrity is highly valued and that the dysutility consequent upon violation of this is not well compensated other than by other spiritual/philosophical gains such as acting in an altruistic fashion.[25]

More hard-nosed commentators note the existence of a global capitalist consumer society in which financial exchanges are viewed as a legitimate norm. To those that argue that paid organ donation will inevitably become exploitative comes the response that exploitation is a (regrettably) widespread norm. People work in dangerous underpaid jobs, as professional boxers, in prostitution – is there a moral difference between this and selling one's organs?

The issue of consent **freely given** is important. It is likely that there will be a considerable power gradient between recipient and donor. The circumstances of procurement may not be in facilities with standards comparable to those in the developed world. In unrestricted organ trading it is likely that organs will flow from the young to the old, from the poor to the rich, from females to males, and from the black and brown races to the white and yellow races. In this sense the principles of justice and autonomy are violated, although supporters of paid donation claim that autonomy is more hampered by prohibition.

In developed countries, including the UK, there is a prohibition on involvement in any aspect of organ trading. The surgeon in the first of the above case studies could not arrange for his colleague's father to have an operation of the kind proposed performed in the UK. The plight of this family is disturbing, and how one may help is not clear. The second case is interesting in that the principle of living related donation is non-problematic but the exchange of money between brothers appears on the surface unacceptable while the reimbursement by the regional health authority is allowed. The Human Organ Tissue Act, 1989 permits reimbursement that is reasonable but does not define or set limits on this. Furthermore the Act does not limit the act of reimbursement to the health authority. Provided that such reimbursement may be defended as being 'reasonable' then the Act is not contravened (suspicion as to an 'unreasonable' reimbursement could lead to prosecution on the advice of the Director of Public Prosecutions). Such apparent double standards represent real problems and need to be dealt with on a case-by-case basis. The prin-

ciple of non-payment for organs is important, and some have sought to suggest alternative strategies to minimise risks to the donor.

Harris and Erin have suggested a system where organs could be ethically purchased from individuals.[26] They propose that the market would be made ethically defensible by being 'monopsonistic', that is by having a nationally limited system in which there is a sole purchaser, such as the National Health Service (NHS), thereby avoiding potential donor exploitation. It is important to note that the NHS is an unusual healthcare delivery system, being 'free of charge at the point of delivery'. This model may, therefore, not be applicable in other contexts – and it is in these contexts (i.e. the developing world) that the greatest 'need to purchase' and greatest 'need to sell' exists. This argument should not be allowed to slide into justification of such a market in a mixed healthcare system where the wealthy can purchase organs with the risk of exploitation of the vulnerable donor.[27]

Even if the monopsonistic broker is an NHS-like beast, there is no guarantee that it would not still prey on the vulnerable, but at a state rather than an individual level. The poor are those most likely to sell their organs. Furthermore, a system similar to that described may be controlled locally, but could lead to major problems if applied on a wider scale.[28] Financial compensation for donors would probably differ between countries, thereby encouraging 'transplant tourism'.

It is important to acknowledge the potential for harm to the donor, and this highlights the moral difference between the sale of organs and voluntary donation. To expose an individual to harm for the benefit of another violates the principle of non-maleficence. It is accepted as 'allowable' in altruistic organ donation. Is it equally acceptable in a transaction that is commercial? Multidisciplinary teams looking after a donor may be uncomfortable with involvement in paid-donation; bodily integrity is highly valued and its violation is not well compensated for except by spiritual/philosophical gains. Recently published guidelines on living-donor transplantation emphasise the paucity of information on long-term consequences of living kidney donation and urge lifelong follow-up for donors.[22] Presumably the monopsony would also provide this aspect of care?

Fair distribution among recipients is an important principle of organ allocation. Whilst nodding to this, Harris and Erin immediately break the equity of access principle by suggesting a 'special' future priority to be awarded to those living-donors who subsequently require transplantation. This argument can easily slip into the more general awarding of 'special category status' on the basis of other sociodemographic discriminators.

Some have condemned the attitude of developed-world clinicians towards commercial organ trading in the developing world. Prohibiting it in countries without extensive dialysis facilities may condemn patients, such as the doctor's father in the above case, to death.[29] A utilitarian view, heavily weighted to account for the unique context of the problem, argues that paid donation is the only option with a potential for welfare maximisation.[30] On the other hand, it is in precisely these countries that governments are seeking to prohibit commercial dealings in organs.

The United Nations Bellagio Principles on Sustainable Development[31] have been endorsed by most sovereign states in the world. Organ trading and the sale of organs were specifically identified as activities in violation of these principles. Much media attention has focused on the alleged activities of criminal gangs running networks for organ trading, on the use of organs from executed prisoners in the People's Republic of China, and on Indian peasants selling kidneys to raise money for their daughters' dowries.

For the present, it is likely that paid donation will remain an item of academic discussion (with some strong advocates) within mainstream transplant circles, whilst continuing to occur in less well-regulated societies, probably with criminal associations. It is interesting to speculate that, if paid donation did become more acceptable, the poor of the developing world could become a vast reservoir of organs for the elderly with degenerative disease in the developed world. This is very distasteful and unlikely, but follows as a logical progression from many of the arguments of those who advocate liberalisation of the organ trade. If society chooses the road to paid organ donation, it is essential that the accompanying debate is transparent and complete. Furthermore, the debate has been predominantly abstract – very considerable legal, administrative and logistical measures would be needed to introduce and run a genuinely regulated 'trade' in organs; such blueprints would require acceptance by substantial political, social, ethical and medical constituencies.

A related, but slightly different issue, is the notion of financial incentives to **promote** procurement.[32,33] Some US commentators feel that transplantation is an activity with financial rewards (clinicians' salaries, for-profit institutions, drug companies, etc.) for all bar the donor and his or her heirs. 'Future contracts' in which the estate or heirs of an organ donor will receive some financial reward should he or she become a donor at some point in the future have been developed. The defraying of funeral expenses has been suggested.

As these are **incentives** rather than **payments**, they avoid the (probably important) semantic distinction between **donor** and **vendor**. It is likely that more schemes of these kinds will develop.

Other schemes of reward or incentives to donation have been suggested that do not involve exchange of money but offer preferential access to transplantation. One such scheme has suggested that individuals who make an agreement to donate should they ever be declared brainstem dead will have preferential access to organs should they ever require a transplant. It is difficult to imagine how such a system could be considered legally binding and why individuals should not renege from such a deal. It is also difficult to imagine how donor rates would be improved by such a scheme since presumably there would be a flood of people with impending organ failure wanting to register as potential future donors.

XENOTRANSPLANTATION

Enormous endeavour and resources have been allocated to research on overcoming the immunological and technical barriers to transplantation across the species barrier (xenotransplantation). It is probable that some clinical activity in this field will occur in the not too distant future. Are we ready to deal with the ethical dimension to this?

General principles

Xenotransplantation poses numerous ethical questions, of which the following are crucial:

- Is it ethically (and culturally) acceptable to utilise sentient non-human species for research into human disease?
- What new issues arise when these are subjected to genetic modification?
- Is it acceptable to transplant across species barriers – especially from non-human species to humans?
- Should different non-human species be viewed differently in these contexts?

These are difficult questions, addressing issues of animal welfare and animal rights. Extensive arguments exist on the general morality of exploiting other species to human benefit. Some[34] argue (in classically deontological fashion) that animals have unique rights independent of the consequences of recognition of these upon human outcomes. Others[35] have stressed the need to assess, in a proportionate sense, the balance between human benefits and animal harm.

Animal experimentation (in common with other exploitative uses) remains widespread and broadly acceptable to the medical community and to society in general. Vigorous opposition is provided by many organisations such as PETA (People for the Ethical Treatment of Animals) – claiming a membership in excess of 500 000 – and others.

In the UK, the legal basis for experimental activity is addressed by the Animals (Scientific Procedures) Act, 1986. This is largely concerned with the minimisation of suffering and distress, and is largely utilitarian in tone. For the immediate future, it is likely that experimentation will continue, and its entanglement with the drive to try to match organ supplies to ever-increasing demands will be a prominent area of controversy.

Current scientific advances using genetically modified pigs to overcome some of the technical barriers to successful xenotransplantation are well known.[36] To many (often for religious and cultural reasons) this degree of 'interference' in natural genomes is disturbing. However, it seems unlikely that xenotransplantation will be possible (in the medium term) without this approach. Much of its ethical justification will thus be utilitarian, although a vigorous deontological argument to utilise 'all possible means' to 'help sick human beings' also holds currency.

The general issue of genetic modification is one that is topical in all aspects of medicine (as well as agriculture) and is beyond the immediate scope of this discussion. This is likely to be an area of vigorous debate and continuing controversy, and as such it may well lead to an 'unsettled' background ethical climate to xenotransplantation.

With regard to the species of candidate donor animals, two reports are of interest. In 1996 the Nuffield Council for Bioethics[37] expressed a view that a special case might be made to avoid the use of primates (particularly great apes) as organ donors for human xenotransplantation (although it acknowledged that a limited number might be used as experimental recipients). This, in part, reflected safety concerns and concerns regarding the risk of extinction to species such as chimpanzees. However, the notion that the 'intellectually higher' species might be viewed as having different 'rights' is suggested. A similar conclusion was reached by the UK Advisory Group on the Ethics of Xenotransplantation, chaired by Professor Ian Kennedy, in its 1997 report *Animal Tissue into Humans*. Some may see this as no more than pragmatism in the avoidance of potential controversy.

The issue of 'animal rights' is undoubtedly a theme for our time and one that will not be as easily avoided or resolved as in the past. To engage in constructive debate requires explicit description of the principles in conflict. It is unlikely that an appeal, such as was attempted in the past, to the opening lines of the Book of Genesis as a source of blanket justification will, in future, convince other than a minority of the disputants.

Patenting organs and purchasing organs

The 'Holy Grail' of the adventure into xenotransplantation is that there might be a potentially limitless supply of organs for use in transplantation. Furthermore, the potential to genetically modify candidate organ–donor animal models might allow for 'customised' tissues to become available. Such an outcome could be viewed as 'solving' the principal current problem of access to organs (insufficient supply due to limited cadaveric and live donor sources). However, this problem may be replaced by another.

The development costs of transgenic animals are enormous and ultimately those who have invested in these endeavours will (legitimately) seek a return and, perhaps, a profit on their outgoing. This will represent a major paradigm shift in transplant practice. It is unlikely that such organs will be inexpensive, and there will probably be considerable anxiety on the long-term safety of these organs. How much will we be prepared to spend on xenografts? How will we decide who gets a human living-donor allograft, a human cadaveric-donor allograft, or a xenograft? **The need to answer these questions and to justify the answers may be closer than we think.**

Consent and the unknown risks of xenotransplantation

CASE STUDY

Xenotransplantation is not without its potential hazards. Apart from the general risk of organ rejection and the side effects of (possibly more intensive) immunosuppression there is the worrying possibility of development/transmission of currently unknown xenozoonoses.[38] Consider the following (although maybe not so) imaginary scenario.

The regulatory authority for xenotransplantation in a country has consented to allow a clinical trial of kidney transplantation from a commercially developed transgenic pig model to humans. As part of the protocol, trial participants will be asked not to conceive/father a child and asked to use barrier contraception for the rest of their lives. Known sexual partners will be asked to consent to regular microbiological screening. The biotechnology company that has developed the xenograft will fund the trial.

This may not be as bizarre as it seems. One of the greatest fears with xenotransplantation is the possibility that the combination of genetic manipulation, immunosuppression and transplantation may lead to new xenozoonoses. Much attention has focused on porcine endogenous retroviruses (PERVs) and potential problems from these. To date little experimental evidence has emerged to give substance to these fears. However, as part of its remit, the UK Xenotransplantation Interim Regulatory Authority (UKXIRA) has published a consultation document from its infection surveillance team, which lays out in detail potential concerns similar to those expressed above. Proposals for lifelong surveillance and counselling of partners have been submitted. A host of new ethical issues emerges from these.

In order to obtain informed consent from a recipient of a xenotransplant, there must be some sharing with the patient of future potential risks. In the current state of uncertainty about potential infectious risks this is difficult (especially so if one is contemplating the options of live donor, cadaver donor and xenodonor for an individual patient). The earliest xenografts will obviously be done within trial conditions and this will doubtless be a factor to which the attention of Ethics Committees will be directed.

The advice to avoid conception or fertilisation seems prudent, as does the advice to avoid bringing others into contact with one's bodily fluids. This is a very utilitarian approach with heavy emphasis on non-maleficence, of extended scope (contacts of patients included). In effect, the desire is to avoid introducing a new zoonosis **to the human race**. The autonomy of the patient (and by extension, sexual partners of the patient) is being curtailed. As was commented in the Steering Group's Report, ensuring compliance with these limitations may be difficult. The history of humanity is littered with the broken vows of those who have attempted to control sexual intercourse by issuing a guideline!

CONCLUSION

Transplantation is awash with ethical dilemmas. Just as we are catching up with the new developments of yesterday, we face even more strange scenarios, for which we have no precedent. In this context, therefore, we believe that the structured application of the general principles of medical ethics and bioethics is more than a casual intellectual adornment. It is a tool that helps us to describe our dilemmas, analyse the important elements and formulate strategies to deal with these real-life issues in everyday practice.

REFERENCES

1. American Medical Association. Principles of medical ethics. http://www.ama-assn.org/ama/pub/category/2512.html

2. Bierce A. The enlarged devil's dictionary. London: Penguin, 1990.

3. Gillon R. Philosophical medical ethics. Chichester: Wiley, 1985.

4. Boyd KM, Higgs R, Pinching AJ (eds) The new dictionary of medical ethics. London: BMJ Publishing, 1997.

5. General Medical Council. Good medical practice, 2nd edn. London: GMC, 1998.

6. Davies M. Textbook on medical law, 2nd edn. London: Blackstone Press, 1998.

7. General Medical Council. Seeking patients' consent: the ethical considerations. London: GMC, 1999.

8. Mason JK, McCall Smith RA. Law and medical ethics. London: Butterworth, 1994.

9. Daar AS. Transplantation in developing countries. In: Morris PJ (ed.) Kidney transplantation, 4th edn. Philadelphia: Saunders, 1994; pp. 478–503.

10. Collins CH. Elective ventilation for organ donation – the case in favour. Care Crit Ill 1992; 8:60.

11. Willetts SH. Transplantation and interventional ventilation on the intensive therapy unit. BMJ 1995; 310:714–18.

12. Youngner SJ. Respect for the dead body. Transplant Proc 1990; 22:1014.

13. Anaise D, Rapaport FT. Use of non heart beating cadavers in clinical organ transplantation – logistics, ethics and legal considerations. Transplant Proc 1993; 25:2153–5.

14. Kootsra G. Non-heart beating donor programmes. Transplant Proc 1995; 27:2965.

15. Dossetor JB. Ethics in transplantation. In: Morris PJ (ed.) Kidney transplantation, 4th edn. Philadelphia: Saunders, 1994; pp. 524–31.

16. Andrews LB. My body, my property. Hastings Centre Report 1986; 16:28.

17. Cahn E, cited by Calabresi G, Bobbitt P. Tragic choices. New York: Norton, 1978.

18. Doyal L. The role of the public in health care rationing. Crit Pub Health 1993; 4:49–53.

19. Rawls J. A theory of justice. Oxford: Oxford University Press, 1976.

20. Michielsen P. Medical risk and benefit in renal donors: the use of living donation reconsidered. In: Land W, Dossetor JB (eds) Organ replacement therapy: ethics, justice and commerce. Berlin: Springer-Verlag, 1991.

21. Najarian JS, Chavers BM, McHugh LE et al. 20 years or more of follow up of living donors. Lancet 1992; 340:807–10.

22. The British Transplantation Society and The Renal Association. United Kingdom guidelines for living donor kidney transplantation. London: British Transplantation Society, 2000.

23. Russell S, Jacob RG. Living related organ donation: the donor's dilemma. Patient Educ Counselling 1993; 21:89–99.

24. Department of Health. An investigation into conditional organ donation (http://www.dh.gov.uk/assetRoot/04/03/54/65/04035465.pdf), 2000.

25. Wilkinson S, Garrard E. Bodily integrity and the sale of human organs. J Med Ethics 1996; 22:334–9.

26. Harris J, Erin C. An ethically defensible market in organs. BMJ 2002, 325:114–15.

27. Wigmore SJ, Lumsdaine JA, Forsythe JLR. Ethical market in organs – defending the indefensible? BMJ 2002; 325:835

28. Schlitt HJ. Paid non-related living donation: Horn of plenty or Pandora's box? Lancet 2002, 359:906–7.

29. Bignall J. Kidneys: buy or die. Lancet 1993; 342:45.

30. Davies I. Live donation of human body parts: a case for negotiability? Med Legal J 1991; 59:100

31. Bellagio Task Force. Report on transplantation, bodily integrity and the international traffic in organs. Transplantation Proceedings 1997, 29:2739–45.

32. Financial incentives for organ donation. Payment Subcommittee, UNOS Ethics Committee, 1993 (http://www.unos.org/resources/bioethics.asp?index=3)

33. Wigmore SJ, Forsythe JLR. Incentives to promote organ donation. Transplantation 2004; 71:159–61.

34. Regan T, Singer P (eds) Animal rights and human obligations. Englewood Cliffs, NJ: Prentice Hall, 1989.

35. Smith JA, Boyd KM (eds) Lives in the balance: the ethics of using animals in biomedical research. Oxford: Oxford University Press, 1991.

36. Cozzi E, White DJG. The generation of transgenic pigs as potential organ donors for humans. Nature Med 1995; 333:1498–501.

37. Nuffield Council on Bioethics. Animal-to-human transplants: the ethics of xenotransplantation, 1996 (http://www.nuffieldbioethics.org/go/browseablepublications/xenotransplantation/report_87.html).

38. Chapman LE, Folks TM, Salomon DR, et al. Xenotransplantation and xenogeneic infections. New Engl J Med 1995; 333:1498–501.

Two

The acute shortage of donors: a UK and European perspective

Rafael Matesanz and
Christopher J. Rudge

● Part 1 ●

The situation in Europe

Rafael Matesanz

Organ transplantation is the best technique for the treatment of end-stage failure of most essential organs (kidney, liver, heart and lungs). Over 1 million people worldwide have benefited from successful organ transplantation. A number of transplant patients have survived well over 25 years, and 5-year survival rates for most organ transplant programmes are over 70%.[1] However, the shortage of cadaveric organ donors imposes a severe limit on the number of patients who can benefit from transplantation, while there is an ever-increasing demand for cadaveric solid organs in most countries.

The situation in Europe with respect to cadaveric organ donation is very heterogeneous, from very low levels in Eastern European countries – under 5 donors per million population (pmp) in most of them – to over 30 donors pmp in Spain[2] and some regions of Italy, France and Austria. Even in the European Union, cadaveric organ donation can range from 5.9 donors pmp in Greece to 33.7 in Spain (i.e. a ratio of roughly 1:6). The reasons for this variability are multiple although it is clear that it cannot be attributed to differences in the public willingness to donate organs but rather to differences in health structure, hospital facilities and

especially in the organisation of the organ donation system, as analysed below. The only common point to all the European countries is the ever-increasing gap between the number of available organs and the waiting list: wherever more solid organs are obtained, more and more patients are accepted as candidates to be transplanted. The shortage of organs means that only the patients most likely to benefit are chosen for these therapies. To put patients on a waiting list who have no hope of receiving an organ is both pointless and highly questionable ethically.[3]

The terms employed in this section of the chapter are defined in **Box 2.1** according to the definitions agreed by the Transplant Committee of the Council of Europe and used in the European consensus document 'Meeting The Organ Shortage'.[1]

THE STATISTICS OF SHORTAGE

Table 2.1 and Fig. 2.1 show the official organ donation and transplantation rates of the European countries (and some non-European for reference) for the year 2002.[2] Table 2.2 gives the official

Box 2.1 • Definition of terms

Death confirmed by brainstem tests

Complete and irreversible cessation of all cerebral and brainstem functions that, from the scientific, ethical and legal point of view, is accepted as equivalent to the death of the individual. Strict testing according to agreed protocols is required to establish brain death beyond doubt.

Potential donor

Any person diagnosed as dead by brainstem testing, by means of clinical examination, following the elimination of any absolute contraindications to donation, i.e. conditions representing a risk for recipients.

Effective donor

A potential donor from whom at least one solid organ (or tissue) has been retrieved for transplantation.

Potential and/or effective donor rates can be expressed either by reference to the catchment population – donors per million population (pmp) – or by reference to hospital parameters (e.g. donors as a percentage of overall hospital mortality; of intensive care mortality or as a rate per hundred hospital beds, etc.

Retrieval

Removal of an organ or tissue intended for transplantation whether subsequently transplanted or not.

Key donation person

A person responsible for organ donation in a specific area or hospital. He/she may or may not be the transplant coordinator.

Organ sharing office (OSO)*

A bureau responsible for the collection and management of data from donors and recipients and allocation of organs according to agreed criteria.

Organ exchange organisation (OEO)*

An organisation responsible for the organ and/or tissue allocation in a specific region/country.

Organ procurement organisation (OPO)*

A body or organisation responsible for organ donation and procurement in a specific region/country.

*In some countries one organisation may perform more than one or all of these functions within a region or country.

waiting lists for solid organ transplants in those European countries where these data are available. **Fig. 2.2** shows the number of effective solid organ donors in Western European countries during the period 1989–2002.

From these data we can draw several conclusions, which we will try to analyse and explain together with areas for possible improvement.

- There are great differences from country to country. Only Spain is over 30 donors pmp, six countries are over 20 (Austria, Belgium, Republic of Ireland, Estonia, Latvia and France) while most other Western European countries (including the UK) are between 12 and 15 donors pmp. There are still many Eastern European countries where organ donor rates are under 5 pmp and sometimes there are no statistics available.
- Waiting lists far exceed the number of available organ donors. At the end of 2002, at least 45 308 patients were waiting for a kidney in Europe (53 880 in the USA), 5715 for a liver (USA 16 963), 2146 for a heart (USA 3787) and 1667 for a lung (USA 3804). As a whole, 55 962 European patients were waiting for a solid organ while the total number of transplants performed during 2002 was just 24 055, that is 43%. Figures for the USA were 82 445 and 24 368 respectively (or 29.5%).
- The number of solid organ donors increased only slightly in Western European countries (from 5443 in 1989 to 6861 in 2002, i.e. by only 2% per year).
- As a consequence of this gap, at least 3330 European patients died in 2002 while waiting for an organ transplant. However, this number is no doubt an underestimate as not all suitable patients are included on the waiting list. Moreover, many countries do not record these data, especially in non-life-saving transplants such as renal or pancreatic.
- The number of living donors for kidney and liver has, however, steadily increased in recent years as an alternative to the shortage of cadaveric organ donors. Up to 14.2% of renal transplants in Europe and 42% in the USA come from living donation whereas the corresponding figures for liver transplants are 4.9 and 6.7%.

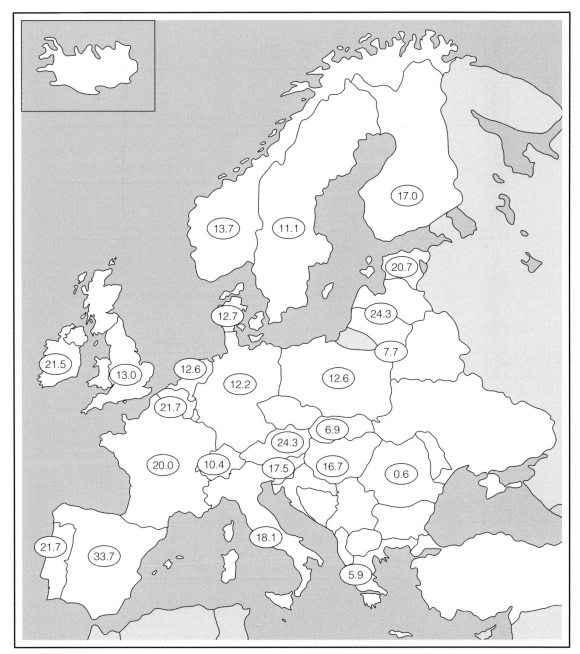

Figure 2.1 • Organ donation rates in donors per million population (pmp) in the main countries, or organ exchange organisations in Europe during 2002.

Table 2.1 • Organ donation and transplantation of solid organs in Europe during 2002. Data from the Council of Europe

Countries	Austria	Belgium	Bulgaria	Croatia	Cyprus	Denmark	Estonia	Finland	France	Georgia	Germany
Population (million inhabitants)	8.04	10.3	7.79	4.38	0.65	5.7	1.40	5.2	59.9	5.50	82.2
DONATION											
Cadaveric donors	195	223	8	41	7	73	29	89	1198	0	1001
Rate (pmp)	24.3	21.7	1.02	9.4	10.7	12.7	20.7	17	20	0	12.2
Paediatric <15 years	1	13	0	1	1	4	0	1	45	0	40
Percent multiorgan donors	76.9	75.8	–	73.2	65	72.6	–	65.2	–	–	67.3
TRANSPLANTATION											
Kidney											
Cadaveric transplants	368	334	16	77	13	132	50	169	2147	0	1742
Rate (pmp)	45.8	32.4	2.05	17.5	20	23	35.7	32.5	35.8	0	21.2
Paediatric <15 years	9	9	0	0	1	2	0	9	59	–	74
Living transplant	42	15	15	4	33	39	0	3	108	6	442
Rate (pmp)	5.2	1.5	1.92	0.91	50.7	6.8	0	0.6	1.8	1.1	5.4
Paediatric <15 years	3	3	–	0	1	4	0	1	6	0	33
Liver											
Transplants (including all combinations)	155	226	–	25	–	39	0	47	882	0	756
Rate (pmp)	19.3	21.9	–	5.71	–	6.8	0	9	14.7	–	9.2
Paediatric <15 years	7	16	–	1	–	3	0	2	62	–	71
Split-liver transplants	1	9	–	0	–		0	0	65	0	75
Split-liver paediatric	0	1	–	0	–		–	0	29	–	42
Domino liver transplant	0	2	–	0	–		0	0	12	0	4
Domino liver paediatric	0	0	–	0	–		–	0	0	–	0
Living liver transplant	4	30	–	1	–	1	0	0	45	0	85
Living liver paediatric	3	14	–	1	–	1	–	0	3	–	35

Table 2.1 • (Cont'd) Organ donation and transplantation of solid organs in Europe during 2002. Data from the Council of Europe

Countries	Austria	Belgium	Bulgaria	Croatia	Cyprus	Denmark	Estonia	Finland	France	Georgia	Germany
Heart											
Transplants (including heart–lung transplants)	72	85	–	9	–	30	0	18	339	0	395
Rate (pmp)	9	8.3	–	2.05	–	5.2	–	3.5	5.6	–	4.8
Paediatric <15 years	0	3	–	0	–	1	–	4	6	–	33
Heart–lung											
Transplants	2	5	–	0	–	1	0	0	20	0	15
Rate (pmp)	0.2	0.5	–	–	–	0.1	–	0	0.3	–	0.2
Paediatric <15 years	0	0	–	–	–	–	0	0	–	–	0
Lung											
Single lung	24	12	–	1	–	37	0	0	33	0	43
Rate (pmp)	3	1.2	–	0.23	–	6.4	–	0	0.5	–	0.5
Double lung	66	37	–	0	–	10	0	4	54	–	0
Rate (pmp)	8.2	3.6	–	–	–	1.7	–	0.8	0.9	–	156
S+D lung (rate) (including heart–lung transplants)	90 (11.2)	49 (4.8)	–	–	–	47 (8.1)	–	4 (0.8)	87 (1.4)	–	1.9
Paediatric < 15 years	2	0	–	–	–	–	–	0	2	–	1
Pancreas											
Kidney–pancreas transplants	35	20	–	0	–		0	0	53	0	140
Rate (pmp)	4.4	1.9	–	–	–		–	–	0.9	–	1.7
Isolate pancreas (rate)	17 (2.1)	66 (6.4)	–	0	–		0	–	6 (0.1)	0	34 (0.4)
Organ combinations (rate)	0	2 (0.3)	–	0	–		0	–	0	0	1 (0.01)
Small bowel											
Isolated small bowel transplant (rate)	5 (0.6)	–	–	0	–		0	0	6 (0.1)	0	4 (0.5)
Isolated small bowel transplant (paediatric) (rate)		–	–	–	–		–	–	6 (0.1)	–	0
Organ combinations (rate)	–	–	–	0	–		0	–	3 (0.05)	0	1 (0.01)
Organ combinations (paediatric) (rate)	–	–	–	–	–		–	–	3 (0.05)	–	0

Table 2.1 • (*Cont'd*) Organ donation and transplantation of solid organs in Europe during 2002. Data from the Council of Europe

Countries	Greece	Hungary	Israel	Italy	Latvia	Luxembourg	Malta	The Netherlands	Norway	Poland	Portugal
Population (million inhabitants)	11	10	6.5	56.3	2.30	0.4	0.40	16	4.53	38.6	10
DONATION											
Cadaveric donors	65	167	64	1019	56	3	6	202	62	490	217
Rate (pmp)	5.9	16.7	9.84	18.1	24.3	7.5	15	12.6	13.7	12.6	21.7
Paediatric <15 years	5	6	3	–	0	0	0	12	8	15	–
Percent multiorgan donors	83	24.6	92.2	–	–	100	100	56.9	64.5	37	76
TRANSPLANTATION											
Kidney											
Cadaveric transplants	107	289	97	1464	71	5	12	361	115	910	367
Rate (pmp)	9.7	28.9	14.92	26	30.8	12.5	30	22.6	25.4	23.5	36.7
Paediatric <15 years	5	9	8	–	4	0	0	20	1	2	10
Living transplant	85	10	68	124	0	0	3	199	98	25	23
Rate (pmp)	7.7	1	10.4	2.2	0	–	7.5	12.4	21.6	0.6	2.3
Paediatric <15 years	0	0	2	–	0	0	0	7	9	–	–
Liver											
Transplants (including all combinations)	21	17	53	863	0	–	1	109	25	148	191
Rate (pmp)	1.9	1.7	8.15	15.3	–	–	10	6.8	5.6	3.8	19.1
Paediatric <15 years	0	0	6	80	–	–	0	10	4	13	13
Split-liver transplants	0	0	1	–	–	–	–	2	4	–	2
Split-liver paediatric	0	0	1	–	–	–	–	1	0	–	–
Domino liver transplant	0	0	–	–	–	–	–	2	0	–	32
Domino liver paediatric	0	0	–	–	–	–	–	0	0	–	–
Living liver transplant	0	0	1	33	–	–	–	0	0	13	1
Living liver paediatric	0	0	1	–	–	–	–	0	0	–	–

Table 2.1 • (Cont'd) Organ donation and transplantation of solid organs in Europe during 2002. Data from the Council of Europe

Countries	Greece	Hungary	Israel	Italy	Latvia	Luxembourg	Malta	The Netherlands	Norway	Poland	Portugal
Heart											
Transplants (including heart–lung transplants)	9	9	24	312	1	–	0	43	26	111	13
Rate (pmp)	0.8	0.9	3.69	5.5	0.43	–	0	2.7	5.7	2.8	1.3
Paediatric <15 years	0	0	–	–	–	–	–	3	0	–	1
Heart–lung											
Transplants	0	0	2	1	–	–	–	2	0	2	–
Rate (pmp)	0	0	0.3	0.02	–	–	–	0.1	0	0.05	–
Paediatric <15 years	0	0	–	–	–	–	–	0	0	–	–
Lung											
Single lung	0	3	16		0	–	–	14	3	–	–
Rate (pmp)	0	0.3	2.4		–	–	–	0.9	0.6	–	–
Double lung	0	16	1		0	–	–	29	9	–	1
Rate (pmp)	0	1.6	0.15		–	–	–	1.8	2	–	0.1
S+D lung (rate) (including heart–lung transplants)	0	19 (1.9)	17 (2.6)	59 (1.1)	0	–	–	43 (2.7)	12 (2.6)	–	1 (0.1)
Paediatric < 15 years	0	1	–	–	–	–	–	2	0	–	–
Pancreas											
Kidney–pancreas transplants	0	7	5	50	0	–	–	17	15	12	8
Rate (pmp)	0	0.7	0.7	0.9	–	–	–	1.1	3.3	0.31	0.8
Isolate pancreas (rate)	0	0	–	16 (0.3)	0	–	–	0	2 (0.4)	–	–
Organ combinations (rate)	0	0	–	10 (0.2)	0	–	–	0	0	–	–
Small bowel											
Isolate sb tx. (rate)	0	0	–	5 (0.1)	0	–	–	0	0	–	–
Isolate sb ped. (rate)	0	0	–	–	–	–	–	0	–	–	–
Organ combinations (rate)	0	0	–	2 (0.04)	0	–	–	0	0	1	–

26

Table 2.1 • (Cont'd) Organ donation and transplantation of solid organs in Europe during 2002. Data from the Council of Europe

Countries	Ireland	Romania	Slovak Republic	Slovenia	Spain	Sweden	Switzerland	UK	USA	Canada	Australia
Population (million inhabitants)	3.80	21	5.3	2	41.84	8.9	7.2	59.01	287.4	31.26	19.4
DONATION											
Cadaveric donors	78	13	37	35	1409	98	75	765	6184	411	206
Rate (pmp)	20.5	0.62	6.9	17.5	33.7	11.1	10.4	13	21.5	13.1	10.6
Paediatric <15 years	10	0	3	1	74	2	4	37	935	–	20
Percent multiorgan donors	83.3	85	48.6	77.1	83	87	85	85.5	–	–	81
TRANSPLANTATION											
Kidney											
Cadaveric transplants	130	24	58	55	1998	194	131	1202	8490	627	374
Rate (pmp)	34.2	1.14	10.8	27.5	47.7	21.7	18.2	20.4	29.5	20.1	19.3
Paediatric <15 years	7	0	3	0	62	6	5	51	327	23	–
Living transplant	3	151	15	0	34	114	73	371	6232	391	238
Rate (pmp)	0.8	7.19	2.8	0	0.8	12.8	10.1	6.3	21.6	12.5	12.3
Paediatric <15 years	–	9	1	0	4	8	0	33	441	19	–
Liver											
Transplants (including all combinations)	37	16	3	11	1033	102	83	702	5573	381	153
Rate (pmp)	9.7	0.76	0.6	5.5	24.7	11.4	11.5	11.9	19.3	12.1	7.9
Paediatric <15 years	–	4	0	0	70	7	6	81	555	2	22
Split-liver transplants	–	2		0	22	12	4	85	–	0	0
Split-liver paediatric	–	2		0	9	–	2	51	–	0	0
Domino liver transplant	–	0		0	14	2	0	4	–	0	–
Domino liver paediatric	–	0		0	0	0	0	0	–	0	–
Living liver transplant	–	2		0	41	5	10	2	358	42	1
Living liver paediatric	–	2		0	18	2	0	1	72	0	–

Table 2.1 • (Cont'd) Organ donation and transplantation of solid organs in Europe during 2002. Data from the Council of Europe

Countries	Ireland	Romania	Slovak Republic	Slovenia	Spain	Sweden	Switzerland	UK	USA	Canada	Australia
Heart											
Transplants (including heart–lung transplants)	15	6	7	3	310	20	32	174	2567	168	87
Rate (pmp)	3.9	0.29	1.3	1.5	7.4	2.2	4.4	2.9	8.9	5.4	4.5
Paediatric <15 years	–	1	0	0	19	3	2	24	294	–	–
Heart–lung											
Transplants	–	–	0	0	6	1	1	16	33	7	8
Rate (pmp)	–	–	0	0	0.14	0.11	0.1	03	0.11	0.2	0.4
Paediatric <15 years	–	–	0	0	0	0	0	1	6	–	–
Lung											
Single lung	–	–	0	0	38	37	6	54		36	26
Rate (pmp)	–	–	0	–	0.90	4.1	0.8	0.9		1.2	1.3
Double lung	–	0	0	0	123	14	28	73		105	73
Rate (pmp)	–	–	0	–	2.9	1.5	3.9	1.2		3.4	3.8
S+D lung (rate) (including heart–lung transplants)	–	–	0	–	161 (3.8)	51 (5.6)	34 (4.7)	127 (2.1)	1077 (3.7)	141 (4.6)	99 (5.1)
Paediatric < 15 years	–	–	0	–	7	1	3	1	51	–	–
Pancreas											
Kidney–pancreas transplants	9	–	0	0	56	8	11	52	903	41	24
Rate (pmp)	2.4	–	0	–	1.3	0.8	1.5	0.9	3.1	1.3	1.2
Isolate pancreas (rate)	1 (0.3)	–	1 (0.2)	0	11 (0.2)	0	2 (0.3)	8 (0.1)	546 (1.8)	33 (1.1)	1 (0.05)
Organ combinations (rate)	–	–	0	0	2 (0.04)	0	22 (3)	–	30 (0.10)	0	1 (0.05)
Small bowel											
Isolate sb tx. (rate)	–	–	0	0	2 (0.04)	0	1 (0.1)	–	107 (0.37)	0	0
Isolate sb ped. (rate)	–	–	0	–	1 (0.02)	0	–	1	68	–	–
Organ combinations (rate)	–	–	0	0	1 (0.02)	4 (0.4)	–	1	59 (0.20)	0	0

*included all combination (10 domino heart transplant)

Table 2.2 • Waiting lists of solid organ transplantations in Europe during 2002. Data from the Council of Europe

Countries	Austria	Belgium	Bulgaria	Croatia	Cyprus	Denmark	Estonia	Finland	France	Georgia	Germany
Population (million inhabitants)	8.04	10.3	7.79	4.38	0.65	5.7	1.40	5.2	59.9	5.50	82.18
Kidney											
No. transplant centres	5	7	–	–	–	4	1	1	44	2	41
Patients admitted to the waiting list during 2002	539	549	119	180	30	194	40	223	2637	–	3372
Patients waiting for a transplant by end 2002	774	876	689	821	110	375	24	214	5227	–	9623
Patients dead while on the WL during 2002	36	38	46	–	15	7	5	6	109	–	418
Liver											
No. transplant centres	3	6	–	–	–	1	1	1	24	0	25
Patients admitted to the waiting list during 2002	228	338	–	43	–	48	1	48	1051	–	1451
Patients waiting for a transplant by end 2002	112	159	–	26	–	10	0	9	438	–	994
Patients dead while on the WL during 2002	29	37	–	–	–	0	1	3	98	–	277
Heart											
No. transplant centres	3	7	–	–	–	2	0	1	27	0	28
Patients admitted to the waiting list during 2002	103	112	–	11	–	35	–	15	470	–	622
Patients waiting for a transplant by end 2002	39	40	–	10	–	22	–	7	355	–	359
Patients dead while on the WL during 2002	17	17	–	–	–	2	–	1	74	–	131

Table 2.2 • (Cont'd) Waiting lists of solid organ transplantations in Europe during 2002. Data from the Council of Europe

Countries	Austria	Belgium	Bulgaria	Croatia	Cyprus	Denmark	Estonia	Finland	France	Georgia	Germany
Lung											
No. transplant centres	2	3	–	0	–	1	0	1	14	0	11
Patients admitted to the waiting list during 2002	114	71	–	4	–	36	–	4	169	–	336
Patients waiting for a transplant by end 2002	41	51	–	3	–	50	–	1	158	–	347
Patients dead while on the WL during 2002	11	9	–	–	–	17	–	1	36	–	86
Pancreas											
No. transplant centres	3	6	–	0	–		0	0	14	0	27
Patients admitted to the waiting list during 2002	63	90	–	–	–		–	–	86	–	273
Patients waiting for a transplant by end 2002	38	56	–	–	–		–	–	193	–	181
Patients dead while on the WL during 2002	0	1	–	–	–		–	–	8	–	22
Small bowel											
No. transplant centres		1	–	0	–		0	0	4	0	5
Patients admitted to the waiting list during 2002		2	–	–	–		–	–	4	–	11
Patients waiting for a transplant by end 2002		1	–	–	–		–	–	8	–	6
Patients dead while on the WL during 2002		0	–	–	–		–	–	0	–	2

Table 2.2 • (Cont'd) Waiting lists of solid organ transplantations in Europe during 2002. Data from the Council of Europe

Countries	Greece	Hungary	Israel	Italy	Latvia	Luxembourg	Malta	The Netherlands	Norway	Poland	Portugal	Ireland
Population (million inhabitants)	11	10	6.5	56.3	2.30	0.4	0.40	16	4.53	38.6	10	3.8
Kidney												
No. transplant centres	4	4	6	39	1	1	1	7	1	18	8	1
Patients admitted to the waiting list during 2002	198	342	172	3711	153	8	30	803	195		–	146
Patients waiting for a transplant by end 2002	956	998	594	8434	381	17	93	1287	195		–	213
Patients dead while on the WL during 2002	41	60	25	144	15	0	10	124	14		–	7
Liver												
No. transplant centres	1	1	4	19	1	0	–	3	1	7	4	1
Patients admitted to the waiting list during 2002		50	61	1270	3	0	–	156	33		–	43
Patients waiting for a transplant by end 2002	67	41	143	1183	–	0	–	94	8		–	17
Patients dead while on the WL during 2002		22	15	126	–	0	–	15	5		–	–
Heart												
No. transplant centres	3	1	3	17	1	0	1	3	1	4	3	1
Patients admitted to the waiting list during 2002	20	23	36	496	3	0		53	25		–	1
Patients waiting for a transplant by end 2002	4	16	112	698	2	0	4	26	6		–	23
Patients dead while on the WL during 2002	2	9	13	109	0	0	0	10	0		–	–

Table 2.2 • (Cont'd) Waiting lists of solid organ transplantations in Europe during 2002. Data from the Council of Europe

Countries	Greece	Hungary	Israel	Italy	Latvia	Luxembourg	Malta	The Netherlands	Norway	Poland	Portugal	Ireland
Lung												
No. transplant centres	2	–	2	10	–	0	–	2	1	–	1	1
Patients admitted to the waiting list during 2002	1	9	15	153	–	0	–	84	27	–	–	–
Patients waiting for a transplant by end 2002	2	1	38	253	–	0	–	66	40	–	–	–
Patients dead while on the WL during 2002	0	3	7	54	–	0	–	7	8	–	–	–
Pancreas												
No. transplant centres	0	1	–	15	–	0	–	2	1	3	1	1
Patients admitted to the waiting list during 2002	0	6	–	127	–	0	–	28	19	–	–	10
Patients waiting for a transplant by end 2002	0	19	–	287	–	0	–	15	11	–	–	16
Patients dead while on the WL during 2002	0	0	–	13	–	0	–	3	1	–	–	–
Small bowel												
No. transplant centres	0	0	–	1	–	0	–	1	0	–	1	–
Patients admitted to the waiting list during 2002	0	0	–	8	–	0	–	1	0	0	–	–
Patients waiting for a transplant by end 2002	0	0	–	17	–	0	–	1	–	0	–	–
Patients dead while on the WL during 2002	0	0	–	0	–	0	–	0	–	0	–	–

Table 2.2 • (Cont'd) Waiting lists of solid organ transplantations in Europe during 2002. Data from the Council of Europe

Countries	Romania	Slovak Republic	Slovenia	Spain	Sweden	Switzerland	Turkey	UK	USA*	Canada	Australia
Population (million inhabitants)	21	5.3	2	41.8	8.9	7.2	68.61	59.01	287.4	31.26	19.4
Kidney											
No. transplant centres	4	3	1	40	4	6		27	1368	–	–
Patients admitted to the waiting list during 2002	378	204	52	NG	370	352		2438	22 603	–	–
Patients waiting for a transplant by end 2002	1114	796	76	4014	445	498		6419	53 880	2963	1490
Patients dead while on the WL during 2002	55	98	2	NG	8	16		247	3204	89	49
Liver											
No. transplant centres	1	1	1	23	–	4		7	695	–	–
Patients admitted to the waiting list during 2002	71	17	14	1455	110	135		801	8942	–	–
Patients waiting for a transplant by end 2002	97	16	7	546	26	94		168	16 963	559	78
Patients dead while on the WL during 2002	26	4	0	181	8	20		56	1766	82	
Heart											
No. transplant centres	2	2	1	17	3	5		7	1464	–	–
Patients admitted to the waiting list during 2002	58	14	–	423	23	36		239	3153	–	–
Patients waiting for a transplant by end 2002	101	10	–	96	14	24		175	3787	103	70
Patients dead while on the WL during 2002	11	3	–	35	1	7		35	551	35	

Table 2.2 • (*Cont'd*) Waiting lists of solid organ transplantations in Europe during 2002. Data from the Council of Europe

Countries	Romania	Slovak Republic	Slovenia	Spain	Sweden	Switzerland	Turkey	UK	USA*	Canada	Australia
Lung											
No. transplant centres	–	0	0	9	2	3		6	1509	–	–
Patients admitted to the waiting list during 2002	–	0	–	231	33	36		233	1839	–	
Patients waiting for a transplant by end 2002	–	0	–	98	24	24		343	3804	150	112
Patients dead while on the WL during 2002	–	0	–	25	7	7		52	470	26	
Pancreas											
No. transplant centres	–	1	0	8	4	2		4	1436	–	–
Patients admitted to the waiting list during 2002	–	10	–	105	12	33		94	1688	–	
Patients waiting for a transplant by end 2002	–	12	–	47	20	27		154	3828	161	35
Patients dead while on the WL during 2002	–	1	–	1	–	1		6	229	3	
Small bowel											
No. transplant centres	–	0	0	3	2	1		1	1494	–	–
Patients admitted to the waiting list during 2002	–	0	–	15	–	1		–	195	–	0
Patients waiting for a transplant by end 2002	–	0	–	7	–	0		–	183	2	0
Patients dead while on the WL during 2002	–	0	–	4	–	0		–	52	0	0

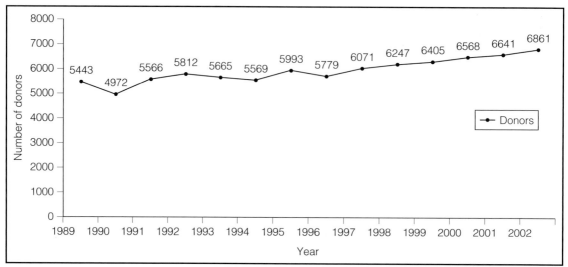

Figure 2.2 • Evolution of the total number of organ donors in selected European countries with available data during the period 1989–2002 (viz. Austria, Belgium, Denmark, Finland, France, Germany, Greece, Hungary, Republic of Ireland, Italy, Luxembourg, Norway, Poland, Portugal, Spain, Sweden, Switzerland, The Netherlands and the UK).

THE SITUATION IN SPAIN

Partial strategies in many countries, designed to improve cadaveric organ donation, have resulted in small or transient increases of donor numbers or even no improvement at all.[4,5] In the early 1990s, Spain started an original, integrated approach specifically designed to improve cadaveric organ donation.[6,7] The Spanish National Transplant Organisation (ONT) was created in 1989, and resulted among other measures in the establishment of a national network of specifically trained, part-time but strongly motivated hospital physicians in charge of the whole process of organ donation.[8,9] Since then, Spain has gone from 14 to 33.7 organ donors pmp (a 140% increase), by far the highest donor rate ever reached by a single country.[2] This is the only example in the world of a large country (41 million inhabitants) with a continuous increase in cadaveric organ donation sustained over a period of more than 10 years,[10] with parallel increases in the number of all solid organ transplants.

All the actions introduced in Spain in order to improve cadaveric organ donation during the 1990s are known at an international level as the 'Spanish Model' of organ donation,[6–10] and have been extensively described in the medical literature. The points that (taken together) define the Spanish Model are:

- A transplant coordination network at three levels: national, regional and hospital.
- The first two levels, nominated and paid by the national and regional authorities, are real interfaces between the political and the professional levels. All the technical decisions about transplants are taken by consensus in a Regional Council formed by the appropriate national and regional personnel.
- The third level, the hospital coordinator, should be a medical doctor (although helped by nurses in big hospitals), working preferentially on a part-time basis, and based within the hospital. These individuals are nominated by, and report to, the hospital director (not the head of the transplant units), although functionally linked with the regional and national coordinators.
- Most hospital coordinators are anaesthetists/intensivists, which results in the active participation of these physicians in organ donation. Part-time commitment allows them to continue working in their principal speciality and, importantly, to be present even in the smaller hospitals.

- Continuous audit of potential donors is performed by the transplant coordinators.[11]
- The central office of the ONT acts as the support agency in charge of organ sharing, transport, waiting list management, transplant registries, statistics, general and specialised information, and action that can improve the whole process of organ donation and transplantation. As a significant percentage of organs are retrieved in small hospitals without neurosurgery (up to 15% in the national 2001 brain death audit[11]), regional and national offices give external support to those centres where resources for the whole process are not easily available.
- A great effort in continuous medical training and education for new and existing transplant coordinators financed and directed by the central Health Administration. Development of various training programmes for health professionals, specifically dedicated to every step of the process (donor detection and management, legal aspects, family approach, organisational aspects, management of resources, etc.) have been promoted.
- Hospital reimbursement by the regional or national health administrations, which finances adequately the procurement and transplant activity. Otherwise, the sustained procurement activity, especially from small non-university and non-transplant hospitals becomes practically impossible.
- Much attention is devoted to the important role of the mass media and to improve the level of information of the Spanish population on these topics. Examples include a 24-hour transplantation hotline, periodic meetings between journalists and opinion leaders, training courses in communication for hospital and regional coordinators, and management of adverse publicity. Systematic communication, via the media, to the medical and lay community[12] has also been implemented.
- An adequate legal background, technically similar to that of other Western countries.[13] There is a definition of death after brainstem testing. Organ retrieval only takes place after obtaining the consent of the family and no compensation can be paid either for donation or transplanted organs. Spain has a theoretical

'presumed consent' law, but from a practical point of view, family consent is always asked and the wishes of the relatives are always respected, as is the case in practically all the EU countries. In fact, the family refusal rate has remained stable at between 20 and 25% during the last years.[10,13] What is clear is that the increase in organ donation during the 1990s cannot be attributed to any change of the Spanish legislation, which has remained unmodified since 1979.

These measures are of course far more than just appointing transplant coordinators and are not easy to integrate. The results can be heavily influenced by undue weight paid to any one factor alone or the structural differences from country to country. Furthermore, before trying to adapt this model of organisation to other countries or regions, several structural characteristics should be analysed:[14]

- **Number of doctors available in each country and the average basic pay per year for these professionals.** It is easy to understand that a system like the Spanish one, based on a network of medical doctors, would be very difficult or very expensive to implement in countries with a low index of physicians to population or in those with very high incomes for the doctors. A low number of doctors, with high incomes not related to objectives but linked to the concept of 'availability', is probably the worst possible scenario.
- **Number of acute beds and ICU facilities available.** Among the different rates that are relevant for organ donation, the number of intensive care unit (ICU) beds per million population and the ratio of ICU beds/total acute beds seem to be the most relevant ones. Differences from country to country can explain some of the difficulties found in the detection of potential donors and their continued management until the full process of organ procurement is completed.
- **Epidemiology of the population.** The results of an integrated approach to increase cadaveric organ donation such as that in Spain demonstrate an expansion of the organ donor pool thanks to the acceptance of older and

more difficult donors.[5,14] The percentage of Spanish donors over 60 years increased during the last ten years from 10 to 33.9%. In the same way, most of donors now die following intracerebral bleeding, whilst traffic deaths accounted for just 17.5% of all donors during 2002. Therefore marked differences from country to country, or even from region to region, in the age distribution of the population can explain relevant differences in the potential for organ donors as these differences are linked to other epidemiological data (intracerebral bleeding, cancer deaths, etc.). All these data, together with the road traffic accident mortality rate and perhaps other factors, form a clear definition of the basic situation in a country/region, a necessary prerequisite when considering an approach like the Spanish Model.

THE PROCESS OF ORGAN DONATION AND TRANSPLANTATION

The organ donation/transplantation process is necessarily complex. There are a number of important steps, each of which needs to be recognised, and an effective system must be put in place to manage every part of the process if potential donor organs are not to be lost. The steps are:[1]

1. **Donor identification** – all potential donors should be identified at as early a stage as possible. This will facilitate donor screening and donor management (see below).

2. **Donor screening** – donors should not be used if there is a significant risk of transmission of serious disease (cancer, infection) to the recipient. Guidance has been prepared by the Council of Europe and some member states on the serological and other screening methods that should be used to minimise the risk of transmission of infectious or malignant diseases to the recipient.[15] Whenever possible, screening should include a social history taken from the relatives to exclude recent high-risk behaviour, which might indicate risk of a transmissible disease at an early stage, in the 'window' between acquisition of the virus and a positive screening test.

3. **Donor management** – it is essential that all organs procured are in good condition prior to retrieval. The management of the potential donor's physiological state while in intensive care, prior to and during retrieval can make a major difference to the condition of the organs. Poor donor management can make organs unusable.

4. **Consent/authorisation** – appropriate consent or authorisation has to be obtained before organs can be removed. Countries have different legal requirements; in some consent is presumed while in others specific consent has to be sought from either the donor's relatives or an official body. Whatever the system, it is advisable to discuss donation with any relatives as part of the screening process. There is evidence that the approach to the relatives can affect their willingness to agree to donation. Staff seeking to obtain the agreement of relatives should be appropriately trained.

5. **Organ retrieval** – the surgical technique for removing organs from the body and the way those organs are subsequently handled and preserved prior to and during transportation are critical to the successful outcome of the transplant. Each year a number of organs are damaged during removal and/or transportation. Some can be repaired but a few will have to be discarded.[16]

6. **Organ allocation** – for some organs, particularly kidneys, the successful long-term outcome of the transplant depends partly on appropriate HLA (human leucocyte antigen) matching between donor and recipient. A well-organised system for allocating and transporting donated organs to the most appropriate recipient is important. In some cases, optimum allocation will require exchange of organs or tissues between transplant organisations and countries. Cooperation between countries is increasingly important.

AREAS AND STRATEGIES FOR IMPROVEMENT: THE QUALITY PROGRAMMES

Figure 2.3 represents graphically all the steps of the process of organ donation and transplantation,

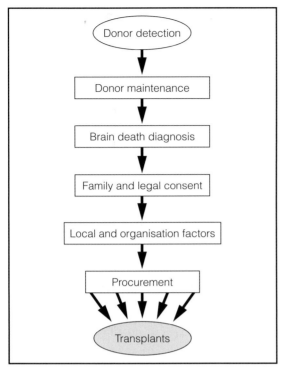

Figure 2.3 • Organ donation and transplantation process.

which has been described as being like 'a chain of events that can be always broken by the weakest link'. Each step should be analysed whenever there is a problem in organ donation, in order to detect the weak points of the chain and determine strategies for improvement.

As is always the case in medicine it is almost impossible to prescribe an adequate therapy if we do not have first a correct diagnosis. Probably the best way to evaluate in a continuous way the process of organ donation is the establishment of one of the so-called 'Quality Improvement Programmes'. The objectives of these programmes are:[11,17]

• Definition of the theoretical potential for organ procurement depending on the characteristics of the hospital.
• Detection of any obstacles in the process of organ donation and procurement and an analysis of the causes of the potential donor losses, as a tool to identify the areas for improvement.
• Description of hospital factors that can influence the donation and transplantation process.

The Spanish programme of quality improvement was the first to be described and implemented during the mid-1990s, and has served as a basis for other international programmes such as Donor Action and that adopted in the Italian region of Tuscany[18] or (more recently) in Argentina. The programme is based on a systematic review of all medical records of patient deaths in intensive care units (ICUs), carried out at least every three months. For the purpose of this programme an intensive care bed is defined as a hospital bed with mechanical ventilation and intensive care facilities where a patient can be admitted for more than 12 hours.

Three kinds of datasets should be completed periodically. An individual dataset should be completed for every patient with the clinical diagnosis of death by brainstem testing, and a compilation of all these should be sent to the central office at least every three months. Secondly, an ICU dataset with the total number of deaths, number of brain deaths and number of organ donors should be completed for every ICU of the hospital and sent to the central office every three months. Finally, general data on every hospital about the total number of deaths, number of available beds, neurosurgery procedures and patients admitted to the ICU and emergency rooms should be collected each year. Individual, ICU and hospital data are maintained in a database with an application that can automatically calculate the different indices accepted internationally.

Hospitals are classified according to the presence or absence of a neurosurgical department as this has been the main factor in establishing differences with respect to the number of patients with death diagnosed by tests of brain, or brainstem, function.[13] Although it is possible to calculate many indices to evaluate the efficiency of the process, the two most useful and the published 'gold standards' in Spain are:

• Number of brain deaths/deaths in ICU – an index of the process of potential donor detection (the first part of the process).
  Hospitals with neurosurgery   15.1%
  Hospitals without neurosurgery   7.5%
• Number of actual donors/brain deaths – an index of the efficiency of the process of organ donation (the final part of the process).
  Hospitals with neurosurgery   49%
  Hospitals without neurosurgery   37.8%

These are, however, mean values and great variation has been observed, even among hospitals with the same characteristics.[13] As a consequence, these standards should be redefined for every country/ region/hospital.

Several authors in different geographical areas and with different methodologies have suggested that the potential donor pool is probably close to or even exceeds 50 donors pmp.[9,13,19,20] In these studies, as many as one third of the potential donors remain unidentified or poorly managed, and another third are lost due to family or coroner refusal: the actual number of donors may therefore be less than one-third of the potential.[9] Thus, the problem is not only a lack of suitable donors but also a failure to turn potential donors into actual donors.[20]

That is one of the reasons why the Council of Europe has approved a European Consensus Document ('Meeting the Organ Shortage'[1]) where every one of these steps is analysed and after detecting the possible problems, strategies for improvement are suggested. For example, if the percentage of brain deaths/number of deaths in a particular ICU is clearly under the norm, a problem of under-detection becomes evident. All efforts should be addressed to establishing the criteria adopted in this particular ICU to define a potential donor, and determining the outcome of patients with intra-cerebral bleeding. Up-to-date protocols may need to be established in close agreement with the clinician responsible for the ICU. If, however, a high family refusal rate is the diagnosis, training courses in communication skills should be considered for all staff of the ICU and emergency rooms, among other measures.

'Meeting the Organ Shortage': Summary of recommendations

The recommendations included in this document are:

1. The transplant process is long and complex and cannot be left to chance. Protocols should be developed for each step. A key person should be made responsible in each area/hospital for managing and monitoring the process with the power to determine where efforts and resources should be directed.

2. Published national or regional figures cannot be extrapolated to provide local rates of potential versus effective donors (although marked differences from published rates for potential donors should be considered as suggestive of underdetection). A donor detection gap should be established for each hospital/area and systems for monitoring the rates established.

3. A means should be developed to evaluate the size and characteristics of the potential donor pool to measure and monitor potential donor detection rates. To ensure reliability, data should be collected prospectively and analysed retrospectively as recommended in the 'Donor Action Programme'.

4. Proactive donor detection programmes should be instituted in every acute hospital using specially trained professionals (key donation persons) working to agreed protocols and ethical rules.

5. A 'key donation person', independent from transplant teams, should be appointed in every acute hospital, with a clearly defined role and responsibility for establishing, managing and auditing systems for donor identification and identifying potential areas for improvement.

6. Protocols should be developed setting out the criteria for screening potential donors and their organs for the risk of disease transmission and potential viability. All appropriate steps should be taken to avoid the transmission of infectious and neoplastic diseases.

7. The incidence of irreversible cardiac arrest, sepsis and other contraindications to organ donation relating to management of potential donors should be monitored and audited to detect and correct any problems identified. Involvement of ICU staff in research and/or educational programmes on donor management should help raise standards.

8. An appropriate legal framework for donation and transplantation is required, which adequately defines:
   • brain death;
   • the type of consent or authorisation required for retrieval (see below);

- the means of organ retrieval that ensures traceability but maintains confidentiality and bans organ trafficking.

9. Law professionals should be fully aware of the transplant process, and the cooperation of those most closely involved, i.e. judges and coroners, should be sought to reduce legal refusals to a minimum.

10. It is advisable to ascertain the opinion of the public and health professionals about presumed or informed consent for organ donation before considering legal changes that might be potentially detrimental. The key donation person appointed in each centre/area must be aware of all local legal criteria and should be responsible for meeting these requirements. There should be a system for the safe custody of all certificates and test results required by the law.

11. Because both positive and negative messages can affect the public's willingness to donate organs, there is a need for a professional attitude to communications, which may require support from experts. They should help to minimise the impact of 'bad news', and maximise the communication of 'good news' about transplantation to health professionals, the media and the public. Special attention should be paid to both the content of the message and the best means of dealing with the most controversial topics. The preparation of specific briefing materials should be considered.

12. The most cost-effective means of increasing the public's willingness to donate seems to be improving the knowledge of health professionals (not directly involved in transplantation) and the media about transplantation issues. Continuing education should form an essential element of any communication strategy. A transplant 'hotline' manned by appropriately trained professionals should be considered.

13. People should be encouraged to speak about organ donation and transplantation and to communicate their wishes to their relatives. As a donor's wishes will not always be known, staff in a position to make requests for agreement to organ donation to relatives should be properly trained for the purpose. If such requests are well handled the rate of donation refusals can be reduced.

14. Organ retrieval procedures should be well planned to minimise delay and disruption to the donor hospital. Retrieval teams should be led by experienced surgeons trained, where appropriate, in multiorgan retrieval. Organ damage during retrieval should be reported and monitored and further training provided as necessary to minimise damage during retrieval or transportation.

15. An organ sharing/allocation organisation is essential but its roles and responsibilities must be clearly defined, particularly if it is to have a role in organ donation and procurement (see below).

16. Attention should be paid to ensuring that hospitals are properly resourced and, if necessary, reimbursed for maximising organ procurement.

17. In order to optimise organ donation there is need for a supra-hospital transplant organisation, appropriate in size and structure to the local situation with specific responsibilities for the whole process of organ procurement.

18. The most effective organisational approach is one that balances the requirements for effective organ procurement (small, local) with those for organ allocation (large, national/ multinational) (see below). The aim should be to optimise organ procurement whilst ensuring the most clinically effective allocation of organs and tissues.

19. Health administrations are responsible for ensuring that there is proper organisational support for organ donation and distribution and should guarantee the fairness, transparency and safety of the whole system.

20. International cooperation on the promotion of organ donation is desirable to help maximise organ donation and equalise access to transplantation between countries. Governments should actively promote such cooperation.

21. Priority should be given to international cooperation that improves standards of training, exchange of experience, and helps

guarantee the safety of organs and the ethical standards by which they are retrieved and transplanted.

ALTERNATIVES TO CONVENTIONAL CADAVERIC ORGAN DONATION

Even when the process of conventional cadaveric organ donation (after the diagnosis of death) becomes fully optimised, it seems unlikely that the need for organ donors can be met.[1–3] Consequently, other possible additional sources of organ procurement must be considered. This chapter will not discuss future possibilities such as xeno-transplantation,[21] but as a real option for patients on the waiting list for a kidney, liver or lung, non-heart-beating and living organ donation will be discussed.

Non-heart-beating donors

Thanks to the pioneer work of García-Rinaldi and others,[22] kidneys removed from non-heart-beating donors (NHBD) were used in the early days of solid organ transplants. During the 1980s, except in a very limited number of units, this technique fell into disuse with the progressive increase of brainstem-dead donors. During the 1990s, however, the concern of the international transplant community about the organ shortage created a growing interest in this technique, especially after the Maastricht conference in 1995.[23] The results published about the viability of kidneys procured in this way (and to a lesser extent livers and even lungs) are encouraging,[24] although a very 'positive selection' with respect to the age criteria and other risk factors should be considered when evaluating the results.

There are great differences in Europe from country to country with respect to the legal consideration of this kind of donation.[13] Some countries like Germany forbid the use of organs procured in this way. In others, such as Italy, it is neither forbidden nor permitted, whilst countries such as Spain have regulated the process in a very strict way. The exact potential of NHBD is not known. It is true that some successful programmes have more than doubled the number of organs procured in a specific

hospital. These figures, however, cannot be extrapolated to a whole country because these programmes are very time consuming and require a great effort of many well-trained staff (coordinators, surgeons, emergency department, etc.) 24 hours a day. Despite the great development of the Spanish transplant coordinators' network the only structured programme of NHBD is in Madrid. However, this technique accounted for only 2–3% of organ donors in Spain during recent years.

Non-heart-beating donation can be a significant step in the process of increasing organ donation for transplantation. However, the technique has a high cost–benefit ratio and should be considered only in those hospitals where conventional organ donation has been fully optimised.

Living donation

Living kidney donation was historically the first procedure used for kidney transplantation, 50 years ago. As happened with NHBD this modality fell into disuse with the progressive increase of brainstem-dead donors in developed countries. However, live donor numbers started to grow again during the 1990s due to the lack of organs, and also to the availability of new drugs to prevent rejection, which made possible living transplants from non-genetically related persons. The number of living kidney donors has steadily increased during recent years, as an alternative to cadaveric organ shortage, and now represents 14.2% of renal transplants in Europe and 42% in USA. There is, however, a very great variation from country to country, ranging from 46% in Norway or 44% in Greece to 1.5% in Spain.

Liver transplants for children using a left lobe of an adult donor started in 1989. The use of adult-to-child living donor liver transplantation has helped to diminish waiting list mortality with a risk of death for the donor, which is considered to be less than 0.2%. Adult-to-adult living liver donation is, however, a relatively new area that has developed rapidly in Europe, USA and Japan in recent years. For an adult recipient, more liver must be removed from the donor, and the risk for adult-to-adult donation is significantly higher than for adult-to-child donation. The estimated risk of dying is between 0.5 and 1%. Up to seven deaths have been reported in the medical literature (and probably more have occurred) among previously healthy living liver donors. In addition, there is about a 20% risk to the adult-to-adult donor of other complications, such as wound infection, bile duct leaks, etc.

During 2002, a total of 274 living liver transplants were performed in 15 European countries (4.9% of total liver transplants), and 358 in the USA (6.7%) and these numbers look set to grow.

CONCLUSIONS

The shortage of cadaveric donors is a universal problem and imposes a severe limit on the number of patients who can benefit from transplantation. At the same time there is an ever-increasing demand for cadaveric solid organs all over the world. Organ shortage is not due to a lack of potential donors, but rather to a failure to turn many potential into actual donors. Spain is the only example in the world of continuous improvement in cadaveric organ donation recorded in a large country during more than a ten-year period. A proactive donor detection programme performed by well-trained transplant coordinators, the introduction of systematic death audits in the hospitals and the combination of a favourable public attitude, effective management of mass-media relations, and adequate economic reimbursement for the hospitals accounted for this success. This model can be partially or totally adapted to other countries or regions if basic conditions are guaranteed. An adequate and careful study of local characteristics, which can influence organ donation in a direct or indirect way, should be done before planning any specific action to improve organ donor rates.

Key points

- The shortage of cadaveric donors is a universal problem, while there is an ever-increasing worldwide demand for organs.
- Organ shortage is not due to a lack of potential donors, but rather to a failure to turn many potential into actual donors.
- Spain is the only large country to show continuous improvement in cadaveric organ donation over a more than 10-year period. This has been accomplished by a combination of: a proactive donor detection programme run by well-trained transplant coordinators; systematic death audits in hospitals; positive public attitudes, effective mass media relations; and adequate reimbursement for the hospitals.
- This model can be partially or totally adapted to other countries or regions if basic conditions are guaranteed.
- An adequate and careful study of local characteristics, which can influence organ donation in a direct or indirect way, should be done before planning any specific action to improve organ donor rates.

Part 2

The acute shortage of donors – a UK perspective

Christopher J. Rudge

INTRODUCTION

Since organ transplantation became recognised as the definitive form of treatment for patients with end-stage heart, lung, liver and kidney failure there has probably never been a time when there **wasn't** a shortage of suitable donors in the UK. However, this shortage has become ever more apparent and important over the past 10–15 years as the success rates for all forms of transplantation have steadily increased. Initially, in the 1960s and 1970s, the shortage was almost certainly the result of ignorance and uncertainty about organ donation on the part of both the medical profession and the general public. Donor numbers generally rose throughout the 1980s, despite occasional setbacks such as the infamous Panorama programme on BBC television: 'Transplants – are the donors really dead?' (Oct 1980), helped in part by a number of high-profile public appeals for a liver or heart donor and by a much wider (although not universal) acceptance of organ donation by public and profession alike. The Organ Donor Card was introduced in 1974. However, UK solid organ donor numbers reached an annual peak of 875 in 1995, and have declined slowly but steadily thereafter until 2000–02 (**Fig. 2.4**).

Whilst the full explanation for this falling donor rate is not clear there are a number of factors that are probably relevant. First, there have been significant falls in the UK death rates from both road traffic accidents (RTA) and cerebrovascular haemorrhage (the two main causes of death of solid organ cadaver donors) over the past 20 years.[25,26] Indeed, the UK now has one of the lowest RTA mortality rates in Europe[27] – one of the many things that make international donor rate comparisons difficult to interpret.

Secondly, the UK has an ageing population and it would appear that UK transplant centres were well behind the Spanish in accepting that for many patients transplantation of an organ (particularly a kidney) from an older donor may be better than no transplantation at all.[28] Even in 2002 only 15% of UK donors were over 60 years of age[29] compared with 33.9% in Spain. Part of the Spanish success story is undoubtedly the willingness of transplant units to remove organs from older donors even though this may lead to more kidneys that are donated being discarded compared with the UK.

This is a good example of a third factor that many feel became increasingly relevant during the 1990s but for which the evidence is no more than anecdotal – an increasing reluctance on the part of transplant surgeons and other clinicians to accept organs from donors with any perceived risk of disease transmission or poor organ function. Official documents from both the UK and Europe[30,31] contained guidelines designed to eliminate, or at least reduce to an absolute minimum, the risk of transmitting malignant or infective diseases (particularly hepatitis B and C and HIV) from donor to recipient. There is a widespread perception that this advice, or its interpretation, was unnecessarily restrictive. Indeed, a more recent UK document gave much more balanced advice that for all transplant recipients there is an informed decision to be made between the potential risks and benefits of any proposed transplant.[32]

Poor organ function may be associated with increasing donor age, and there are also organ-specific

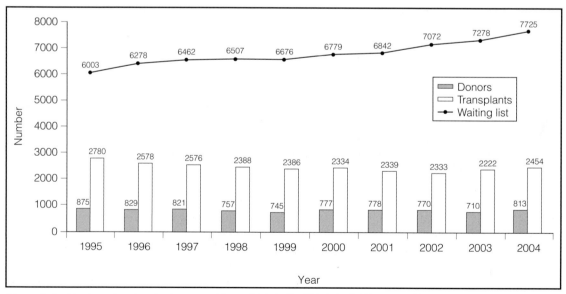

Figure 2.4 • Number of cadaveric donors and transplants in the UK, 1 April 1995 to 31 March 2004, and patients on the active and suspended waiting lists at 31 March for each year.

comorbidities, such as a history of hypertension or diabetes for kidney donors and a 'fatty' liver for liver donors, that have in the past been considered by some as contraindications to donation and transplantation. With increased emphasis on monitoring outcomes and awareness of clinical governance issues clinicians have been understandably reluctant to use 'marginal' donors or organs. However, as evidence increases that such organs may be transplanted with acceptable outcomes and that the patient and clinician can take an informed decision on the risk/benefit analysis it is to be hoped that such organs will increasingly be accepted in appropriate circumstances.

There are two other factors thought to be associated with the UK's falling donor rate, but again evidence to support these is limited. First, there have been changes in neurosurgical practice.[33] The selection of appropriate (i.e. potentially treatable) patients for transfer to neurosurgical centres has become more refined with the possible result that patients with more severe lesions do not receive active (intensive care) treatment. They are therefore likely to die in circumstances that mitigate against organ donation. In addition, surgical developments have reduced the extent and consequences of raised intracranial pressure[34,35] and thus the likelihood that the patient will 'cone' and suffer death that can be confirmed by brainstem tests.

Secondly, there is an increasing number of local studies suggesting that 40–50% or more of the relatives of potential organ donors are refusing permission for donation, and the first year's results of the UK Potential Donor Audit (see below) lead to a similar conclusion. This compares with the 30% relatives refusal rate found in the study by Gore et al.[36] and the much lower figure of 20–25% quoted earlier in this chapter for Spain.[10] The reasons for this apparent increase in the UK refusal rate are not clear but it seems quite possible that public medical 'scandals' such as the Alder Hey organ retention story and Dr Harold Shipman's conviction for the murder of a number of his patients[37] have contributed to an increasing distrust of the medical profession in general rather than any specific opposition to organ donation and transplantation.

It should be emphasised that much of the preceding section is little more than speculation, thus stressing the need for a detailed analysis of the national potential for organ donation and the current obstacles.

REGIONAL VARIATIONS IN DONOR RATES

Not only has there been a falling UK donor rate but there is also clear evidence of marked regional variation. Solid organ donor rates varied in 1999–2000 between the 21 kidney retrieval areas from 8 pmp to 27.4 pmp, and Wight and Cameron have recently carried out a detailed study of possible factors leading to this variation.[38] They obtained data from UK Transplant and the UK's Offices of Statistics, Health Departments, Intensive Care Societies and other professional bodies. The study was designed geographically to compare the donor rate pmp with a number of factors that might reasonably be expected to affect it: deaths from road traffic accidents, intracerebral haemorrhage and other trauma; the number of general and neurosurgical intensive care unit (ICU) beds; co-location of transplant and neurosurgical units in the same hospital; the proportion of the population from minority ethnic groups; the proportion of the population on the organ donor register; the number of transplant coordinators working in organ retrieval; and the number of transplant units. Their results showed a weak link between the number of general ICU beds and the donor rate ($P = 0.065$). In areas with more neurosurgical ICU beds, and those with a higher proportion of the population from ethnic minority origin, the donor rate was significantly lower – more neurosurgical ICU beds, fewer donors. This is clearly counterintuitive and appears to differ from the earlier findings from Spain. If confirmed it requires further investigation to understand the mechanisms. There was no significant association with any of the other variables. Overall a substantial amount of the variation (possibly as much as 80%) remains unexplained. The national Potential Donor Audit (see below) may provide the information to answer many of these questions.

THE CURRENT SITUATION

The years 2000–2003 appear to have seen the UK donor rate stabilise, with 770, 710 and 813 donors per year (a rate of 13.0 pmp). Virtually all donors donate kidneys, and 88% also donate the liver. Heart and lung donation rates are much lower, with only 30% of donors donating one or more cardio-thoracic organs.[39] In part this is due to the more rigorous clinical criteria (including age) that affect the suitability of these organs for transplantation. Once again there are regional variations, with the proportion of multiorgan donors ranging from 71% to 100%. There may still be aspects of organisation or attitude that influence local practice. Clearly, part of the process of maximising organ donation rates is to introduce best practice across all areas of the country, and this requires not only an effective donor identification and coordination process but also optimal donor management and an efficient organ retrieval service.

To document donor and transplant numbers is straightforward. To identify the true need for transplantation is more difficult, and it is necessary to consider each organ separately.

In April 2005 there were 5333 patients on the active national renal transplant list and the median waiting time for a cadaveric transplant was 558 days (with wide variation depending on factors such as recipient blood group and ethnic origin). In 2004 a total of 1821 kidney transplants were performed and 2808 new patients were added to the list. A transplant rate of 50 pmp, which means 2950 transplants per year, would therefore meet the needs of all new patients and progressively reduce the backlog. Whether more patients would be accepted onto the list if more kidneys were available is not clear (see below). There are now national guidelines for transplant waiting list assessment[40] and it is to be hoped that all suitable patients are being assessed and placed on the list. There are also agreed criteria for combined kidney–pancreas transplantation for diabetic patients, and a recent assessment suggested that there is potentially a need for approximately 350 such transplants per year (C. Watson, personal communication).

The true need for liver transplantation was discussed at a UK meeting in January 2003.[41] It seems clear that the current practice of limiting access to the liver list to patients expected to have at least a 50% chance of surviving 5 years after transplantation denies this option to a number of patients who could nonetheless benefit from a transplant. Although there are insufficient data to give a precise estimate of need it may be reasonable to suggest that the liver transplant rate needs to double. Even with current criteria, 12% of patients accepted for routine (i.e. non-urgent) liver transplants die before an organ becomes available.

It is also the case that approximately 12% of patients accepted for cardiac transplantation die on the waiting list but the situation is complex. Intensive medical management of end-stage heart failure has probably reduced the number of potential recipients, and a recent study by Dark into the non-use of donor hearts demonstrated that some were not used because there were no suitable recipients in the UK (J. Dark, personal communication). This was particularly true in the case of smaller, blood group A donors. However, it is also the case that the current national criteria for both heart and lung recipient selection would be relaxed, and more recipients identified, if the donor supply were consistently greater than at present.

THE UK MODEL TO INCREASE ORGAN DONATION

UK Transplant was established as a Special Health Authority in 2000, and for the first time in the UK a single organisation was given responsibility – and a certain amount of funding – to increase organ donation rates, thus adopting the first requirement of the Spanish model for a national transplant coordination network. A 5-year Business Case was approved by the UK Health Departments in April 2001, and a number of developments have been introduced since then, based in part on the Spanish model but drawn up in the context of what is realistic and appropriate for the UK. It is too early to assess the impact of these developments, but the financial year 2002–3 saw a 4% increase in solid organ donors, a 6% increase in corneal donors and small increases in the number of kidney, liver, kidney–pancreas and lung transplants. Time alone will tell whether this progress can be maintained.

There are a number of components of the UK model.

1. Transplant coordinators

It is very important to recognise that the term 'transplant coordinator' is used in very different ways in different countries. The Spanish transplant coordinators described earlier in this chapter are almost all doctors and they work within a single hospital. Whilst there has been considerable variation across the UK, transplant coordinators have generally been nurses, have usually been based within a transplant unit, and in many units have combined the roles of encouraging and organising organ donation from local donor hospitals with a degree of responsibility for potential transplant recipients. The result has been a somewhat variable service, often inadequately staffed and funded and with wide differences in the level of contact between coordinators and their local hospitals and intensive care units. Working with the existing coordinators, UK Transplant has been able to fund extra posts in the most hard-pressed areas, to introduce a more clearly defined structure for coordinators that includes local and regional leadership, has clarified the separate roles and responsibilities of donor and recipient coordinators and is progressively introducing best practice into all donor coordinator teams in order to focus efforts on improving the profile and practice of organ donation across all intensive care units in the UK. There is also much greater cooperation with, for example, the Intensive Care Society and the Critical Care networks in order to understand the possible obstacles to donation as seen from the ICU perspective. These changes are still evolving but there are encouraging signs of a more coherent approach that will put donor coordination in a very much stronger position than before.

2. Donor liaison nurses

It was not felt possible to introduce doctors as coordinators in the UK, but a pilot study is under way of the use of experienced intensive care nurses in a somewhat similar role. Called donor liaison nurses (DLNs), 35 of these posts are currently funded. Each post involves the donor liaison nurse working within either a single ICU, several ICUs within a single NHS trust or, in one or two cases, within an ICU network in several closely linked local hospitals. Each DLN is supported by a nominated intensive care clinician. Their role is to work closely with the local donor coordinator team in raising the profile of organ donation from their individual

hospital and to ensure that all necessary training and education needs of local staff are met. Any local problems with organ donation can be identified and, hopefully, resolved. In particular the DLNs can work towards establishing the optimal approach to the relatives of potential donors in the light of the experience and wishes of the ICU staff and the donor coordinator teams. To date the impact of these posts has been varied, but it would appear that in a number of hospitals there has been a positive effect on the number of referrals of both solid organ and tissue potential donors. The DLNs have been particularly effective in the introduction of the Potential Donor Audit into their local ICUs (see below).

The new donor transplant coordinator system and the donor liaison nurse schemes are designed principally to improve organ donation from heart-beating donors in intensive care units. The Intensive Care Societies in the UK have been supportive of these developments, and recognise the need to do everything possible – their support is crucial and very welcome.

However, options to increase organ donation are not limited to heart-beating donors, and there are also developments designed to increase both non-heart-beating and living donation in the UK.

3. Non-heart-beating organ donors (NHBDs)

Despite the considerable contribution to donor numbers made by NHBDs reported from units such as Maastricht, only three UK transplant centres continued to retrieve such organs throughout the 1980s and 1990s.[42] The main emphasis was on so-called 'uncontrolled' donors from Accident and Emergency departments and the programmes were extremely demanding in terms of the availability of both coordinators and surgical staff. Initial anxieties about the clinical outcome using kidneys from such donors were resolved with data showing equivalent graft survival and function compared with kidneys from heart-beating donors.[43] Accordingly, funding has been provided to nine units to start or to develop further their NHBD programmes. The emphasis has moved largely, although not exclusively, towards 'controlled' NHBDs from intensive care units where the logistical problems, whilst still considerable, are perhaps less than for uncontrolled donors. Suitable patients are those who whilst not meeting the criteria for the diagnosis of death by brainstem testing have suffered a devastating and irreversible brain injury and where the decision to withdraw further treatment – because it is futile – has been made. A number of aspects of this practice have raised possible legal and ethical concerns (see below) but in certain centres it appears to be developing strongly with the support of all concerned. Whilst in most units organ removal is limited to the kidneys, several centres are developing experience in liver transplantation from NHBDs, with encouraging preliminary results, and to date four lung transplants have also been performed. This latter is a particularly interesting development as there is evidence to suggest that the lung may be relatively resistant to warm ischaemia, and may indeed benefit from the absence of the damaging effects of the major physiological consequences following death of the brainstem.

4. Living donation

Whilst there is currently a debate in liver transplant circles about the possibility of starting a UK programme of living donor liver transplantation for adults, in effect living donation is restricted to kidney donation. However, at least one programme in the UK is set to start adult-to-adult living donation soon. The number of living donor kidney transplants carried out in the UK stayed under 100 per year (i.e. about 6–7% of all transplants) until 1993, since when it has increased steadily and in 2004 had reached 463, or 25% of transplants. This figure is still lower than in Norway and the USA, but it is clear that there is an increasing willingness on the part of transplant units to carry out these procedures, supported by detailed professional advice.[44] A large part of the increase in numbers is accounted for by non-genetically related (mainly spouse/partner) donors. There is a considerable workload involved in the assessment and investigation of potential living donors, with a significant number being found to be unsuitable at some stage of the process. Experience from one or two of the larger centres has shown that the appointment of a full-time living donor coordinator can streamline the process, shorten the time taken, increase the number of suitable donors that are identified, and also improve the way in which potential donors are counselled at all stages of the assessment. Such appointments have now been made in virtually all transplant units, although regrettably central funding is not currently available for the larger dialysis centres that carry out living donor work-up locally before referring patients to the transplant unit for surgery.

5. Potential Donor Audit

The Spanish model incorporates a regular assessment of the potential for organ donation from each hospital carried out by the in-house transplant coordinator, and the Council of Europe document 'Meeting the Organ Shortage' recommends that a 'donor detection gap monitoring system' should be established for each hospital. A major review of the number of potential organ donors from intensive care units in the USA has recently been published.[45,46] In the UK there have in the past been several studies of the national potential for organ donation, most importantly that of Gore et al.,[36] and many local studies. An important component of the new UK initiatives is the national Potential Donor Audit (PDA), which builds on previous work and started as a pilot project in June 2002. It has now collected data on virtually all patients who have died in intensive care in the United Kingdom since January 2003. This provides a detailed picture of the true potential for organ donation from ICUs (from both heartbeating and non-heart-beating donors) and will help to identify the main obstacles to increasing the donor rate.

Unlike a number of previous UK donor audits the PDA data is collected primarily by donor transplant coordinators and donor liaison nurses, supported by link nurses within the ICUs. The audit attempts to identify:

- all patients who die in intensive care;
- those in whom the diagnosis of death is made following tests of brainstem function (and those who were not tested when this may have been appropriate);

- those with absolute contraindications to organ donation (currently a positive test for HIV and known or suspected CJD);
- those with other medical contraindications to donation such as uncontrolled sepsis or cancer.

Additionally, whether or not the next of kin were approached, and the outcome of such a request for donation is recorded, as is the response (if required) of the coroner or procurator fiscal. The audit is contemporaneous with data normally collected and reported every 1–2 weeks and it is intended that it should continue indefinitely. It should go considerably further than the basic epidemiological data described earlier in this chapter, in that it should be possible to describe, for each ICU, the donor rate as a 'percentage of the potential'. No unit, region or country can do more than achieve its maximum potential for donation,[47] and that will be influenced by many of the factors mentioned earlier such as death rates from trauma and cerebrovascular haemorrhage, intensive care facilities and practice, and consent rates for donation. If all potential donors become actual donors that is success – whether it translates to a donor rate of 5 pmp or 55 pmp.

The results from the first year of the PDA to date suggest that in the UK a major limiting factor to increased donation is a remarkably high rate of relatives' refusal of permission for donation – approximately 42% across the UK. If confirmed, this finding alone could explain the UK's relatively low donor rate compared with other European countries. A relatives' refusal rate of only 25% (as in Spain) with the current number of identified potential donors would result in a donor rate of 19–20 pmp, almost on a par with the best in Europe with the inevitable exception of Spain. Such a finding would also give a clear indication of possible steps to improve the donor rate, such as a trial of 'collaborative requesting' – a joint approach involving both ICU staff and donor coordinators in the approach to a potential donor's next of kin.

6. Public opinion and the Organ Donor Register

It is axiomatic that a successful national donation programme depends on the support of the general public. Whilst there has always been a large majority of the UK population in favour of donation in principle, and many millions of donor cards were distributed, attention is now being focused on the Organ Donor Register (ODR) as a means of raising the profile of donation and encouraging individuals to consider, and then register, their own views. The ODR was established in 1994 and is purely an 'opting in' register. Individuals can register on it directly, but the principal routes for registration are through the General Practitioner system (when patients register or change their GP), the driving licence process and local electoral lists. There are currently 12 million names on the ODR (approximately 21% of the population), and since April 2003 the ODR has been made much more accessible to donor coordinators and senior medical and nursing staff in ICUs. It is now possible at any time of day or night to establish whether a potential donor has registered their wishes on the ODR, and it is clear that when the patient's positive wishes are known the relatives almost invariably give their permission.

UK Transplant has commissioned a public opinion survey in order to identify barriers to joining the ODR.[48] The encouraging initial finding was that 90% of those surveyed were in favour in principle of organ donation, with no significant differences between socioeconomic groups and people of different age, gender, work status or ethnicity.

The main barriers to joining the register were lack of awareness of the ODR itself and the ways of joining it, a belief that carrying a donor card means there is no need to join the ODR, fear of commitment and distrust of medical professionals leading to anxiety as to 'whether they'll try as hard if you're going to be a donor'. Of those asked, 26% had never thought about the register and 17% just 'haven't got round to it'. Thus increased awareness and knowledge of the ODR, together with easier ways of registering may lead to more people doing so, and work is now under way to achieve these aims. One key long-term aim is to incorporate teaching about organ donation and transplantation into the school education system. A detailed teaching pack has been produced and introduced in Scotland, and it is hoped that this can also be made available in the remainder of the UK. The main priority for governmental media campaigns intended to raise awareness of donation issues in recent years has been directed towards the Asian and black communities, principally because there is a 3–4-fold higher incidence of end-stage renal failure in people from these ethnic minorities, and a real need to improve donation rates to increase the availability of blood group and HLA-matched kidneys for these patients.

7. The legal framework in the UK

The removal of organs after death for transplantation is carried out under the Human Tissue Act, 1961. In one sense the wording of this Act could be interpreted as an 'opting out' system, in that the requirement is that a lack of objection on the part of the deceased patient is to be established and there is no absolute need to obtain positive consent from either the patient or the next of kin. However, in every aspect of custom and practice the system operates as 'opting in' and organs are only removed with the express agreement of the patient, the next of kin or, in the absence of any known relatives, the hospital authorities. If the death would normally be reported to the coroner or (in Scotland) the procurator fiscal, their permission for organ removal must be obtained.

The Human Organ Transplant Act, 1989 governs living donor transplantation and makes it an offence to buy, sell or be involved in any way in the buying or selling of an organ for transplantation.

Several aspects of this legislative framework are felt to require clarification or amendment, and in England and Wales a very wide-ranging consultation document covering virtually every aspect of donation and transplantation was published in 2002.[49] In November 2004 the Human Tissue Act was passed, and it will become law in April 2006. Much detail will be provided by the regulations and codes of practice yet to be written. However, several general themes have emerged. First, in the case of cadaveric donation, it would appear that much greater emphasis may be given to any known views of the potential donor (e.g. if the person had registered on the ODR), with perhaps greater freedom to carry out appropriate procedures necessary to preserve the option of organ donation. Specifically, either legislation or professional Codes of Practice to

clarify uncertainties about several aspects of non-heart-beating donation are anticipated. Secondly, there is likely to be some form of supervision of all forms of living donor transplantation (extending or modifying the law in unrelated living donor transplants), which may be accompanied by a more permissive approach to paired live donor exchange and altruistic stranger donation.

SUMMARY

For too long organ donation has been dependent on the goodwill and hard work of a limited number of intensivists, coordinators and transplant surgeons. It has not received the priority and funding necessary, and it has not been recognised more widely as a responsibility of the whole NHS. The government has now committed itself to raising the profile of organ donation and transplantation,[50] and it is to be hoped that this commitment together with current and future steps to increase donor rates will produce real improvements in the not-too-far-distant future.

REFERENCES

1. Meeting the organ shortage: Current status and strategies for improvement. Council of Europe. http://www.social.coe.int/en/qoflife/publi/donation.htm

2. International figures on organ donation and transplantation – 2002. In: Matesanz R, Miranda B (eds) Newsletter transplant – Council of Europe. Madrid: Aula Medica, 2003.

3. Matesanz R, Miranda B. Need for liver transplantation. Lancet 1995; 346:1170.

4. First MR. Transplantation in the nineties. Transplantation 1992; 53:1–11.

5. Hou S. Expanding the donor pool: Ethical and medical considerations. Kidney Int 2000; 58(4):1820–36.

6. Matesanz R. Organ procurement in Spain. Lancet 1992; 340:733.

7. Matesanz R, Miranda B, Felipe C. Organ procurement in Spain: The impact of transplant coordination. Clin Transplant 1994; 8:281–6.

8. Matesanz R, Miranda B, Felipe C et al. Continuous improvement in organ donation. Transplantation 1996; 61(7):1119–21.

9. Miranda B, Matesanz R. International issues in transplantation. Setting the scene and flagging the

urgent and controversial issues. Ann New York Acad Sci 1998; 862:129–43.

10. Matesanz R, Miranda B. A decade of continuous improvement in cadaveric organ donation: The Spanish Model. J Nephrol 2002; 15(1):22–8.

11. Organizacion Nacional de Transplantes. http://www.msc.es/ont/esp/calidad/f_calidad.htm

12. Matesanz R. Organ donation, transplantation and mass media. Transplant Proc 2003; 35:987–9.

13. Matesanz R. Cadaveric organ donation: comparison of legislation in various countries of Europe. Nephrol Dial Transplant 1998, 13:1632–5.

14. Matesanz R. Factors influencing the adaptation of the Spanish model of organ donation. Transplant Int 2003; 16:736–41.

15. Council of Europe. Guides to safety and quality assurance for organs, tissues and cells. http://book.coe.int/GB/SEL/fr_index.htm

16. Wigmore SJ, Seeney FM, Pleass HP et al. Kidney damage during organ retrieval: data from UK National Transplant Database. Lancet 1999; 354:1143–6.

17. Cuende N, Cañón JF, Miranda B et al. The organ donation process: a program for its evaluation and improvement. Organs and Tissues 2002; 5(2):109–18.

18. Bozzi G, Saviozzi AR, Matesanz R. The quality improvement programme in organ donation of the Tuscany Region. Transplant Proc 2004; 36.

19. Miranda B, Matesanz R. The potential organ donor pool. International figures. In: Matesanz R, Miranda B (eds) Organ donation for transplantation: the Spanish Model. Madrid: Aula Medica; pp. 128–35.

20. Gortmaker SL, Beasley C, Brigham HG et al. Organ donation potential and performance: size and nature of the organ donor short fall. Crit Care Med 1996; 24:432–9.

21. Council of Europe: Recommendation Rec(2003)10, of the Committee of Ministers to member states on xenotransplantation. (Adopted by the Committee of Ministers on 19 June 2003 at the 844th meeting of the Ministers' Deputies.)

22. García-Rinaldi R, Le Frak EA, de Fore WW et al. In situ preservation of cadaver kidneys for transplantation. Ann Surg 1975; 182:576–84.

23. Kootstra G, Daemen JHC, Oomen APA. Categories of non-heartbeating donors. Transplant Proc 1995; 27:2893–5.

24. Sánchez-Fructuoso AI, Prats D, Torrente J et al. Renal transplantation from non-heartbeating donors: a promising alternative to enlarge the donor pool. J Am Soc Nephrol 2000; 11:350–8.

25. Department of the Environment, Transport and the Regions. Road accident statistics 1996, HMSO. www.dft.gov.uk

26. Office of Population, Censuses and Surveys (now Office of National Statistics). 1976–1996, mortality statistics: cause. 1997, HMSO.

27. World Health Organization. WHO European HFA Database. http://www.euro.who.int/hfadb

28. Ojo AO, Hanson JA, Meier-Kriesche H et al. Survival in recipients of marginal cadaveric donor kidneys compared with other recipients and wait-listed transplant candidates. J Am Soc Nephrol 2001; 12:589–97.

29. UK Transplant. National Transplant Database. www.uktransplant.org.uk

30. Advisory Committee on the Microbiological Safety of Blood and Tissues for Transplantation (MSBT). Guidance on the microbiological safety of human organs, tissues and cells used in transplantation. London: Department of Health, 1996.

31. Council of Europe. Standardisation of organ donor screening to prevent transmission of neoplastic diseases. Strasbourg: Council of Europe, 1997.

32. Advisory Committee on the Microbiological Safety of Blood and Tissues for Transplantation (MSBT). Guidance on the microbiological safety of human organs, tissues and cells used in transplantation. London: Department of Health, 2000.

33. Royal College of Surgeons of England. Report of the Working Party on the management of patients with head injuries. London: Royal College of Surgeons of England, 1999.

34. Whitfield PC, Patel H, Hutchinson PJA et al. Bifrontal decompressive craniectomy in the management of post traumatic intracranial hypertension. Br J Neurosurgery 2001; 15(6):500–7.

35. Patel HC, Menon DK, Tebbs S et al. Specialist neurocritical care and outcome from head injury. Intensive Care Medicine 2002; 28;547–53.

36. Gore SM, Cable DJ, Holland AJ. Organ donation from intensive care units in England and Wales; two-year confidential audit of deaths in intensive care. BMJ 1992; 302:349–55.

37. Baker R. Harold Shipman's clinical practice 1974–1998. London: Stationery Office, 2001.

38. Wight J, Cameron JS. A study of variation in the organ donor rates in the United Kingdom. Peterborough: The National Kidney Research Fund, 2002.

39. UK Transplant. Activity report, calendar year 2002. www.uktransplant.org.uk

40. UK Transplant. Waiting list criteria for potential renal transplant recipients. www.uktransplant.org.uk

41. Neuberger J, Price D. Role of living liver donation in the United Kingdom. BMJ 2003; 327:676–9.

42. Nicholson M. Kidney transplantation from non-heartbeating donors. Peterborough: The National Kidney Research Fund, 2002.

43. Weber M, Dindo D, Demartines N et al. Kidney transplantation from donors without a heartbeat. N Engl J Med 2002; 347:248–55.

44. British Transplantation Society/Renal Association. United Kingdom guidelines for living donor kidney transplantation. www.bts.org.uk

45. Sheehy E, Conrad SL, Brigham LE et al. Estimating the number of potential organ donors in the United States. N Engl J Med 2003; 349:667–74.

46. Langone AJ, Helderman JH. Disparity between solid organ supply and demand. N Engl J Med 2003; 349:704–6.

47. Baxter D. Beyond comparison: Canada's organ donation rates in an international context. The Urban Futures Institute Report 51. Vancouver: Urban Futures Institute, 2001.

48. Market research into barriers to joining the NHS Organ Donor Register. Commissioned for UK Transplant, February 2003.

49. Department of Health. Human bodies, human choices – the law on human organs and tissue in England and Wales – a consultation report. London: Department of Health, July 2002.

50. Department of Health. Saving lives, valuing donors. A transplant framework for England. London: Department of Health, July 2003.

Three

Immunology of graft rejection

Simon T. Ball and
Margaret J. Dallman

INTRODUCTION

The optimal treatment of end-stage renal failure is transplantation, since it enhances both quality of life and survival compared with dialysis.[1,2] The combination of pancreatic and renal transplantation has similar benefits,[3] whilst transplantation of other organs is truly life saving since no long-term biomechanical support is available.

In clinical practice, organ donor and recipient are genetically distinct, excepting identical twins (see **Box 3.1** for terminology). The genetically encoded immunologically mediated barrier to transplantation was recognised and defined over the course of the last century. This study of transplantation has played a pivotal role in understanding immunity, and immunology has provided rationale for the development of clinical transplantation.

The first successful renal transplant was between identical twins,[4] but the development of transplantation as an important facet of modern medical therapy required the introduction of immunosuppression to prevent and treat rejection of allogeneic organs.[5–7] Clinical transplantation developed alongside an appreciation that rejection of foreign tissue belonged 'to the general category of actively acquired immunity'[8] and this was consequent upon differences in genetically encoded histocompatibility antigens.[9,10] The process of

Box 3.1 • Transplant terminology

Autograft (autologous transplant)
Transplantation of an individual's own tissue to another site, e.g. the use of a patient's own skin to cover third-degree burns or a saphenous vein femoro-popliteal graft.
Isograft (syngeneic or isogeneic transplant)
Transplantation of tissue between genetically identical members of the same species, e.g. kidney transplant between identical twins or grafts between mice of the same inbred strain.
Allograft (allogeneic transplant)
Transplantation of tissue between genetically non-identical members of the same species, e.g. cadaveric renal transplant or graft between mice of different inbred strains.
Xenograft (xenogeneic transplant)
Transplantation of tissue between members of different species, e.g. baboon kidney into a human.

rejection was shown to be caused by infiltrating leucocytes; it exhibits specificity and memory and is prevented by lymphocyte depletion.[11] The major histocompatibility complex (MHC) was identified as encoding the dominant transplantation antigens, and these were shown to be identical to serologically defined human leucocyte antigens (HLA)[12] and subsequently to the elements responsible for self-restriction of immunological responses to conventional antigen.[13]

These fundamental observations form the scientific basis of transplantation, and there is now a highly sophisticated understanding of the molecular and cellular events that lead to graft rejection or acceptance, the subjects of this chapter (**Fig. 3.1**).

BEFORE TRANSPLANTATION

Inflammation lies at the centre of the afferent and efferent arms of rejection. This begins prior to transplantation in the haemodynamic and neuro-endocrine responses to brainstem death, in the process of multiorgan retrieval and the act of cold preservation. The transplant surgical procedure then adds a period of warm ischaemia and reperfusion. The consequent injury may result in delayed graft function and generates an inflammatory response, which may itself promote and shape alloantigen-specific immunity.

The importance of these aspects of transplantation is illustrated by:

- the superior outcome of live donor transplants even in the face of significant MHC mismatch;[14]

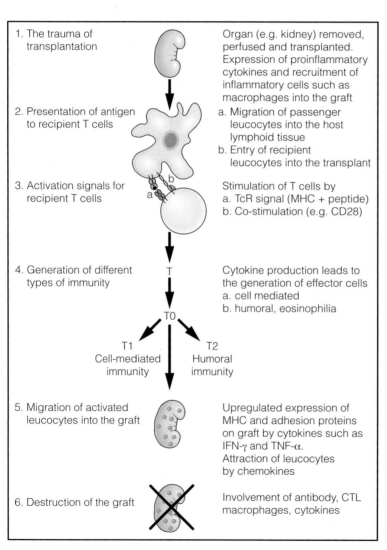

1. The trauma of transplantation

Organ (e.g. kidney) removed, perfused and transplanted. Expression of proinflammatory cytokines and recruitment of inflammatory cells such as macrophages into the graft

2. Presentation of antigen to recipient T cells

a. Migration of passenger leucocytes into the host lymphoid tissue
b. Entry of recipient leucocytes into the transplant

3. Activation signals for recipient T cells

Stimulation of T cells by
a. TcR signal (MHC + peptide)
b. Co-stimulation (e.g. CD28)

4. Generation of different types of immunity

Cytokine production leads to the generation of effector cells
a. cell mediated
b. humoral, eosinophilia

T
T0
T1
Cell-mediated immunity
T2
Humoral immunity

5. Migration of activated leucocytes into the graft

Upregulated expression of MHC and adhesion proteins on graft by cytokines such as IFN-γ and TNF-α. Attraction of leucocytes by chemokines

6. Destruction of the graft

Involvement of antibody, CTL macrophages, cytokines

Figure 3.1 • The evolution of the immune response following kidney transplantation. TCR, T-cell receptor; MHC, major histocompatibility complex; IFN, interferon; TNF, tumour necrosis factor; CTL, cytotoxic T lymphocyte.

- the importance of cold ischaemia time in graft outcome;[15]
- reportedly higher rates of rejection observed in individuals with delayed graft function.[16]

Indeed, in experimental syngeneic transplantation, graft histology very similar to that seen in chronic allograft nephropathy may be reproduced by prolonged ischaemia.[17]

Early following reperfusion, vascular endothelium is activated and several immunologically active soluble proteins (or their transcripts) such as interleukins 1 and 6 (IL-1 and IL-6), have been demonstrated in transplanted organs. There is an early infiltrate of inflammatory cells including macrophages. This is apparent even in syngeneic transplants in which alloimmunity is absent.

The severity of this initial injury and the nature of the subsequent inflammatory infiltrate are likely to be important in the stimulation of specific alloimmunity: a maximally damaged organ generates a maximal 'danger signal',[18] which initiates productive immunity manifested as rejection. The relationship between cellular infiltration and outcome is not simple in that this also occurs during the acquisition of tolerance in many animal models of transplantation. The context of such an initial encounter with alloantigen must therefore be important in determining the subsequent nature of any response. The mechanisms by which innate immunity shapes the immune response are increasingly defined, for example the role of Toll-like receptors (TLRs)[19] and γ-interferon (IFN-γ), produced by natural killer (NK) cells,[20] in activating dendritic cells (DCs).

It is also likely that non-immunological mechanisms directly influence long-term graft outcome.[15,16] For example, accelerated replicative senescence of parenchymal cells may play a role in the development of chronic allograft nephropathy, and this may be promoted by prolonged ischaemia.[21]

HISTOCOMPATIBILITY

Histocompatibility antigens were defined on the basis of their preventing transplantation between outbred members of the same species. In vertebrates they can be classified into the major histocompatibility complex (MHC) and numerous minor histocompatibility (miH) systems. Differences between

histocompatibility antigens stimulate rejection, and by far the most vigorous response arises from discordance at the MHC. This arises in part from the extreme polymorphism of MHC antigens and their physiological role in immune recognition. This role as the self-restricting element in engagement of the T-cell receptor (TCR) by antigenic peptide will be described in the next section.

Although differences in multiple minor histocompatibility antigens alone can result in allograft rejection in rodents,[22] in clinical solid organ transplantation the MHC is of overwhelming importance. However, this is not the case in bone marrow transplantation, in which grafts between HLA-identical siblings may be rejected or cause graft versus host disease[23] due to differences in only a limited number of minor antigens.

Antigens stimulating rejection by T lymphocytes

MHC CLASS I AND II

The MHC is divided into three regions, namely the class I, II and III regions, and these are described in detail in Chapter 4. A large array of genes has been localised to the MHC by sequencing, but two major classes of transplantation antigens were those first mapped by classical genetic techniques. The structure of these molecules is shown in **Fig. 3.2**.

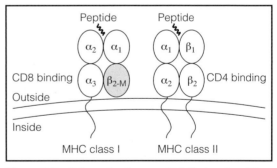

Figure 3.2 • Schematic diagram of MHC class I and II proteins showing their basic structure, membrane association and peptide-binding groove. α1, α2 and α3 of MHC class I are membrane integral and form a non-covalent bond with β2-microglobulin, which is not membrane bound. MHC class II is formed from α and β chains, each with two domains and each membrane integral. β2-M, β2-microglobulin.

MHC class I proteins are cell-surface glycoproteins comprising a heavy chain (~45 kDa), which is highly polymorphic, and a less variable light chain, β_2-microglobulin (~12 kDa), which is encoded outside of the MHC. The β_2-microglobulin is not anchored in the membrane and binds non-covalently to the heavy chain. MHC class I proteins are expressed on most nucleated cells and generally engage T lymphocytes bearing the cell-surface protein CD8. CD8 is required for effective T-cell receptor engagement of MHC class I protein and resultant intracellular signalling.

MHC class II proteins consist of two membrane-anchored glycoproteins (α-chain, ~35 kDa; β-chain, ~28 kDa),[24] which are both encoded within the MHC. The tissue distribution of MHC class II proteins is more restricted than that of MHC class I. MHC class II is expressed constitutively by B lymphocytes and dendritic cells, which have specialised functions in the generation of the immune response. It is also expressed on some endothelial cells in humans and can be induced by inflammation on many cell types. MHC class II generally engages T lymphocytes bearing the CD4 surface protein. CD4 is required for effective T-cell receptor engagement of MHC class II protein and resultant intracellular signalling.

In humans these transplantation antigens were defined serologically on leucocytes and so are referred to as human leucocyte antigens (HLAs).[25]

Structure of MHC class I and II proteins

MHC class I and II proteins have a similar three-dimensional structure forming a 'peptide-binding groove' between two alpha helices (**Fig. 3.2**). The amino acids that constitute this groove are those that vary most between allotypes. During synthesis and transport of MHC class I and class II proteins to the cell surface the groove binds a wide range of short peptides. The groove in MHC class I has closed ends and the peptides bound are 8–10 amino acids long.[26] The groove in MHC class II is open and can accommodate peptides of considerably greater length. The sequences flanking those bound within the groove, whilst not contributing to antigen specificity, may contribute to the physicochemical stability of the complex.[27] The peptides bound to MHC class I are primarily derived from intracellular proteins (but see Indirect allorecognition below) and those from MHC class II primarily from extra-cellular proteins (**Fig. 3.3**). This difference arises from their distinct intracellular trafficking. In the presence of infection, foreign protein is processed to generate peptides bound to MHC forming a compound antigenic determinant, which engages the T-cell receptor (TCR) and stimulates T-lymphocyte activation.[28,29] This compound determinant is the structural basis for self-restricted antigen recognition by a T-cell repertoire that is skewed, by thymic selection, toward the engagement of peptide presented in the context of self-MHC. In the absence of foreign protein, all peptides are derived from self-proteins, to which the individual is, to varying degrees, tolerant. A significant proportion of self-peptides are derived from MHC proteins themselves and this has consequences for allorecognition.

CD8+ T lymphocytes engage antigenic peptide bound to MHC class I and are typically cytotoxic. The normal function of these lymphocytes is to lyse cells infected intracellularly with, for example, virus. CD8+ cells also produce a range of cytokines and some have regulatory properties.[30]

CD4+ T lymphocytes engage antigenic peptide bound to MHC class II. Antigen generally derives from extracellular source proteins. These cells have a variety of functions, summarised in their designation as 'helper cells'. These functions include help for cytotoxic T-cell generation, B-cell maturation, and promotion of delayed type hypersensitivity (DTH) inflammation. CD4+ T-cell responses are evidently central to many forms of allogeneic rejection, and their activation by dendritic cells is an important component of this response. In some rodent models absence of CD4+ T-cell stimulation can abolish rejection despite the presence of CD8+ T cells and fully allogeneic MHC class I mismatches.[31] In such cases tolerance to alloantigen may emerge rather than productive immunity, illustrating the crucial importance of CD4+ T-cell responses in rejection.

The specific structure of the binding groove determines the peptide that can be bound by any given MHC, and only a limited number of peptides from any given protein can form a stable complex. The ontogenetic drive for extreme polymorphism in the MHC is therefore likely to reflect the need to counter a wide variety of infectious organisms that rapidly mutate and could evolve a sequence that does not bind an individual's MHC repertoire. This is unlikely to occur across an entire species if there is the full range of polymorphism observed in

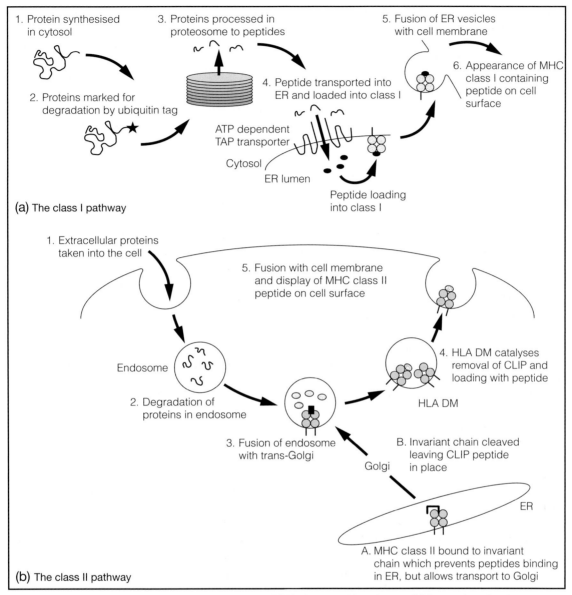

1. Protein synthesised in cytosol

2. Proteins marked for degradation by ubiquitin tag

3. Proteins processed in proteosome to peptides

4. Peptide transported into ER and loaded into class I

ATP dependent TAP transporter

Cytosol

ER lumen

Peptide loading into class I

5. Fusion of ER vesicles with cell membrane

6. Appearance of MHC class I containing peptide on cell surface

(a) The class I pathway

1. Extracellular proteins taken into the cell

5. Fusion with cell membrane and display of MHC class II peptide on cell surface

Endosome

2. Degradation of proteins in endosome

3. Fusion of endosome with trans-Golgi

Golgi

HLA DM

4. HLA DM catalyses removal of CLIP and loading with peptide

B. Invariant chain cleaved leaving CLIP peptide in place

ER

A. MHC class II bound to invariant chain which prevents peptides binding in ER, but allows transport to Golgi

(b) The class II pathway

Figure 3.3 • Antigen processing and presentation in the MHC class I and II pathways. **(a)** Processing of endogenous antigens occurs primarily via the class I pathway. Peptides are produced and loaded into MHC class I proteins as shown in steps 1–4. During the synthesis of MHC class I proteins (steps 1–3) the α chain is stabilised by calnexin before β_2-microglobulin binds. Folding of the MHC class I–β_2-microglobulin remains incomplete but the complex is released by calnexin to bind with the chaperone proteins tapaisin and calreticulin. Only when the TAP transporter delivers peptide to the MHC class I–β_2-microglobulin can folding of this complex be completed and transport to the cell membrane occur (steps 5 and 6). **(b)** Processing of exogenous antigens occurs primarily via the class II pathway. Antigens are taken up into intracellular vesicles where acidification aids their degradation into peptide fragments (steps 1–2). Vesicles containing peptides fuse with trans-Golgi, containing CLIP–MHC class II complexes (step 3). HLA-DM aids removal of CLIP and loading of peptide before the class II peptide complex is displayed on the cell surface (steps 4–5). MHC class II proteins are synthesised in the endoplasmic reticulum where peptide binding is prevented by the invariant chain. Invariant chain is cleaved leaving the CLIP peptide still in place (steps A and B) before fusing with acidified vesicles containing peptide. In B lymphocytes and epithelial cells of the thymus an atypical class II protein, HLA-DO, is expressed; this is a dimer of HLA-DMα and HLA-DOβ. It, like HLA-DM, is not expressed at the cell surface and inhibits the action of HLA-DM. Its precise role is unknown. TAP, transporters associated with antigen processing; ER, endoplasmic reticulum; MHC, major histocompatibility complex; ATP, adenosine triphosphate; CLIP, class II-associated invariant chain peptide.

humans. Certain species with limited polymorphism at either MHC class I or II can be devastated by infections that, in closely related species with polymorphic MHC, do not threaten the population.[32]

It is now possible to predict the sequences of peptides likely to bind to a given MHC from its structure and to then confirm this from peptide elution and peptide-binding studies. The peptide can be orientated in the groove and those amino acids in contact with MHC and those in contact with the T-cell receptor can be predicted. This is likely to be a powerful tool in future vaccine development.

Assembly of the MHC–peptide complex

The assembly of the MHC–peptide complex (**Fig. 3.3**) involves sophisticated mechanisms of antigen uptake, processing to peptide and, in the case of MHC class I, transport into the endosomal compartment.[33] The proteasome components (LMP, low-molecular-mass polypeptide) and transporters associated with antigen processing (TAP), responsible for these aspects of processing, are encoded within the MHC. In the case of classical MHC class II, assembly requires the initial presence of an invariant chain from which a peptide, CLIP, combines with α and β chains to form a nascent complex. CLIP is subsequently exchanged for antigenic peptide.[24,34]

NON-CLASSICAL MHC

The MHC locus is large and it encodes a wide range of proteins other than the classical histocompatibility antigens described above. Some of these have a structure similar to classical histocompatibility antigens but are not polymorphic. They may present specialised antigens, such as lipids (e.g. mycolic acid and lipoarabinomannan from mycobacteria) or peptides of various sequences but with common characteristics (e.g. with *N*-formylated amino termini).[35] The relevance of these molecules to transplantation is uncertain but they do not behave as classical transplantation antigens.

Molecules such as HLA-DM, TAP and LMP, which have a role in antigen processing and are referred to above, are encoded within the large MHC locus along with other molecules more broadly involved in immunity, for example tumour necrosis factors α and β (TNF-α and TNF-β) and complement components C2 and C4. Polymorphisms linked to these genes have been implicated in disease expression and transplantation responses.[36]

MINOR HISTOCOMPATIBILITY ANTIGENS

The study in rodents of genetic loci determining organ rejection identifies a range of sites encoding transplant antigens that are distinct from the MHC. These minor histocompatibility (miH) antigens are less polymorphic and typically induce a weaker response than disparities in the MHC. It is almost impossible to raise antibodies to these antigens although they induce a well-defined cellular response.

The crystallographic structure of the MHC with bound peptide provides a structural explanation for these properties of miH antigens. They are peptides derived from proteins of limited polymorphism that, when bound to syngeneic MHC, constitute an antigenic determinant in the same way as any conventional antigen.[23,37,38] This explains why it is difficult to raise antibodies to miH antigens, since antibodies typically engage conformational determinants on proteins and the B lymphocyte is less discriminatory of subtle differences in the structure of peptide–MHC composites than is the T lymphocyte.

The most easily defined miH antigen is the male-specific H-Y antigen, which is in fact a series of antigenic peptides derived from proteins encoded on the Y chromosome, accounting for its consistent detection across a wide range of background MHC (although in certain strain combinations there is a single dominant antigen[37]). In rodent studies the role of miH antigens can be readily demonstrated, particularly when there has been prior sensitisation to the relevant antigen.

In rare cases of rejection in renal transplants between HLA-identical siblings miH are thought to be the inciting antigens but their importance in other forms of solid organ transplantation is generally limited. This is not true, however, in bone marrow transplantation, in which rejection is easily stimulated by such differences causing graft vs. host or graft vs. tumour response.[39]

Recognition of alloantigen

The T-cell receptor can engage MHC in two distinct ways, either **directly** on antigen-presenting cells

(APCs) derived from the graft, or **indirectly** as processed peptides in the context of self MHC on self APCs.

DIRECT ALLORECOGNITION

Allogeneic MHC on dendritic cells (DCs) derived from the graft will be occupied by any number of different endogenous peptides (**Fig. 3.4**). The frequency of alloreactive T lymphocytes stimulated through this pathway is high, in the order of $1/10^2$. Although this appears to contradict the principles of 'self-MHC' restriction resulting from thymic education, it emerges as a consequence of the vast array of endogenous peptides that occupy the MHC generating an equivalent number of compound epitopes. It also arises from the relatively limited differences in the structure of MHC alloantigens outside the peptide-binding groove and the corresponding fact that T lymphocytes can distinguish subtle differences in the kinetics of TCR–peptide–MHC interactions. These facts also apply to the response to recall antigens: that is to say, other than in immunologically naive animals any direct alloresponse will include cross-reactions with self-restricted secondary responses to conventional antigens.[40–46] As most studies on experimental transplantation, particularly those on the induction of tolerance, use naive rodents these are unlikely to accurately reflect the alloresponse observed clinically. Indeed, strategies to induce transplantation tolerance that succeed in the naive animal are unsuccessful in previously infected animals[45,46] – providing one possible explanation for the difficulties in translating such strategies into preclinical models.

INDIRECT ALLORECOGNITION

Proteins from extracellular infectious organisms are generally processed by antigen-presenting cells (APCs) and presented in the context of MHC class II. As discussed above, only a small proportion of potential peptide sequences from a protein will be processed, bind MHC and generate a response.[47,48]

In the setting of allogeneic transplantation any donor protein can be processed and presented in the context of MHC by recipient APCs. As most proteins have little or no polymorphism within a

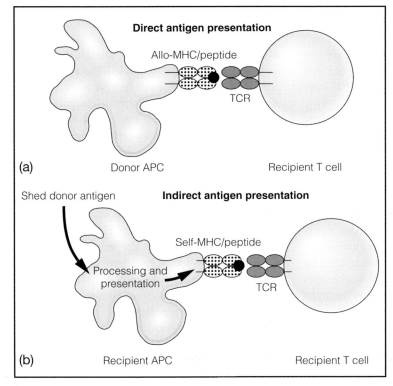

Figure 3.4 • Direct and indirect pathways of antigen presentation. Sensitisation of the recipient can occur by antigen presentation delivered through passenger leucocytes or dendritic cells of donor origin **(a)** or recipient origin **(b)**. APC, antigen-presenting cell; MHC, major histocompatibility complex; TCR, T-cell receptor.

species they will not always initiate an alloimmune response, and even if they do, the response may not result in graft rejection. However, polymorphic proteins such as those of the MHC can stimulate an immune response via this conventional or 'indirect pathway' of antigen presentation (**Fig. 3.4**).[49–53]

The potential importance of this route of allorecognition is demonstrated by experiments in which immunisation with MHC class I peptides prime for subsequent rejection of a skin allograft bearing the intact class I antigens from which the peptides were derived.[51] Studies in other models have demonstrated that priming with MHC class I- and II-derived peptides leads to chronic allograft rejection, with accelerated vasculopathy.[54,55] These peptides are most likely to be presented in the context of recipient class II since they are extracellular for the self APCs. However, there is now clear evidence of crossover, or 'cross-presentation', between the two pathways so there may also be presentation of such peptides in the context of MHC class I.[56–59] The importance of indirect presentation of alloantigen is also illustrated by transplantation of skin allografts from MHC class II-deficient onto normal mice. Donor APCs are unable to stimulate recipient CD4+ T cells and yet rejection remains dependent upon CD4+ T cells. It is likely that this reflects recipient CD4+ T cell stimulation through indirect presentation of donor alloantigens by self MHC.[56,58,60] In this latter case, peptides are not artificially introduced into the recipients but produced by normal processing of MHC from apoptosed donor-derived cells.

In longstanding renal transplant recipients there is evidence of donor-specific hyporesponsiveness of peripheral blood lymphocytes to directly presented alloantigen,[61–63] and this may be true even in those who have suffered allograft failure.[61] There is increasing evidence for the association of indirect pathway alloreactivity in peripheral blood lymphocytes with chronic rejection in solid organ transplants.[62,64–66] The interpretation of peripheral responses as indicative of tissue responses must be guarded but these observations suggest strategies for monitoring patient responses[66] and assessing the effects of treatment[67] for chronic rejection.

Allorecognition via the indirect pathway has also been linked to regulation of alloimmune responses, and this is discussed in a later section.

INITIATION OF THE IMMUNE RESPONSE: DC–T-CELL INTERACTIONS

'Passenger leucocytes' in transplantation

In rodent models of transplantation allogeneic MHC can be more or less immunogenic according to the context in which it is encountered by the recipient immune system. Following transplantation, 'passenger leucocytes' – tissue-resident immature dendritic cells (DCs) – migrate to secondary lymphoid organs, mature and there deliver a powerful stimulus to the recipient immune system. Mature DCs express high levels of MHC class I and II and can therefore stimulate both CD8+ and CD4+ T lymphocytes. They also have other properties, including efficient co-stimulatory activity, which render them uniquely powerful stimulators of naive T cells[68–70] and earn them the title of 'professional' APCs. A number of experimental systems have been used to dissect the role of donor DCs in stimulating allograft rejection.

Allografts can be depleted of donor-derived passenger leucocytes by irradiation, a period of tissue culture or by exchange with DCs of recipient type whilst 'parked' in an immunoincompetent animal of recipient origin.[71,72] These organs when retransplanted into immunocompetent animals often fail to induce rejection. These experiments suggest that DCs are required for the initiation of the immune response that leads to acute rejection. After such successful transplantation, rejection can frequently be induced by the infusion of donor origin leucocytes.[73]

Clear data implicating the DC as the primary or only stimulus of graft rejection in all donor-recipient pairs are lacking. Also, application of these findings to the immunology of clinical transplantation must be cautioned against by the fact that in many experimental models of long-term graft survival an active regulatory immune response plays a role in the failure of organ rejection. DCs may themselves be important for the induction of a regulatory response rather than rejection,[74,75] although this may be more important for recipient DCs presenting via the indirect pathway than for donor DCs via the direct pathway of allorecognition. Further, DCs are highly important in the stimulation of primary T-cell responses but seem less important for secondary responses. In clinical transplantation a major component of the T-cell response is likely to be heterologous,[40,45] that is arising from the cross-reaction of a primed, self-restricted pathogen-specific T lymphocyte with an allogeneic MHC–peptide complex. These primed cells will be significantly less dependent upon DCs for activation. Nevertheless, the stimulation of lymphocytes through the 'direct' pathway of allorecognition by the migration of 'passenger' DCs seems to provide a powerful early stimulus to acute graft rejection,[76,77] whether this be a primary or secondary response.

In humans, vascular endothelium constitutively expresses MHC class II and it too may play a greater role in stimulating alloimmunity than is the case in rodents.[78–81]

ACTIVATION OF DENDRITIC CELLS

Although the immunostimulatory properties of dendritic cells are most apparent in the experimental data described above it is now evident that marked phenotypic and functional differences exist between dendritic cells, depending upon the context in which they are studied. The factors that contribute to acquisition of such properties include:

- lineage;[82]
- maturity;[83,84]
- activation by infection[85,86] and inflammation;[20,87]
- interaction with T cells[84,85,88] and T-cell-derived cytokines.[89]

The precise mechanisms of dendritic cell differentiation and maturation are currently undergoing intense investigation. For example, Toll-like receptors (TLRs) are pattern recognition receptors that detect both microbial infection[86,90] and inflammation-induced release of endogenous ligands.[91,92] They are not only important components of innate immunity but also, by activating DCs, play a role in stimulating and shaping adaptive, antigen-specific immune responses. Dendritic cell phenotype may, for example, determine the pattern of cytokine secretion by T cells upon antigenic stimulation and therefore the type of effector immunity that is generated.[93,94] Immature dendritic cells may play a role in maintaining peripheral tolerance[88,95,96] by both deletional[97] and regulatory mechanisms.[96,98–100] These properties may themselves be regulated by T lymphocytes.[88,101] The relevance of these interactive and dynamic properties of DCs to transplantation has recently been reviewed.[102–104]

Co-stimulation

Evidently, engagement of the TCR can result in a range of outcomes depending upon context provided by, for example, co-stimulatory molecules and soluble cytokines. The fate of the T lymphocyte following TCR engagement can include proliferation, apoptosis, anergy, acquisition of different regulatory phenotypes, acquisition of different effector phenotypes or differentiation into memory cells.

The importance of co-stimulation was first evident from experimental models in which its inhibition was achieved by various means, including the fixation of APCs, presentation by purified MHC in lipid bilayers and by 'non-professional' APCs transfected with MHC class II.[105] In these studies CD4[+] T cells that engaged with cognate antigen in the absence of co-stimulation did not proliferate; furthermore, they often acquired a stable change in phenotype: they became 'anergic', failing to proliferate on restimulation with competent APCs. This generated a model in which TCR was said to provide 'signal 1' and co-stimulatory molecule engagement 'signal 2'. Together these signals resulted in proliferation but signal 1 in the absence of signal 2 resulted in anergy. In many in vitro systems signal 2 was found to be the engagement of CD28 by B7 (CD80 or CD86).[106,107]

The field of co-stimulation has since become considerably more complex, in that large numbers of molecules with signal 2 properties have been identified in different experimental systems, and some of these act as 'negative co-stimulation' – the engagement of cell surface molecules that have a dominant negative effect on T-cell activation and promote the acquisition of anergic/regulatory phenotypes or cell death. The most important examples of such negative co-stimulation include CTLA4 (CD152[108–114]) and more recently PD1.[115–117]

Co-stimulatory interactions can be broadly separated into those of the CD28–B7 family and those of the tumour necrosis factor receptor (TNFR)/tumour necrosis factor (TNF) family (or CD40 ligand–CD40 family), summarised in **Table 3.1**. The relative importance of different co-stimulatory pathways and the way in which they interact remains to be fully elucidated. In alloimmunity it is not yet clear whether different pathways are functionally redundant or whether they play specialised roles relevant to different aspects of successful transplantation. The most studied members of each family are CD28–CD80/86 interactions and CD154–CD40, described below.

CD28–B7

The role of CD28 has perhaps been that most intensively investigated in the field of co-stimulation.[107,118,119] CD28 is a homodimeric glycoprotein present on the surface of T cells and interacts with two counter-receptors, CD80 and CD86 (the B7 proteins), expressed on the surface of APCs. CD80 and CD86 are of similar structure although they have different patterns of expression and bind with distinct affinities to CD28.[120]

CD86 is expressed constitutively at low level by APCs and is upregulated rapidly following interaction with the T lymphocyte. It has a rather low affinity for CD28 whereas CD80, which is not constitutively expressed and is upregulated with slower kinetics, has an approximately ten-fold greater binding affinity for CD28.[121]

The result of ligation of CD28 by either CD86 or CD80 appears to be increased cytokine synthesis and proliferation through various intracellular signalling pathways.[111,122] The results of their respective engagement do not appear to be qualitatively distinct. The reason for this apparent redundancy is as yet uncertain but may relate to differences in their interaction with other ligands such as CTLA4 (CD152). It may be that this 'positive' CD28-dominated signal switches to a 'negative' CTLA4-dominated

Table 3.1 • Members of the CD28 and CD40–ligand (CD154) families of molecules expressed on T lymphocytes and their corresponding ligands

	CD28–B7 family			
	CD28	**CTLA-4**	**ICOS**	**PD-1**
Expression	Constitutive on T cells	Induced on T cells	Induced on T cells	Induced on T, B and dendritic cells Constitutive on NK cells
Ligand	B7-2 > B7-1	B7-1 > B7-2	B7RP-1	PD-L1 and PD-L2
Activity	Blockade promotes allograft survival and tolerance in some models[111,123–125,149,295]	Blockade promotes graft survival/complex effects[111,296–298]	Blockade inhibits tolerance induction and ligation inhibits activation[111,275,299,300]	Activation promotes and blockade inhibits allograft survival[179,301,302]
	CD40 ligand–CD40 family			
	CD154	**CD137 (4-1 BB)**	**CD134 (OX-40)**	**CD27**
Expression	Induced on T cells, NK cells and eosinophils	Induced on T cells	Induced on T cells	Constitutive on T cells and on APCs
Ligand	CD40	CD137 ligand	CD134 ligand	CD70
Activity	Blockade promotes graft survival/ tolerance[133–135,303]	Blockade inhibits CD8+ T-cell-mediated rejection[304]	Blockade inhibits CD28/CD154-independent rejection, inhibition of primed responses[305–30]	Effector and memory cell generation (B cell and T cell)[308–310]

Activity refers to the consequences of blockade or of stimulation through engagement of these molecules, assessed from the outcome in various experimental models of transplantation.

signal as the immune response progresses and the relative amounts of CD80 and CD86 change.

Blocking the CD28 pathway in normal rodents can have dramatic effects on the generation of primary immune responses and may result in prolonged graft survival or even tolerance of grafts in some experimental models,[123,124] but mice with a disrupted CD28 gene can make productive immune responses albeit with sometimes altered kinetics.[125] This may in part be due to redundancy of co-stimulatory pathways including other recently identified members of the B7 and CD28 families. (The severe phenotype of CTLA4 –/– mice, which die from uncontrolled lymphoid proliferation shortly after birth,[108] suggests that there is less redundancy in this aspect of immune regulation.)

The most widely used method to block CD28–B7 interactions has been CTLA4-Ig, but this will also block the CTLA4–B7 interaction. The inhibition of negative CTLA4 signalling may account for diverse observations on immune responses in different experimental systems using CDA4-Ig, as may the recent observation that B7 cross-linking on APCs by CTLA4-Ig induces indoleamine 2,3-dioxygenase (IDO), which itself inhibits local T-cell activation.[126–128]

Reagents such as CTLA4-Ig are notably less effective in large animal models than in rodents, although prolongation of graft survival has been observed, particularly in combination with other immunoregulatory agents or drugs.[129] Perhaps most important to the setting of clinical transplantation is the relative lack of requirement for CD28 signals in CD8[+] T-cell responses and in secondary CD4[+] T-cell responses. Virus-reactive CD8[+] cells may not require co-stimulation through CD28 or CD28-dependent help,[130,131] although they may require a high concentration of cognate peptide–MHC generated by replicating virus, which is less likely to occur in other immune responses. Furthermore, heterologous CD4[+] T-cell secondary responses, which are likely to be important in clinical alloimmune responses, are evidently significantly less responsive to the inhibition of co-stimulation than are primary responses.[44,45] An unanswered question is whether other recently identified co-stimulatory pathways can be used to specifically target T-cell memory.[132] More selective approaches that are designed to block co-stimulation whilst leaving the CTLA4–B7 interaction intact are certainly also of interest in

view of the critical negative signalling potential of this interaction.

CD154–CD40

Upon activation T cells express CD154 (CD40 ligand, gp39). Interaction of this protein with its counter-receptor, CD40, appears to be critical for the activation of B cells, dendritic cells and monocytes. This activation is itself crucial to subsequent T-cell stimulation. In dendritic cells, CD40 ligation upregulates interleukin 12 (IL-12) production and in macrophages it results in the production of a range of proinflammatory cytokines, including TNF-α and IL-8, whilst in B cells it provides signals for proliferation, maturation, isotype switching and generation of memory.

In a murine cardiac transplant model, blockade of CD40–CD154 interactions prolongs graft survival,[133] and combined block of CD28 and CD40 interactions can induce permanent survival of an allogeneic skin graft in mice with no long-term deterioration of graft integrity.[134] The latter is a rigorous marker of non-responsiveness but, interestingly, these animals did not exhibit tolerance to a second allograft. In short this combination seems to be highly effective for immunosuppression in the setting of experimental allogeneic transplantation but without evidence of tolerance induction.

A recent report suggests that CD154–CD40 interaction plays a role in promoting dendritic cell maturation in the presence of CD4[+]CD25[+] regulatory lymphocytes, whilst these cells promote the maintenance of immaturity.[101] This reiterates the importance of DC activation not only by innate immune mechanisms but also by activated T cells, in driving productive immunity.

These actions underlie significant beneficial effects for anti-CD154 in preclinical models of transplantation;[135] unfortunately its clinical application has as yet been prevented by prothrombotic effects – a probable consequence of the expression of CD154 on platelets.

The DC–T-cell synapse

It is evident that on TCR engagement multiple cell-surface proteins (**Fig. 3.5**) become highly organised within the two dimensions of the cell membrane forming a structure referred to as the immunological synapse. This depends upon cytoskeletal–cell

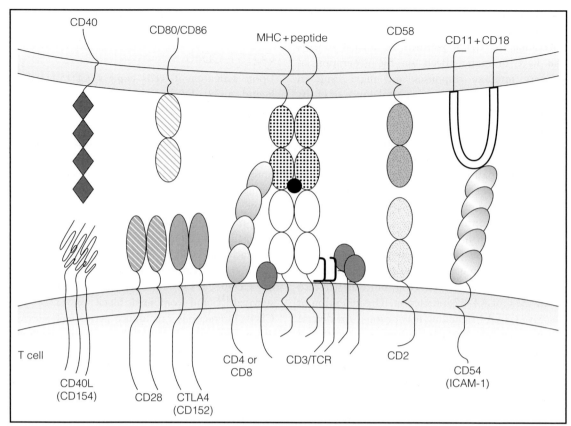

Figure 3.5 • Cell-surface protein–protein interactions important in T-cell activation. Receptors on the T cell are shown with their ligands on the antigen-presenting cell (APC). Immunoglobulin (Ig) domains are common amongst cell-surface proteins of leucocytes and are denoted in this diagram by ovals. Several of these interactions are important in delivering signals to both T cell and APC.

membrane interactions and is in part orchestrated by the coordinated movement of proteins congregated within lipid rafts.[136] The orderly congregation of molecules has been referred to as a supramolecular activation complex (SMAC).[137] Studied in vitro it varies in its precise organisation over the period of cell–cell interaction, but the initial response is a rapid accumulation of TCR and MHC to a central (c)SMAC surrounded by cell adhesion molecules like LFA-1 in the peripheral (p)SMAC. The nature of the synapse in vivo requires further investigation, as there is some evidence to suggest considerably greater motility of T cells in lymph nodes than would be suggested from the kinetics observed in vitro.[138,139]

Although the signal 1–signal 2 model of co-stimulation proved useful it is increasingly apparent that the distinction between adhesion and co-stimulation is not strict. Thus the kinetics of TCR binding, non-antigen-specific interactions between T cell and APC, the presence of cytokines, and the state of T-cell maturation will all determine cell fate following TCR engagement. This integration of antigen-specific and non-specific signals is manifest in the T-cell synapse, which controls and amplifies TCR signalling. Thus molecules previously considered as having a predominantly structural role in T-cell–APC binding may in certain circumstances play an important role in determining intracellular events in the same way as molecules initially defined as providing a second signal in experimental models.

TCR signalling

The majority of T cells bear a TCR of two chains, the alpha and beta chains, complexed with various other proteins, in particular those of the CD3 complex (γ, δ, ε) and ζ chains. The phosphorylation of ζ chains results in zap-70 recruitment[140,141] and subsequent congregation of other signalling elements around membrane scaffold protein linker for activation of T cells (LAT), which is located in lipid rafts.[142,143]

Diverse signalling pathways are activated, which ultimately lead to transcriptional activation and the de novo expression of a range of genes, including those encoding cytokines and new cell surface proteins. These pathways are highly complex but in broad terms, those relevant to T-cell activation include:

- phospholipase C-γ1 (PLC-γ1) → Ca^{2+} influx → activation through nuclear factor of activated T cells (NFAT);
- protein kinase C-θ (PKC-θ) → activation through nuclear factor-κB (NF-κB) and activator protein 1 (AP1);
- RAS-guanosine releasing protein (GRP) and the growth factor receptor-bound protein 2 (GRB2)–SOS complex → activation through RAS;
- VAV1–SLP76 complex → activation through Rho family GTPases.

These signalling pathways coordinate to drive proliferation and differentiation of the T lymphocyte and are therefore targets or potential targets of pharmacological intervention.[144]

It is apparent that activation of all these intracellular signalling pathways can be influenced by various co-stimulatory molecules.

Differential cytokine production, CD4+ and CD8+ T cells

As described above the interaction of T cell and APC is central to initiation of the alloimmune response. The default for such a response following transplantation is the generation of productive immunity manifest as rejection mediated through a variety of effector pathways. A productive immune response generally results in proliferation and differentiation of 'helper' T cells, which drive and direct antigen-specific immune responses through various effector pathways. They are mostly CD4+ T lymphocytes but in certain situations CD8+ T lymphocytes perform similar functions.[145,146] The type of effector response is determined, in part at least, through the elaboration of particular patterns of cytokines, which (as described above) are themselves determined by the signals delivered to cells of the innate immune system. The effector mechanisms are orchestrated to deliver effective host defence but at the same time maintain self-tolerance in the face of an adaptive immune system of immense potential diversity.

The original model of Mosmann and colleagues describes the association of cell-mediated immunity with the elaboration of T1 cytokines (hallmarked by IFN-γ) and humoral immunity with T2 cytokines (IL-5, IL-13). Differential cytokine production is, however, central also in the maintenance of tolerance to self via peripheral regulatory mechanisms dependent on cytokines like IL-10 and TGF-β (transforming growth factor β),[147,148] and it is clear, therefore, that the model must be broadened along the lines indicated in **Fig. 3.6** to accommodate this.

Thus, although the paradigm that effective operational tolerance to solid organ transplants is associated with immune deviation from T1 to T2 responses has proven to be simplistic,[149–154] it identifies broad mechanisms that are involved in controlling various aspects of immune responsiveness. This paradigm evolved from the fact that the experimental models used pathology that was more highly dependent on T1-driven responses as a measure of outcome – for example, rapid graft failure or acute rejection. It has been demonstrated that both Th1 and Th2 clones are capable of initiating graft rejection,[151] although Th1 responses may be of greatest importance when examining short-term allograft survival and Th2 cells may drive chronic graft rejection.[155] The possibility of harnessing the cytokines and cells they control that are normally involved in tolerance to self, for the purposes of transplantation, has not escaped the attention of transplantation immunologists, and this will be discussed in depth later in this chapter.

It is apparent that all sorts of cells, including cytotoxic T cells and DCs as well as T-helper cells, may be skewed in their production of cytokines.

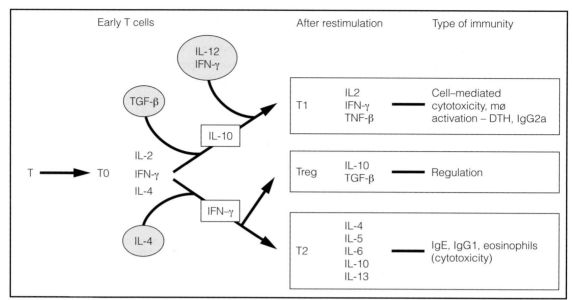

Figure 3.6 • Peripheral T-cell differentiation and cytokine production. Cytokines produced at various stages during the evolution of immune responses are shown. Cytokines that positively or negatively influence the divergence of T1 and T2 cells are shown in ovals or rectangles respectively. Treg cells are those that negatively regulate the immune response and are important in controlling self-reactivity as well as limiting immune responses to pathogens. Their divergence from the T2 pathway is based on data from many groups indicating that T cells can coexpress IL-10 and IL-4 under many conditions. DTH, delayed type hypersensitivity.

This is determined by the inciting stimulus, for example, the nature of an infecting organism,[86,93] by inherited variables determining responsiveness and by prior immune memory. Cytokines[156–158] and cell–cell interactions[100,101,159–162] mediate and integrate information that drives specific effector pathways.

THE EFFECTOR ARM OF THE IMMUNE RESPONSE

The immune system generates many different effector mechanisms depending on the challenge it meets. In certain infections a single mechanism is essential for the clearance of the organism, and the absence of that mechanism renders the host susceptible to disease. For example, in the clearance of lymphocyte choriomeningitis virus infections in mice, cytotoxic cells are absolutely required and disabling this arm of immunity by disrupting the perforin gene leads to death of infected animals.[163] In general, factors such as activation of innate immunity, antigen dose and prior immune stimuli determine which immune effector mechanisms predominate but in clinical transplantation a range of different responses is activated. Unfortunately most of these are capable of damaging a graft such that the obliteration of any single mechanism often has little benefit on graft survival, which is why the prevention of rejection is difficult. It also accounts for the importance of the CD4+ T-cell response since this is involved in the orchestration of many of these mechanisms and for interest in the role of regulatory cells since if it were possible to commandeer a mechanism evolved to control the autoimmunity then abrogation of alloimmunity is likely to be significantly easier than attempts to inhibit multiple different effector pathways.[112]

Migration of activated leucocytes into the graft

In order to enter a site of inflammation leucocytes migrate across vascular endothelium. This is mediated through a variety of chemokines and by cell–cell interactions between the leucocyte and the endothelium. Activated cells and memory cells express a range of chemokine receptors and adhesion molecules that promote migration into peripheral tissues.[164]

CELL–CELL INTERACTIONS

The adhesion of leucocytes to the endothelium is a multistep process, involving a series of interactions between the leucocyte and endothelial cell.[165]

The proteins involved fall into three groups: selectins, integrins and immunoglobulin (Ig) superfamily members along with mucins on a range of glycoproteins. The initial step is attachment and rolling mediated largely by selectins; the cell may then detach or be activated, adhere and subsequently transmigrate.

Rolling of leucocytes along the endothelium allows the leucocyte to sample the endothelial environment whilst maintaining its ability to detach and travel somewhere else. This is largely mediated by selectin binding. Under the appropriate conditions, leucocyte activation ensues and adhesion will be followed by passage through the endothelium in steps largely mediated by integrins and Ig superfamily members – ICAMs (intercellular adhesion molecules) and VCAMs (vascular cell adhesion molecules).

The expression of adhesion molecules involved in these interactions is upregulated by proinflammatory cytokines. The harvesting of a transplanted organ upregulates expression of various cytokines with subsequent upregulation of selectins, ICAM-1 and VCAM-1.[166,167]

Before any alloimmune response has been elicited the transplanted organ is attractive to circulating leucocytes. Although naive cells tend not to enter non-lymphoid sites this is not true of activated and memory cells,[168] therefore there may be early ingress of specific T lymphocytes in the clinical situation (unlike that of experimental transplantation with naive animals). This has implications for therapeutic strategies aimed at reducing trafficking into the graft.[169–171]

CHEMOKINES

Chemokines are small soluble proteins (8–11 kDa), which are responsible for leucocyte recruitment. Specific sequence motifs allow their classification into four groups:

- **CC chemokines**, which are important in the recruitment of mononuclear cells, e.g. macrophage inflammatory protein-1α/β (MIP-1α/β), RANTES and macrophage chemoattractant protein-1 (MCP-1);
- **CXC chemokines**, which are important in neutrophil recruitment (e.g. IL-8 and interferon-γ-inducible protein);
- **C chemokines** and **fractalkine**.

In transplantation chemokines are important in the development of graft infiltrates[172,173] and reperfusion injury.[174–176] They may also enhance the effector functions of leucocytes within the graft.[177] The antagonism of chemokine function is being investigated as a potential therapy in a variety of settings including transplantation.[178,179]

Specificity of rejection

The nature of tissue destruction during rejection tells us about the processes involved – graft destruction can show exquisitely fine specificity for cells carrying donor alloantigens. Mintz and Silvers demonstrated the specificity of donor cell lysis in experiments using allophenic mice as tissue donors.[180,181] Allophenic, or tetraparental, mice are bred by fusing the embryos from mice of two different genetic origins. The tissues of the resulting mosaic offspring are made up of patches of cells from each parental type. If skin from an allophenic donor is grafted to mice of either parental origin only the cells of non-identical type are rejected, leaving cells of recipient type intact. A similar level of specificity has been observed in other experimental situations,[182,183] and it is difficult to envisage how a non-specific mechanism such as DTH could have such specificity.

Nevertheless, 'bystander' destruction of tissue may be observed following specific immune responses to foreign antigens.[184] In the aforementioned experiments of donation from tetraparental animals, if the majority of cells in the graft were allogeneic to the recipient the overwhelming inflammatory response actually led to destruction of the entire tissue. Thus, although the immune system can exhibit fine specificity at the cellular level, once initiated the ongoing inflammation may result in non-directed mechanisms of cell death.

Described below are the effector systems that can damage tissue and their roles in hyperacute, acute and chronic rejection.

Humoral mechanisms

Antibody causes tissue damage through the fixation of complement, but also through antibody-dependent cellular cytotoxicity, although the role of this pathway in allograft rejection has not been fully elucidated.[185]

Patients exposed to MHC antigens through transplantation, blood transfusion or pregnancies often develop antibodies against MHC antigens. These preformed antibodies can cause **hyperacute** rejection, a process in which the organ fails immediately following revascularisation.[186,187] There is deposition of antibody and complement and accumulation of polymorphonuclear leucocytes within the graft.[186] This has been relegated as a significant cause of graft failure because of the success of screening for MHC-directed cytotoxic antibodies and the use of the lymphocyte cross-match with increasing levels of sensitivity. However, in the long term the formation of antibody in waiting-list patients may be the greatest barrier to successful transplantation since this is currently the most difficult to treat. In renal transplantation it creates a group of patients who become virtually 'untransplantable' or in whom transplantation is so delayed as to materially affect outcome[188] or who require novel and potentially hazardous immuno-suppressive protocols.[189–192]

Anti-HLA antibody may develop in the course of acute rejection and this is associated with vascular involvement and a relatively poor response to con-ventional therapy.[193–197] The appearance of donor-specific anti-HLA antibodies following the acute phase of transplantation is not necessarily associated with an acute rejection and this state has been termed 'accommodation'. The mechanisms of accommo-dation are poorly understood[198–200] but are of con-siderable interest particularly in the fields of ABO incompatibility and xenotransplantation.[199,200]

The presence of donor-specific antibodies is associated with poor long-term graft outcome, and deposition in the kidney can be inferred from peritubular capillary staining for C4d (a component of the complement cascade). The causal significance of such antibodies is supported by observations in mice with severe combined immunodeficiency in which infusion of donor-specific antibody causes lesions similar to chronic allograft vasculopathy.[201] On an individual basis these findings may therefore be considered as good evidence for an immunological component to chronic allograft nephropathy.[202]

Interestingly, liver transplantation appears to be an exception to the rules regarding transplantation across a positive cross-match. In fact liver transplants are carried out with little regard to alloimmunity and are performed successfully not only across positive cross-matches but also without MHC matching of donor and recipient (and see below).

The presence of preformed antibodies is also a barrier to xenotransplantation. The predominant antibody specificity is against carbohydrate antigens generated by α-1,3-galactosyltransferase, which is present in many species including pigs, but is absent in primates.[203] These 'natural antibodies' result in hyperacute rejection of pig tissue by the human.[204] The success of xenotransplantation is likely to require the removal of this antigenic barrier achieved by the genetic or other manipulation of the pig.[205,206]

Cellular mechanisms

NATURAL KILLER (NK) CELLS

NK cells are naturally lytic to target cells without prior immune activation (although their activity can be increased by certain cytokines). The activity of NK cells is controlled by the engagement of various receptors with both activating and inhibitory functions.[207] The range and subtlety of these inter-actions arise from an ancient role in host defence and a more recent role in shaping antigen-specific immune responses. One major group of receptors – killer immunoglobulin-like receptors (KIR) – bind self-MHC class I and inhibit NK cytotoxic activity. Thus NK cells may be triggered to kill by 'missing self',[208,209] a property that underlay early obser-vations that these cells preferentially lysed target tumour cells lacking MHC.[210] The role of NK cells as effectors of solid organ transplant rejection is uncertain,[211,212] although it is likely that they play an important role in the initiation and amplification of various immune responses through cytokine secretion. Their role in bone marrow transplantation is complex, encompassing rejection by recipient NK cells[213] and important anti-rejection and graft vs. leukaemia effects by NK cells of donor origin.[214,215]

ANTIGEN-SPECIFIC CYTOTOXIC T CELLS

In cell culture systems, MHC-mismatched lymphocytes proliferate and produce cytokines in response to one another in the mixed lymphocyte reaction (MLR). The resulting cytokine production allows the differentiation of precursor cytotoxic T lymphocytes into effector cells (CTLs) that lyse target cells bearing mismatched MHC antigens.[216,217] The identification of a powerful antigen-specific response, which could be quantified in the MLR, made the CTL a prime suspect as a central effector mechanism of acute graft rejection, the evidence for which is considerable:

- CTLs can be recovered from allografts that are undergoing rejection but they may be present only at low levels in grafts of animals that have been treated with ciclosporin to prevent rejection.[211,218]
- Cloned populations of CTLs can cause the type of tissue damage associated with rejection.[219,220]
- The majority of class I MHC-specific CTLs express CD8, and graft rejection can often be delayed in the absence of CD8$^+$ cells.[221–225]

Conversely, graft destruction may occur in the absence of demonstrable CTL activity, and the presence of such cells within a graft may not always lead to graft destruction. The male-specific miH antigen, H-Y, was first detected by the rejection of male skin grafts by female mice of the same strain, but the correlation between rejection and the presence of CTLs is not consistent.[226–228] Furthermore, alloantigen-specific CTL activity may be recovered from a non-rejected graft, and high alloantigen-specific CTL activity has been demonstrated in splenocytes in rats in whom prolonged allograft survival has been induced by donor-specific pre-operative blood transfusion.[229,230] This suggests that in vitro cytotoxic activity does not necessarily correlate with the destruction of allogeneic cells.

CTLs kill their targets in a variety of ways including through the action of perforins and granzymes, which directly attack membrane integrity, through Fas-mediated apoptosis and the secretion of TNF-α. However, perforin knockout mice are able to reject tumour,[231] skin[232] and solid organ[233] grafts, even when the grafts are resistant to Fas and TNF-α-mediated killing.[231] Nevertheless, grafts mismatched only at MHC class I are rejected more slowly in the absence of perforin, suggesting that cytotoxic T-cell activity does contribute to the efferent arm of rejection, but this is only revealed by excluding other mechanisms.[233]

Although direct cytotoxicity may not be necessary to mediate rejection it is likely to play a role in most cases, and CD8$^+$ T cells are likely to contribute through the elaboration of cytokines that recruit and activate cells involved in more generalised inflammatory responses.

MACROPHAGES AND DTH REACTIONS

T lymphocytes can generate responses that are both exquisitely specific at a cellular level and that non-specifically generate widespread local inflammation – the delayed type hypersensitivity (DTH) reaction (first described by Koch in the cutaneous reaction to tuberculin). The afferent phase of DTH is antigen specific but the efferent phase is not.

DTH involves the production of a wide range of cytokines by CD4$^+$ T lymphocytes, which activate effector cells, the most important of which are macrophages. These cells themselves elaborate a variety of substances, such as oxygen-derived intermediates and TNF-α, that mediate tissue damage. The importance of DTH in rejection is illustrated by acute rejection of H-Y-disparate grafts in which cell-mediated cytotoxicity does not correlate with graft rejection but the DTH response to H-Y antigens does.[234] Furthermore, the reconstitution of irradiated rats with CD4$^+$ T lymphocytes can cause allograft rejection in the absence of detectable cytotoxic T-cell activity.[222]

The changes observed in chronic allograft nephropathy are likely, at least in part, to arise from the elaboration of cytokines by CD4$^+$ T lymphocytes and macrophages.[235,236] Cytokines such as IL-1, TNF-α, TGF-β and PDGF (platelet-derived growth factor) lead to smooth muscle proliferation and increased synthesis of extracellular matrix protein. They are therefore candidate mediators of the vasculopathy and interstitial fibrosis observed in chronic allograft nephropathy.

EOSINOPHILS

Both **acute** and **chronic** kidney allograft rejection are associated with a varying level of eosinophilia,[237,238] but the importance of eosinophils in rejection is uncertain. In a mouse cardiac allograft model, depletion of CD8[+] T lymphocytes results in a dominant T2 response in which rejection is evident and mediated by eosinophils.[239] Other reports have also implicated IL-5 and eosinophils in acute and chronic rejection after the inhibition of other routes of activation.[240,241]

Cytokines

The primary role of cytokines is in the initiation and regulation of immunity as described above, but cytokines may also play an important role in the effector phase of the alloimmune response. This may be the case in both acute and chronic rejection and in non-immune mechanisms of allograft damage such as calcineurin inhibitor toxicity. Thus, TGF-β may play an important intermediate role in alloimmune regulation, chronic rejection and in the nephrotoxicity of calcineurin inhibitors.[242–244]

PRIVILEGED SITES

Privileged sites are those in which tissue allografts appear to elicit a weak immune response and there may consequently be prolonged allograft survival. These sites include the anterior chamber of the eye, the cornea, the brain and the testis.[245,246] They are typified by absent or limited lymphatic drainage. The degree of 'privilege' seems to vary depending on the nature of the transplanted tissue as well as the site of transplantation.

The liver is an unusual vascularised graft in that, despite its extensive blood supply and high immune cell content, it often fails to elicit rejection and may protect co-transplanted organs from rejection despite their usual immunogenicity. Calne et al. demonstrated that outbred pigs often fail to reject orthotopic liver allografts[247] and that simultaneous renal allografts from the same donor show prolonged survival despite the fact that they would otherwise have been rejected. In rat strain combinations in which an orthotopic liver allograft is not rejected the graft may even abrogate an existing state of sensitisation of the host against donor

histocompatibility antigen.[248,249] Similarly, although cross-matching has been demonstrated to be of some relevance in liver transplantation outcome,[250] urgently implanted grafts survive well despite a positive cross-match.

The mechanisms underlying these remarkable properties of the liver are still to be fully explained and may depend on antigenic load, given the liver's size, and its Promethean powers of regeneration. However, if specific mechanisms could be elucidated then they could be applied therapeutically in other solid organs.[251–253] The mechanisms so far identified include induction of regulatory CD4[+] T cells and partial activation followed by apoptosis of CD8[+] T cells as they encounter antigen on liver sinusoidal epithelial cells.

Fas–Fas ligand (FasL) binding initiates the apoptotic pathway of Fas[+] cells, and expression of FasL on certain tissues may be one mechanism of immune privilege; for instance, it may contribute to the relative immune privilege of transplanted corneas.[254,255] In some experimental models the manipulated expression of FasL on cells can,[256] but does not necessarily, confer protection from immune attack.[257]

REGULATORY T CELLS

There is increasing recognition that regulatory cells are important determinants of self-tolerance, that they may play an important role in models of transplantation tolerance, and that an ability to induce or expand such cells in the clinical setting may be of great therapeutic value.

The presence of regulatory or suppressor T cells has been suggested by the work of a number of investigators. The absence of specific T-cell subpopulations can result in autoimmune disease, and their repletion prevents the development of autoimmunity.[258–264] There is good evidence that following their induction, regulatory cells not only suppress activation but can confer a regulatory phenotype on naive cells, a process termed 'infectious tolerance'.[265] Also, tolerance to alloantigen of one type can spread to alloantigen of another type when the two are expressed on the same cell, in what is termed linked suppression.[265–268]

The presence and activity of regulatory cells is frequently demonstrated by the adoptive transfer of cells into naive recipients. However, transfer is usually into lymphopenic or otherwise manipulated recipients so that, in fact, the regulatory cells have a numerical advantage over reactive cells. Indeed, the presence of regulatory cells in allogeneic transplant models, not requiring transfer into lymphopenic hosts, generally involves differences in only minor histocompatibility antigens[267] or inhibition of direct pathway stimulation by prior depletion of dendritic cells (e.g. by 'parking' the organ in an immuno-incompetent host or short courses of immuno-suppression).[269] This may be because the expression of regulatory activity requires that the alloreactive population be of limited size (that is equivalent to the clonal frequency generated by conventional antigen or by autoantigen rather than the vast frequency stimulated by direct recognition of allo-MHC). Nevertheless, it is clear that regulatory T cells can be induced across full MHC incompatibilities, suggesting that reinforcement of such activity or expansion of the relevant cells may be of use in this context.

A considerable amount of interest has been concentrated on the role of CD4+CD25+ regulatory cells. Neonatal rodents undergoing early thymectomy develop autoimmune disease.[261,262] Autoimmunity can be prevented by the infusion of a CD4+CD25+ subpopulation of T lymphocytes from non-thymectomised syngeneic donors.[262,263] A role for such CD4+CD25+ regulatory cells has been demonstrated in a variety of organ-specific model systems including thyroiditis,[259] diabetes mellitus,[270] encephalitis[271,272] and colitis.[273] In the setting of transplantation the generation of de novo CD4+CD25+ immunoregulatory cells has been demonstrated,[274] and these cells can transfer tolerance in combined adoptive transfer using lymphopenic recipients.[275] This model is IL-10 and CTLA-4 dependent. The relevance of these observations to models of transplantation tolerance in treated intact animals (e.g. following antibody induction) remains to be demonstrated. Indeed, the antigen specificity of such CD4+CD25+ regulatory cells remains a matter of controversy.[276,277]

There is also evidence in vivo for regulation by CD4+CD25−[278] and CD8+ T-lymphocyte sub-populations.[30,88] The mechanisms identified are likely to be very incomplete, but they give clues as to relevant pathways. For example, the induction of non-responsiveness in naive cells has been inhibited

by neutralising specific cytokines such as IL-10[264,279,280] and TGF-β,[281,282] and cells whose regulatory activity are so inhibited are referred to as Tr1 and Th3 cells respectively. The relationship between CD4+CD25+ regulatory cells and these cells defined in other systems has yet to be clearly defined.[283]

In vitro studies that mimic such in vivo observations demonstrate suppressor cells that inhibit the proliferation of co-cultured cells with different antigen specificity. These responses require the coexpression of cognate antigen for 'suppressor' and 'responder' cells on the same APC. This shows the 'suppressor' effect to be specific in that it requires specific antigen, and suggests that a 'suppressive' signal is delivered 'laterally' between suppressor and responder or perhaps more plausibly through an intermediate effect on the APC.[88,284] These observations have been extended to the demonstration of altered DC expression of co-stimulatory molecules such as CD40 following their exposure to anergic T-cell clones.[285]

The way in which these findings relate to experimental in vivo models of tolerance is as yet undetermined but the role of the APC recalls the aforementioned observations on linked suppression.[266,276,286] It also recalls human studies in which diminished cytotoxic T-cell activity against allogeneic MHC class I occurred following trans-fusion with HLA-DR (MHC class II)-matched blood, but this was not observed if there was no such match.[287,288]

In summary, these observations on T-regulatory cells offer considerable hope for the induction of dominant tolerance, which may benefit trans-plantation, but the limitations of the experimental models involved need careful consideration before extrapolation to settings more representative of the clinical scenario.

CHRONIC REJECTION

The clinicopathological entity of chronic rejection is perhaps most easily considered from the perspective of renal transplantation. It is apparent that some of the changes associated with deteriorating graft function in established transplants are multifactorial and may relate to donor and recipient factors such as age,[289] peritransplant variables such as cold ischaemia time,[290] nephrotoxic treatment such as calcineurin inhibitors[291] and hypertension. The relevance of these factors is acknowledged in the frequent use of the designation chronic allograft nephropathy (CAN) rather than chronic rejection. It is, though, apparent that immunological factors do impinge on the long-term vascular and tubulointerstitial pathology described as CAN. A history of acute rejection is associated with CAN and whilst this could be a consequence solely of damage established at the time and subsequent changes in calcineurin inhibitor dosing, it is now apparent that CAN is associated with enhanced responses of T lymphocytes through the indirect pathway.[62,64,292] This association has been demonstrated with antigen from disrupted cells and with specific donor-derived HLA-DR peptides.[66] It is apparent that modern immunosuppressive therapy, which has markedly improved early allograft survival and freedom from acute rejection, has had only a limited impact on long-term graft attrition. This may be because conventional immunosuppression has relatively little impact on indirect pathway activation[66] and on B-cell activation, which may both be important.[197,202,293]

A recent report of lung transplant recipients with evidence of humoral chronic rejection failed to detect anti-HLA antibodies, leading to speculation that tissue-specific antibodies may develop in this setting,[294] but these data are limited.

In animal models of chronic rejection there is evidence of upregulation of a wide variety of cytokines, growth factors and lipid mediators of inflammation but their relative importance has yet to be established. Hence, there is no single candidate pathway that might be targeted for therapeutic purposes.

In summary, chronic rejection is likely to largely involve the indirect pathway of allorecognition, resulting in the elaboration of cytokines that interact with non-immunological factors to produce the vasculopathy and tubulointerstitial atrophy and fibrosis typical of chronic allograft nephropathy. This immune response is relatively resistant to conventional immunosuppressive regimes and is therefore a potential target for future prophylactic therapy, which must be safe given the relatively good short- and medium-term results of renal transplantation.

Key points

- The immune response to a transplanted allogeneic organ is multifaceted – and the associated literature is becoming increasingly complex. There is increasing evidence for the importance of indirect allorecognition in chronic rejection and appreciation of the importance of heterologous memory T-cell responses in clinical allorecognition.

- A range of recently characterised molecules, including co-stimulators and chemokines and their receptors, offers potential new targets for therapy.

- The actions of immunoregulatory cells are now the subject of intense study, and commandeering such mechanisms perhaps offers the most attractive prospect of improving graft outcome.

- Finally, it is notable that considerable effort is expended in attempts to improve graft outcome but perhaps the most important group of patients are those who are never or rarely transplanted because they have formed alloreactive antibodies. If mechanisms could be identified to prevent or reverse the formation of such antibodies safely and easily, this would benefit a subgroup of patients with end-stage organ failure who suffer markedly reduced survival because of this failure to be transplanted.

REFERENCES

1. Wolfe RA, Ashby VB, Milford EL et al. Comparison of mortality in all patients on dialysis, patients on dialysis awaiting transplantation, and recipients of a first cadaveric transplant. N Engl J Med 1999; 341(23):1725–30.

2. Meier-Kriesche HU, Ojo AO, Port FK et al. Survival improvement among patients with end-stage renal disease: trends over time for transplant recipients and wait-listed patients. J Am Soc Nephrol 2001; 12(6):1293–6.

3. Reddy KS, Stablein D, Taranto S et al. Long-term survival following simultaneous kidney-pancreas transplantation versus kidney transplantation alone in patients with type 1 diabetes mellitus and renal failure. Am J Kidney Dis 2003; 41(2):464–70.

4. Merrill JP, Murray JE, Harrison JH et al. Successful transplantation of human kidney between identical twins. J Am Med Assoc 1956; 160:277.

5. Calne RY. The rejection of renal homografts: inhibition in dogs by 6-mercaptopurine. Lancet 1960; 1:417.

6. Murray JE, Merrill JP, Dammin GJ et al. Kidney transplantation in modified recipients. Ann Surg 1962; 156:337.

7. Marchioro TL, Axtell HK, LaVia MF et al. The role of adrenocortical steroids in reversing established homograft rejection. Surgery 1964; 55:412.

8. Medawar PB. The behaviour and fate of skin autografts and skin homografts in rabbits (A report to the war wounds committee of the Medical Research Council). J Anat 1944; 78:176–9.

9. Gorer PA. The genetic and antigenic basis for tumour transplantation. J Path Bact 1937; 44:691–7.

10. Snell GD. Methods for the study of histocompatability genes. J Genetics 1948; 49:87–108.

11. Gowans JL. Ann New York Acad Sci 1962; 99:432.

12. van Rood JJ. 1996 Medawar Prize Lecture – looking back and forward. Transplant Proc 1997; 29(1-2):39–42.

13. Zinkernagel RM. The Nobel Lectures in Immunology. The Nobel Prize for Physiology or Medicine, 1996. Cellular immune recognition and the biological role of major transplantation antigens. Scand J Immunol 1997; 46(5):421–36.

14. Mandal AK, Snyder JJ, Gilbertson DT et al. Does cadaveric donor renal transplantation ever provide better outcomes than live-donor renal transplantation? Transplantation 2003; 75(4):494–500.

15. Salahudeen AK, Haider N, May W. Cold ischemia and the reduced long-term survival of cadaveric renal allografts. Kidney Int 2004; 65(2):713–18.

16. Qureshi F, Rabb H, Kasiske BL. Silent acute rejection during prolonged delayed graft function reduces kidney allograft survival. Transplantation 2002; 74(10):1400–4.

17. Tullius SG, Heemann UW, Azuma H et al. Alloantigen-independent factors lead to signs of chronic rejection in long-term kidney isografts. Transplant Int 1994; 7(suppl. 1):S306–7.

18. Matzinger P. Tolerance, danger, and the extended family. Annu Rev Immunol 1994; 12:991–1045.

19. Goldstein DR, Tesar BM, Akira S et al. Critical role of the Toll-like receptor signal adaptor protein MyD88 in acute allograft rejection. J Clin Invest 2003; 111(10):1571–8.

20. Mocikat R, Braumuller H, Gumy A et al. Natural killer cells activated by MHC class I^{low} targets prime dendritic cells to induce protective CD8 T cell responses. Immunity 2003; 19:561–9.

21. Ferlicot S, Durrbach A, Ba N et al. The role of replicative senescence in chronic allograft nephropathy. Hum Pathol 2003; 34(9):924–8.

22. Peugh WN, Superina RA, Wood KJ et al. The role of H-2 and non-H-2 antigens and genes in the rejection of murine cardiac allografts. Immunogenetics 1986; 23(1):30–7.

23. den Haan JM, Meadows LM, Wang W et al. The minor histocompatibility antigen HA-1: a diallelic gene with a single amino acid polymorphism. Science 1998; 279(5353):1054–7.

24. Cresswell P. Assembly, transport, and function of MHC class II molecules. Annu Rev Immunol 1994; 12:259–93.

25. van Rood JJ. HLA and I. Annu Rev Immunol 1993; 11:1–28.

26. Rammensee HG, Falk K, Rotzschke O. Peptides naturally presented by MHC class I molecules. Annu Rev Immunol 1993; 11:213–44.

27. Vignali DA, Strominger JL. Amino acid residues that flank the core peptide epitopes and the extracellular domains of CD4 molecule modulate differential signalling through the T cell receptor. J Exp Med 1994; 179:1945–56.

28. Sherman LA, Chattopadhyay S. The molecular basis of allorecognition. Annu Rev Immunol 1993; 11:385–402.

29. Seth A, Stern LJ, Ottenhoff TH et al. Binary and ternary complexes between T-cell receptor, class II MHC and superantigen in vitro. Nature 1994; 369(6478):324–7.

30. Wong KK, Carpenter MJ, Young LL et al. Notch ligation by Delta1 inhibits peripheral immune responses to transplantation antigens by a CD8+ cell-dependent mechanism. J Clin Invest 2003; 112(11):1741–50.

The Notch signalling pathway is highly conserved from Drosophila to humans and controls cell fate decisions during development. Notch receptors and ligands are widely distributed throughout the haematopoietic system, including on mature leucocytes of most if not all lineages. In this paper overexpressing of one of the Notch ligands, Delta-like1, on alloantigen-bearing cells could, when introduced into animals inhibit the immune response to the same antigen delivered subsequently in the absence of this ligand – this even allowed prolongation of heart allograft survival in an antigen-specific fashion. Interestingly, the immune response was skewed away from the normal T1 type of immunity seen following transplantation towards an IL-10-dominated response, suggesting the activation of Treg in this system, thus providing a possible new opportunity for manipulation of the immune system.

31. Krieger NR, Yin DP, Fathman CG. CD4+ but not CD8+ cells are essential for allorejection. J Exp Med 1996; 184(5):2013–18.

32. O'Brien SJ, Roelke ME, Marker L et al. Genetic basis for species vulnerability in the cheetah. Science 1985; 227(4693):1428–34.

33. Germain RN, Margulies DH. The biochemistry and cell biology of antigen processing and presentation. Annu Rev Immunol 1993; 11:403–50.

34. Roche PA. HLA-DM: an in vivo facilitator of MHC class II peptide loading. Immunity 1995; 3(3):259–62.

35. Vincent MS, Gumperz JE, Brenner MB. Understanding the function of CD1-restricted T cells. Nature Immunol 2003; 4(6):517–23.

36. Turner D, Grant SC, Yonan N et al. Cytokine gene polymorphism and heart transplant rejection. Transplantation 1997; 64(5):776–9.

37. Scott DM, Ehrmann IE, Ellis PS et al. Identification of a mouse male-specific transplantation antigen, H-Y. Nature 1995; 376(6542):695–8.

38. Scott DM, Ehrmann IE, Ellis PS et al. Why do some females reject males? The molecular basis for male-specific graft rejection. J Mol Med 1997; 75(2):103–14.

39. Marijt WA, Heemskerk MH, Kloosterboer FM et al. Hematopoiesis-restricted minor histocompatibility antigens HA-1- or HA-2-specific T cells can induce complete remissions of relapsed leukemia. Proc Natl Acad Sci USA 2003; 100(5):2742–7.

40. Lombardi G, Sidhu S, Daly M et al. Are primary alloresponses truly primary? Int Immunol 1990; 2(1):9–13.

41. 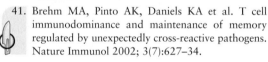 Brehm MA, Pinto AK, Daniels KA et al. T cell immunodominance and maintenance of memory regulated by unexpectedly cross-reactive pathogens. Nature Immunol 2002; 3(7):627–34.

    This paper, which examines viral immune responses, demonstrates the importance of heterologous immunity in determining immunodominance of specific epitopes and the epitopes to which memory is maintained. Evidently, immunity is shaped by the individual's summed history of infection. In the wild this adds further heterogeneity to immune responsiveness to that generated by variation in the MHC, and is likely to thereby contribute to a species' resistance to infection.

42. Nahill SR, Welsh RM. High frequency of cross-reactive cytotoxic T lymphocytes elicited during the virus-induced polyclonal cytotoxic T lymphocyte response. J Exp Med 1993; 177(2):317–27.

43. Selin LK, Vergilis K, Welsh RM et al. Reduction of otherwise remarkably stable virus-specific cytotoxic T lymphocyte memory by heterologous viral infections. J Exp Med 1996; 183(6):2489–99.

44. Brehm MA, Markees TG, Daniels KA et al. Direct visualization of cross-reactive effector and memory allo-specific CD8 T cells generated in response to viral infections. J Immunol 2003; 170(8):4077–86.

45. Adams AB, Williams MA, Jones TR et al. Heterologous immunity provides a potent barrier to transplantation tolerance. J Clin Invest 2003; 111(12):1887–95.

    This paper demonstrates that heterologous immunity, which is virally induced, is a potent barrier to conventional models of tolerance developed in pathogen-free rodents. Although not a new concept this demonstration is both elegant and important, coming from a laboratory that has been at the forefront of investigations in transplantation tolerance.

46. Williams MA, Onami TM, Adams AB et al. Cutting edge: persistent viral infection prevents tolerance induction and escapes immune control following CD28/CD40 blockade-based regimen. J Immunol 2002; 169(10):5387–91.

47. Moudgil KD, Sercarz EE. The self-directed T cell repertoire: its creation and activation. Rev Immunogenet 2000; (1):26–37.

48. Drakesmith H, O'Neil D, Schneider SC et al. In vivo priming of T cells against cryptic determinants by dendritic cells exposed to interleukin 6 and native antigen. Proc Natl Acad Sci USA 1998; 95(25):14903–8.

49. Rock KL, Barnes MC, Germain RN et al. The role of Ia molecules in the activation of T lymphocytes. II. Ia-restricted recognition of allo K/D antigens is required for class I MHC-stimulated mixed lymphocyte responses. J Immunol 1983; 130(1):457–62.

50. Golding H, Singer A. Role of accessory cell processing and presentation of shed H-2 alloantigens in allospecific cytotoxic T lymphocyte responses. J Immunol 1984; 133(2):597–605.

51. Fangmann J, Dalchau R, Fabre JW. Rejection of skin allografts by indirect allorecognition of donor class I major histocompatibility complex peptides. J Exp Med 1992; 175(6):1521–9.

52. Liu Z, Sun YK, Xi YP et al. Contribution of direct and indirect recognition pathways to T cell allo-reactivity. J Exp Med 1993; 177(6):1643–50.

53. Game DS, Lechler RI. Pathways of allorecognition: implications for transplantation tolerance. Transplant Immunol 2002; 10(2-3):101–8.

54. Lee RS, Yamada K, Houser SL et al. Indirect recognition of allopeptides promotes the development of cardiac allograft vasculopathy. Proc Natl Acad Sci USA 2001; 98(6):3276–81.

55. Vella JP, Magee C, Vos L et al. Cellular and humoral mechanisms of vascularized allograft rejection induced by indirect recognition of donor MHC allopeptides. Transplantation 1999; 67(12):1523–32.

56. Lee RS, Grusby MJ, Glimcher LH et al. Indirect recognition by helper cells can induce donor-specific cytotoxic T lymphocytes in vivo. J Exp Med 1994; 179(3):865–72.

57. Malaviya R, Twesten NJ, Ross EA et al. Mast cells process bacterial Ags through a phagocytic route for class I MHC presentation to T cells. J Immunol 1996; 156(4):1490–6.

58. Lee RS, Grusby MJ, Laufer TM et al. CD8+ effector cells responding to residual class I antigens, with help from CD4+ cells stimulated indirectly, cause rejection of 'major histocompatibility complex-deficient' skin grafts. Transplantation 1997; 63(8):1123–33.

59. Iyoda T, Shimoyama S, Liu K et al. The CD8+ dendritic cell subset selectively endocytoses dying cells in culture and in vivo. J Exp Med 2002; 195(10):1289–302.

60. Auchincloss H Jr, Lee R, Shea S et al. The role of 'indirect' recognition in initiating rejection of skin grafts from major histocompatibility complex class II-deficient mice. Proc Natl Acad Sci USA 1993; 90(8):3373–7.

61. Mason PD, Robinson CM, Lechler RI. Detection of donor-specific hyporesponsiveness following late failure of human renal allografts. Kidney Int 1996; 50(3):1019–25.

62. Baker RJ, Hernandez-Fuentes MP, Brookes PA et al. Loss of direct and maintenance of indirect allo-responses in renal allograft recipients: implications for the pathogenesis of chronic allograft nephropathy. J Immunol 2001; 167(12):7199–206.

63. Ng WF, Hernandez-Fuentes M, Baker R et al. Reversibility with interleukin-2 suggests that T cell anergy contributes to donor-specific hyporesponsiveness in renal transplant patients. J Am Soc Nephrol 2002; 13(12):2983–9.

64. Ciubotariu R, Liu Z, Colovai AI et al. Persistent allopeptide reactivity and epitope spreading in chronic rejection of organ allografts. J Clin Invest 1998; 101(2):398–405.

65. SivaSai KS, Smith MA, Poindexter NJ et al. Indirect recognition of donor HLA class I peptides in lung transplant recipients with bronchiolitis obliterans syndrome. Transplantation 1999; 67(8):1094–8.

66. Najafian N, Salama AD, Fedoseyeva EV et al. Enzyme-linked immunosorbent spot assay analysis of peripheral blood lymphocyte reactivity to donor HLA-DR peptides: potential novel assay for prediction of outcomes for renal transplant recipients. J Am Soc Nephrol 2002; 13(1):252–9.

This paper demonstrates indirect alloreactivity of peripheral blood lymphocytes from renal transplant recipients to HLA-DR-derived peptides corresponding to the donor mismatch. The technique used to demonstrate responsiveness was an elispot to γ-interferon. The frequency of responsive cells was greater in those that had undergone an episode of acute rejection (and worse renal function: 'high-risk' patients), than those who had not. It is proposed that this form of 'immunological monitoring' could be used to tailor immunosuppression to the individual but it also suggests that HLA-derived peptides could be used as therapeutic agents.

67. Benichou G, Tam RC, Soares LR et al. Indirect T-cell allorecognition: perspectives for peptide-based therapy in transplantation. Immunol Today 1997; 18(2):67–71.

68. Larsen CP, Morris PJ, Austyn JM. Migration of dendritic leukocytes from cardiac allografts into host spleens. A novel pathway for initiation of rejection. J Exp Med 1990; 171(1):307–14.

69. Steinman RM, Gutchinov B, Witmer MD et al. Dendritic cells are the principal stimulators of the primary mixed leukocyte reaction in mice. J Exp Med 1983; 157(2):613–27.

70. Austyn JM, Weinstein DE, Steinman RM. Clustering with dendritic cells precedes and is essential for T-cell proliferation in a mitogenesis model. Immunology 1988; 63(4):691–6.

71. Lafferty KJ, Bootes A, Dart G et al. Effect of organ culture on the survival of thyroid allografts in mice. Transplantation 1976; 22(2):138–49.

72. Emma DA, Jacobs BB. Prolongation of skin allograft survival following donor irradiation and organ culture explanation. Transplantation 1981; 31(2):138–9.

73. Lechler RI, Batchelor JR. Restoration of immunogenicity to passenger cell-depleted kidney allografts by the addition of donor strain dendritic cells. J Exp Med 1982; 155(1):31–41.

74. Lutz MB, Suri RM, Niimi M et al. Immature dendritic cells generated with low doses of GM-CSF in the absence of IL-4 are maturation resistant and prolong allograft survival in vivo. Eur J Immunol 2000; 30(7):1813–22.

75. Roelen DL, Schuurhuis DH, van den Boogaardt DE et al. Prolongation of skin graft survival by modulation of the alloimmune response with alternatively activated dendritic cells. Transplantation 2003; 76(11):1608–15.

76. Benichou G, Valujskikh A, Heeger PS. Contributions of direct and indirect T cell alloreactivity during allograft rejection in mice. J Immunol 1999; 162(1):352–8.

77. Illigens BM, Yamada A, Fedoseyeva EV et al. The relative contribution of direct and indirect antigen recognition pathways to the alloresponse and graft rejection depends upon the nature of the transplant. Hum Immunol 2002; 63(10):912–25.

78. Rose ML. Endothelial cells as antigen-presenting cells: role in human transplant rejection. Cell Mol Life Sci 1998; 54(9):965–78.

79. McDouall RM, Page CS, Hafizi S et al. Alloproliferation of purified CD4+ T cells to adult human heart endothelial cells, and study of second-signal requirements. Immunology 1996; 89(2):220–6.

80. Page CS, Holloway N, Smith H et al. Allo-proliferative responses of purified CD4+ and CD8+ T cells to endothelial cells in the absence of contaminating accessory cells. Transplantation 1994; 57(11):1628–37.

81. Pober JS, Cotran RS. Immunologic interactions of T lymphocytes with vascular endothelium. Adv Immunol 1991; 50:261–302.

82. Bancereau J, Briere F, Caux C et al. Immuno-biology of dendritic cells. Annu Rev Immunol 2000; 18:767–811.

83. Shreedhar V, Moodycliffe AM, Ullrich SE et al. Dendritic cells require T cells for functional maturation in vivo. Immunity 1999; 11(5):625–36.

84. Moodycliffe AM, Shreedhar V, Ullrich SE et al. CD40–CD40 ligand interactions in vivo regulate migration of antigen-bearing dendritic cells from the skin to draining lymph nodes. J Exp Med 2000; 191(11):2011–20.

85. Boonstra A, Asselin-Paturel C, Gilliet M et al. Flexibility of mouse classical and plasmacytoid-derived dendritic cells in directing T helper type 1 and 2 cell development: dependency on antigen dose and differential toll-like receptor ligation. J Exp Med 2003; 197(1):101–9.

> This paper investigates the effects of antigen dose, state of DC maturation and DC TLR ligation on T1/T2 skewing of primary T immune responses.
>
> Th1 responses were favoured by high and Th2 by low antigen dose. At low antigen dose the stimulation of plasmacytoid DCs through TLR 9 and of myeloid DCs through TLR 4 promoted Th1 responses.
>
> These data illustrate mechanisms by which skewing of immune responses to any given antigen may be integrated at the level of the DC.

86. Reis e Sousa C. Toll-like receptors and dendritic cells: for whom the bug tolls. Semin Immunol 2004; 16(1):27–34.

87. Gallucci S, Lolkema M, Matzinger P. Natural adjuvants: endogenous activators of dendritic cells. Nature Med 1999; 5(11):1249–55.

88. Chang CC, Ciubotariu R, Manavalan JS et al. Tolerization of dendritic cells by T(S) cells: the crucial role of inhibitory receptors ILT3 and ILT4. Nature Immunol 2002; 3(3):237–43.

89. Brandt K, Bulfone-Paus S, Foster DC et al. Interleukin-21 inhibits dendritic cell activation and maturation. Blood 2003; 102(12):4090–8.

90. Medzhitov R, Janeway CA Jr. Innate immunity: the virtues of a nonclonal system of recognition. Cell 1997; 91(3):295–8.

91. Ohashi K, Burkart V, Flohe S et al. Heat shock protein 60 is a putative endogenous ligand of the toll-like receptor-4 complex. J Immunol 2000; 164:558–61.

92. Termeer C, Benedix F, Sleeman J et al. Oligosaccharides of hyaluronan activate dendritic cells via toll-like receptor 4. J Exp Med 2002; 195:99–111.

93. de Jong EC, Vieira PL, Kalinski P et al. Microbial compounds selectively induce Th1 cell-promoting or Th2 cell-promoting dendritic cells in vitro with diverse Th cell-polarizing signals. J Immunol 2002; 168(4):1704–9.

94. Kapsenberg ML. Dendritic-cell control of pathogen-driven T-cell polarization. Nature Rev Immunol 2003; 3(12):984–93.

95. Hawiger D, Inaba K, Dorsett Y et al. Dendritic cells induce peripheral T cell unresponsiveness under steady state conditions in vivo. J Exp Med 2001; 194(6):769–79.

96. Yamazaki S, Iyoda T, Tarbell K et al. Direct expansion of functional CD25+ CD4+ regulatory T cells by antigen-processing dendritic cells. J Exp Med 2003; 198(2):235–47.

97. Lu L, Li W, Zhong C et al. Increased apoptosis of immunoreactive host cells and augmented donor leukocyte chimerism, not sustained inhibition of B7 molecule expression are associated with prolonged cardiac allograft survival in mice preconditioned with immature donor dendritic cells plus anti-CD40L mAb. Transplantation 1999; 68(6):747–57.

98. Lu L, Bonham CA, Liang X et al. Liver-derived DEC205+B220+CD19– dendritic cells regulate T cell responses. J Immunol 2001; 166(12):7042–52.

99. Jonuleit H, Schmitt E, Schuler G et al. Induction of interleukin 10-producing, nonproliferating CD4(+) T cells with regulatory properties by repetitive stimulation with allogeneic immature human dendritic cells. J Exp Med 2000; 192(9):1213–22.

100. Wakkach A, Fournier N, Brun V et al. Characterization of dendritic cells that induce tolerance and T regulatory 1 cell differentiation in vivo. Immunity 2003; 18(5):605–17.

101. Serra P, Amrani A, Yamanouchi J et al. CD40 ligation releases immature dendritic cells from the control of regulatory CD4+CD25+ T cells. Immunity 2003; 19(6):877–89.

102. Hackstein H, Thomson AW. Dendritic cells: emerging pharmacological targets of immuno-suppressive drugs. Nature Rev Immunol 2004; 4(1):24–34.

103. Morelli AE, Thomson AW. Dendritic cells: regulators of alloimmunity and opportunities for tolerance induction. Immunol Rev 2003; 196:125–46.

104. Coates PT, Thomson AW. Dendritic cells, tolerance induction and transplant outcome. Am J Transplant 2002; 2(4):299–307.

105. Schwartz RH. A cell culture model for T-lymphocyte clonal anergy. Science 1990; 248:1349–56.

106. Gimmi CD, Freeman GJ, Gribben JG et al. Human T-cell clonal anergy is induced by antigen presentation in the absence of B7 costimulation. Proc Natl Acad Sci USA 1993; 90:6586–90.

107. Lenschow DJ, Walunas TL, Bluestone JA. CD28/B7 system of T cell costimulation. Annu Rev Immunol 1996; 14:233–58.

108. Tivol EA, Borriello F, Schweizer AN, Lynch WP, Bluestone JA, Sharpe AH. Loss of CTLA-4 leads to massive lymphoproliferation and fatal multiorgan destruction, revealing a critical negative regulatory role of CTLA-4. Immunity 1995; 3:541–7.

109. Perez VL, Van Parijs L, Biuckians A et al. Induction of peripheral T cell tolerance in vivo requires CTLA-4 engagement. Immunity 1997; 6(4):411–17.

110. Ariyan C, Salvalaggio P, Fecteau S et al. Transplantation tolerance through enhanced CTLA-4 expression. J Immunol 2003; 171(11):5673–7.

111. Rudd CE, Schneider H. Unifying concepts in CD28, ICOS and CTLA4 co-receptor signalling. Nature Rev Immunol 2003; 3(7):544–56.

112. Wood KJ, Ushigome H, Karim M et al. Regulatory cells in transplantation. Novartis Found Symp 2003; 252:177–88; discussion 188–93, 203–10.

113. Walunas TL, Lenschow DJ, Bakker CY et al. CTLA-4 can function as a negative regulator of T cell activation. Immunity 1994; 1:405–13.

114. Schneider H, Mandelbrot DA, Greenwald RJ et al. Cutting edge: CTLA-4 (CD152) differentially regulates mitogen-activated protein kinases (extracellular signal-regulated kinase and c-Jun N-terminal kinase) in CD4+ T cells from receptor/ligand-deficient mice. J Immunol 2002; 169(7):3475–9.

115. Salama AD, Chitnis T, Imitola J et al. Critical role of the programmed death-1 (PD-1) pathway in regulation of experimental autoimmune encephalomyelitis. J Exp Med 2003; 198(1):71–8.

116. Ansari MJ, Salama AD, Chitnis T et al. The programmed death-1 (PD-1) pathway regulates autoimmune diabetes in nonobese diabetic (NOD) mice. J Exp Med 2003; 198(1):63–9.

117. Khoury SJ, Sayegh MH. The roles of the new negative T cell costimulatory pathways in regulating autoimmunity. Immunity 2004; 20(5):529–38.

118. Harding FA, McArthur JG, Gross JA et al. CD-28 mediated signalling co-stimulates murine T cells and prevents the induction of anergy in T cell clones. Nature 1992; 356:607–9.

119. Acuto O, Michel F. CD28-mediated co-stimulation: a quantitative support for TCR signalling. Nature Rev Immunol 2003; 3(12):939–51.

This is an excellent review of the role of CD28, which discusses the quantitative and qualitative effects of co-stimulation on the consequences of TcR engagement.

120. Linsley PS, Greene JL, Brady W et al. Human B7-1 (CD80) and B7-2 (CD86) bind with similar avidities but distinct kinetics to CD28 and CTLA-4 receptors. Immunity 1994; 1(9):793–801.

121. van der Merwe PA, Bodian DL, Daenke S et al. CD80 (B7-1) binds both CD28 and CTLA-4 with a low affinity and very fast kinetics. J Exp Med 1997; 185(3):393–403.

122. Thompson CB, Lindsten T, Ledbetter JA et al. CD28 activation pathway regulates the production of multiple T cell derived lymphokines/cytokines. Proc Natl Acad Sci USA 1989; 86:1333.

123. Pearson TC, Alexander DZ, Winn KJ et al. Transplantation tolerance induced by CTLA4-Ig. Transplantation 1994; 57(12):1701–6.

124. Turka LA, Linsley PS, Lin H et al. T-cell activation by the CD28 ligand B7 is required for cardiac allograft rejection in vivo. Proc Natl Acad Sci USA 1992; 89(22):11102–5.

125. Kawai K, Shahinian A, Mak TW et al. Skin allograft rejection in CD28-deficient mice. Transplantation 1996; 61(3):352–5.

126. Grohmann U, Fallarino F, Puccetti P. Tolerance, DCs and tryptophan: much ado about IDO. Trends Immunol 2003; 24(5):242–8.

127. Fallarino F, Grohmann U, Hwang KW et al. Modulation of tryptophan catabolism by regulatory T cells. Nature Immunol 2003; 4(12):1206–12.

128. Grohmann U, Orabona C, Fallarino F et al. CTLA-4-Ig regulates tryptophan catabolism in vivo. Nature Immunol 2002; 3(11):1097–101.

129. Kirk AD, Harlan DM, Armstrong NN et al. CTLA4-Ig and anti-CD40 ligand prevent renal allograft rejection in primates. Proc Natl Acad Sci USA 1997; 94:8789–94.

130. Kundig TM, Shahinian A, Kawai K et al. Duration of TCR stimulation determines costimulatory requirement of T cells. Immunity 1996; 5(1):41–52.

131. Zimmermann C, Seiler P, Lane P et al. Antiviral immune responses in CTLA4 transgenic mice. J Virol 1997; 71(3):1802–7.

132. Gonzalo JA, Tian J, Delaney T et al. ICOS is critical for T helper cell-mediated lung mucosal inflammatory responses. Nature Immunol 2001; 2(7):597–604.

133. Larsen CP, Alexander DZ, Hollenbaugh D et al. CD40-gp39 interactions play a critical role during allograft rejection: Suppression of allograft rejection by blockade of the CD40-gp39 pathway. Transplantation 1996; 61(1):4–9.

134. Larsen CP, Elwood ET, Alexander DZ et al. Long-term acceptance of skin and cardiac allografts after blocking CD40 and CD28 pathways. Nature 1996; 381:434–8.

135. Kirk AD, Burkly LC, Batty DS et al. Treatment with humanized monoclonal antibody against CD154

prevents acute renal allograft rejection in nonhuman primates. Nature Med 1999; 5(6):686–93.

136. Huppa JB, Davis MM. T-cell-antigen recognition and the immunological synapse. Nature Rev Immunol 2003; 3(12):973–83.

137. Monks CR, Freiberg BA, Kupfer H et al. Three-dimensional segregation of supramolecular activation clusters in T cells. Nature 1998; 395(6697):82–6.

138. Miller MJ, Wei SH, Cahalan MD et al. Autonomous T cell trafficking examined in vivo with intravital two-photon microscopy. Proc Natl Acad Sci USA 2003; 100(5):2604–9.

139. Miller MJ, Hejazi AS, Wei SH et al. T cell repertoire scanning is promoted by dynamic dendritic cell behavior and random T cell motility in the lymph node. Proc Natl Acad Sci USA 2004; 101(4): 998–1003.

140. Blanchard N, Di Bartolo V, Hivroz C. In the immune synapse, ZAP-70 controls T cell polarization and recruitment of signaling proteins but not formation of the synaptic pattern. Immunity 2002; 17(4):389–99.

141. Paz PE, Wang S, Clarke H et al. Mapping the Zap-70 phosphorylation sites on LAT (linker for activation of T cells) required for recruitment and activation of signalling proteins in T cells. Biochem J 2001; 356(2):461–71.

142. Viola A, Schroeder S, Sakakibara Y et al. T lymphocyte costimulation mediated by reorganization of membrane microdomains. Science 1999; 283(5402): 680–2.

143. Tanimura N, Nagafuku M, Minaki Y et al. Dynamic changes in the mobility of LAT in aggregated lipid rafts upon T cell activation. J Cell Biol 2003; 160(1):125–35.

144. Gummert JF, Ikonen T, Morris RE. Newer immunosuppressive drugs: a review. J Am Soc Nephrol 1999; 10(6):1366–80.

145. Sprent J, Schaeffer M, Lo D et al. Properties of purified T cell subsets II. In vivo class I vs class II H-2 differences. J Exp Med 1986; 163:998–1011.

146. Rosenberg AS. The T cell populations mediating rejection of MHC class I disparate skin grafts in mice. Transplant Immunol 1993; 2:93–9.

147. Graca L, Cobbold SP, Waldmann H. Identification of regulatory T cells in tolerated allografts. J Exp Med 2002; 195(12):1641–6.

This paper demonstrates the presence of regulatory cells within tolerated skin grafts and that such cells are relatively enriched in the graft. The importance of such cells localised to the graft and their role in immune regulation is likely to be the subject of further investigation.

148. Graca L, Le Moine A, Cobbold SP et al. Antibody-induced transplantation tolerance: the role of dominant regulation. Immunol Res 2003; 28(3): 181–91.

149. Sayegh MH, Akalin E, Hancock WW et al. CD28-B7 blockade after alloantigenic challenge in vivo inhibits Th1 cytokines but spares Th2. J Exp Med 1995; 181(5):1869–74.

150. Strom TB, Roy-Chaudhury P, Manfro R et al. The Th1/Th2 paradigm and the allograft response. Curr Opin Immunol 1996; 8(5):688–93.

151. VanBuskirk AM, Wakely ME, Orosz CG. Transfusion of polarized TH2-like cell populations into SCID mouse cardiac allograft recipients results in acute allograft rejection. Transplantation 1996; 62(2):229–38.

152. Orosz CG, Wakely E, Sedmak DD et al. Prolonged murine cardiac allograft acceptance: characteristics of persistent active alloimmunity after treatment with gallium nitrate versus anti-CD4 monoclonal antibody. Transplantation 1997; 63(8):1109–17.

153. Sirak JH, Orosz CG, Roopenian DC et al. Cardiac allograft tolerance: failure to develop in interleukin-4-deficient mice correlates with unusual allo-sensitization patterns. Transplantation 1998; 65(10):1352–6.

154. Bickerstaff AA, VanBuskirk AM, Wakely E et al. Transforming growth factor-beta and interleukin-10 subvert alloreactive delayed type hypersensitivity in cardiac allograft acceptor mice. Transplantation 2000; 69(7):1517–20.

155. Shirwan H. Chronic allograft rejection. Do the Th2 cells preferentially induced by indirect alloantigen recognition play a dominant role? Transplantation 1999; 68(6):715–26.

156. Swain SL, Weinberg AD, English M et al. IL-4 directs the development of Th2-like helper effectors. J Immunol 1990; 145(11):3796–806.

157. Xu D, Trajkovic V, Hunter D et al. IL-18 induces the differentiation of Th1 or Th2 cells depending upon cytokine milieu and genetic background. Eur J Immunol 2000; 30(11):3147–56.

158. Hsieh CS, Macatonia SE, Tripp CS et al. Development of TH1 CD4+ T cells through IL-12 produced by Listeria-induced macrophages. Science 1993; 260(5107):547–9.

159. Kuchroo VK, Das MP, Brown JA et al. B7-1 and B7-2 costimulatory molecules activate differentially the Th1/Th2 developmental pathways: application to autoimmune disease therapy. Cell 1995; 80(5):707–18.

160. Lenschow DJ, Herold KC, Rhee L et al. CD28/B7 regulation of Th1 and Th2 subsets in the development of autoimmune diabetes. Immunity 1996; 5(3):285–93.

161. Martin E, O'Sullivan B, Low P et al. Antigen-specific suppression of a primed immune response by dendritic cells mediated by regulatory T cells secreting interleukin-10. Immunity 2003; 18(1): 155–67.

162. Witsch EJ, Peiser M, Hutloff A et al. ICOS and CD28 reversely regulate IL-10 on re-activation of human effector T cells with mature dendritic cells. Eur J Immunol 2002; 32(9):2680–6.

163. Kagi D, Seiler P, Pavlovic J et al. The roles of perforin- and Fas-dependent cytotoxicity in protection against cytopathic and noncytopathic viruses. Eur J Immunol 1995; 25(12):3256–62.

164. Ehrhardt C, Kneuer C, Bakowsky U. Selectins – an emerging target for drug delivery. Adv Drug Deliv Rev 2004; 56(4):527–49.

165. Butcher EC, Picker LJ. Lymphocyte homing and homeostasis. Science 1996; 272(5258):60–6.

166. Koo DD, Welsh KI, McLaren AJ et al. Cadaver versus living donor kidneys: impact of donor factors on antigen induction before transplantation. Kidney Int 1999; 56(4):1551–9.

167. Schwarz C, Regele H, Steininger R et al. The contribution of adhesion molecule expression in donor kidney biopsies to early allograft dysfunction. Transplantation 2001; 71(11):1666–70.

168. Valujskikh A, Lakkis FG. In remembrance of things past: memory T cells and transplant rejection. Immunol Rev 2003; 196:65–74.

169. Pinschewer DD, Ochsenbein AF, Odermatt B et al. FTY720 immunosuppression impairs effector T cell peripheral homing without affecting induction, expansion, and memory. J Immunol 2000; 164(11): 5761–70.

170. Troncoso P, Ortiz M, Martinez L et al. FTY 720 prevents ischemic reperfusion damage in rat kidneys. Transplant Proc 2001; 33(1-2):857–9.

171. Kobayashi H, Koga S, Novick AC et al. T-cell mediated induction of allogeneic endothelial cell chemokine expression. Transplantation 2003; 75(4):529–36.

172. Grandaliano G, Gesualdo L, Ranieri E et al. Monocyte chemotactic peptide-1 expression and monocyte infiltration in acute renal transplant rejection. Transplantation 1997; 63(3):414–20.

173. Fairchild RL, VanBuskirk AM, Kondo T et al. Expression of chemokine genes during rejection and long-term acceptance of cardiac allografts. Transplantation 1997; 63(12):1807–12.

174. Yoshidome H, Kato A, Miyazaki M et al. IL-13 activates STAT6 and inhibits liver injury induced by ischemia/reperfusion. Am J Pathol 1999; 155(4): 1059–64.

175. Lentsch AB, Yoshidome H, Kato A et al. Requirement for interleukin-12 in the pathogenesis of warm hepatic ischemia/reperfusion injury in mice. Hepatology 1999; 30(6):1448–53.

176. Lentsch AB, Yoshidome H, Cheadle WG et al. Chemokine involvement in hepatic ischemia/reperfusion injury in mice: roles for macrophage inflammatory protein-2 and KC. Hepatology 1998; 27(4):1172–7.

177. Koga S, Kapoor A, Novick AC et al. RANTES is produced by CD8+ T cells during acute rejection of skin grafts. Transplant Proc 2000; 32(4):796–7.

178. Hancock WW. Chemokine receptor-dependent alloresponses. Immunol Rev 2003; 196:37–50.

179. Lee I, Wang L, Wells AD et al. Blocking the monocyte chemoattractant protein-1/CCR2 chemokine pathway induces permanent survival of islet allografts through a programmed death-1 ligand-1-dependent mechanism. J Immunol 2003; 171(12): 6929–35.

180. Mintz B, Silvers WK. Histocompatibility antigens on melanoblasts and hair follicle cells. Cell-localized homograft rejection in allophenic skin grafts. Transplantation 1970; 9(5):497–505.

181. Mintz B, Silvers WK. 'Intrinsic' immunological tolerance in allophenic mice. Science 1967; 158(807):1484–6.

182. Sutton R, Gray DW, McShane P et al. The specificity of rejection and the absence of susceptibility of pancreatic islet beta cells to nonspecific immune destruction in mixed strain islets grafted beneath the renal capsule in the rat. J Exp Med 1989; 170(3):751–62.

183. Rosenberg AS, Singer A. Cellular basis of skin allograft rejection: an in vivo model of immune-mediated tissue destruction. Annu Rev Immunol 1992; 10:333–58.

184. Snider ME, Steinmuller D. Nonspecific tissue destruction as a consequence of cytotoxic T lymphocyte interaction with antigen-specific target cells. Transplant Proc 1987; 19(1 pt 1):421–3.

185. Tilney NL, Strom TB, Macpherson SG et al. Surface properties and functional characteristics of infiltrating cells harvested from acutely rejecting cardiac allografts in inbred rats. Transplantation 1975; 20(4):323–30.

186. Williams GM, Hume DM, Hudson RP Jr et al. 'Hyperacute' renal-homograft rejection in man. N Engl J Med 1968; 279(12):611–18.

187. Patel R, Terasaki PI. Significance of the positive crossmatch test in kidney transplantation. N Engl J Med 1969; 280(14):735–9.

188. Meier-Kriesche HU, Kaplan B. Waiting time on dialysis as the strongest modifiable risk factor for renal transplant outcomes: a paired donor kidney analysis. Transplantation 2002; 74(10):1377–81.

189. Glotz D, Antoine C, Julia P et al. Intravenous immunoglobulins and transplantation for patients with anti-HLA antibodies. Transplant Int 2004; 17(1):1–8.

190. Glotz D, Antoine C, Julia P et al. Desensitization and subsequent kidney transplantation of patients

using intravenous immunoglobulins (IVIg). Am J Transplant 2002; 2(8):758–60.

191. Zachary AA, Montgomery RA, Ratner LE et al. Specific and durable elimination of antibody to donor HLA antigens in renal-transplant patients. Transplantation 2003; 76(10):1519–25.

192. Warren DS, Zachary AA, Sonnenday CJ et al. Successful renal transplantation across simultaneous ABO incompatible and positive crossmatch barriers. Am J Transplant 2004; 4(4):561–8.

193. Crespo M, Pascual M, Tolkoff-Rubin N et al. Acute humoral rejection in renal allograft recipients: I. Incidence, serology and clinical characteristics. Transplantation 2001; 71(5):652–8.

194. Mauiyyedi S, Crespo M, Collins AB et al. Acute humoral rejection in kidney transplantation: II. Morphology, immunopathology, and pathologic classification. J Am Soc Nephrol 2002; 13(3):779–87.

195. Bohmig GA, Regele H, Exner M et al. C4d-positive acute humoral renal allograft rejection: effective treatment by immunoadsorption. J Am Soc Nephrol 2001; 12(11):2482–9.

196. Halloran PF, Wadgymar A, Ritchie S The significance of the anti-class I antibody response. I. Clinical and pathologic features of anti-class I-mediated rejection. Transplantation 1990; 49(1):85–91.

197. Worthington JE, Martin S, Al-Husseini DM et al. Posttransplantation production of donor HLA-specific antibodies as a predictor of renal transplant outcome. Transplantation 2003; 75(7):1034–40.

198. Salama AD, Delikouras A, Pusey CD et al. Transplant accommodation in highly sensitized patients: a potential role for Bcl-xL and allo-antibody. Am J Transplant 2001; 1(3):260–9.

199. Delikouras A, Fairbanks LD, Simmonds AH et al. Endothelial cell cytoprotection induced in vitro by allo- or xenoreactive antibodies is mediated by signaling through adenosine A2 receptors. Eur J Immunol 2003; 33(11):3127–35.

200. Delikouras A, Dorling A. Transplant accommodation. Am J Transplant 2003; 3(8):917–18.

201. Russell PS, Chase CM, Winn HJ et al. Coronary atherosclerosis in transplanted mouse hearts. II. Importance of humoral immunity. J Immunol 1994; 152(10):5135–41.

202. Mauiyyedi S, Pelle PD, Saidman S et al. Chronic humoral rejection: identification of antibody-mediated chronic renal allograft rejection by C4d deposits in peritubular capillaries. J Am Soc Nephrol 2001; 12(3):574–82.

203. Galili U, Rachmilewitz EA, Peleg A et al. A unique natural human IgG antibody with anti-alpha-galactosyl specificity. J Exp Med 1984; 160(5):1519–31.

204. Auchincloss H Jr, Sachs DH. Xenogeneic transplantation. Annu Rev Immunol 1998; 16:433–70.

205. Cooper DK. Clinical xenotransplantion – how close are we? Lancet 2003; 362(9383):557–9.

206. Piedrahita JA, Mir B. Cloning and transgenesis in mammals: Implications for xenotransplantation. Am J Transplant 2004; 4(suppl. 6):43–50.

207. Colucci F, Caligiuri MA, Di Santo JP. What does it take to make a natural killer? Nature Rev Immunol 2003; 3(5):413–25.

208. Ljunggren HG, Karre K. In search of the 'missing self': MHC molecules and NK cell recognition. Immunol Today 1990; 11(7):237–44.

209. Suzue K, Reinherz EL, Koyasu S. Critical role of NK but not NKT cells in acute rejection of parental bone marrow cells in F1 hybrid mice. Eur J Immunol 2001; 31(11):3147–52.

210. Stern P, Gidlund M, Orn A et al. Natural killer cells mediate lysis of embryonal carcinoma cells lacking MHC. Nature 1980; 285(5763):341–2.

211. Bradley JA, Mason DW, Morris PJ. Evidence that rat renal allografts are rejected by cytotoxic T cells and not by nonspecific effectors. Transplantation 1985; 39(2):169–75.

212. Vampa ML, Norman PJ, Burnapp L et al. Natural killer-cell activity after human renal transplantation in relation to killer immunoglobulin-like receptors and human leukocyte antigen mismatch. Transplantation 2003; 76(8):1220–8.

213. Murphy WJ, Kumar V, Bennett M. Acute rejection of murine bone marrow allografts by natural killer cells and T cells. Differences in kinetics and target antigens recognized. J Exp Med 1987; 166(5):1499–509.

214. Ruggeri L, Capanni M, Casucci M et al. Role of natural killer cell alloreactivity in HLA-mismatched hematopoietic stem cell transplantation. Blood 1999; 94(1):333–9.

215. Ruggeri L, Capanni M, Urbani E et al. Effectiveness of donor natural killer cell alloreactivity in mismatched hematopoietic transplants. Science 2002; 295(5562):2097–100.

216. Hayry P, Defendi V. Mixed lymphocyte cultures produce effector cells: model in vitro for allograft rejection. Science 1970; 168(927):133–5.

217. Hodes RJ, Svedmyr EA. Specific cytotoxicity of H-2-incompatible mouse lymphocytes following mixed culture in vitro. Transplantation 1970; 9(5):470–7.

218. Mason DW, Morris PJ. Inhibition of the accumulation, in rat kidney allografts, of specific – but not nonspecific – cytotoxic cells by cyclosporine. Transplantation 1984; 37(1):46–51.

219. Engers HD, Sorenson GD, Terres G et al. Functional activity in vivo of effector T cell populations. I. Antitumor activity exhibited by allogeneic mixed

leukocyte culture cells. J Immunol 1982; 129(3): 1292–8.

220. Tyler JD, Galli SJ, Snider ME et al. Cloned LYT-2+ cytolytic T lymphocytes destroy allogeneic tissue in vivo. J Exp Med 1984; 159(1):234–43.

221. Tilney NL, Kupiec-Weglinski JW, Heidecke CD et al. Mechanisms of rejection and prolongation of vascularized organ allografts. Immunol Rev 1984; 77:185–216.

222. Lowry RP, Gurley KE, Forbes RD. Immune mechanisms in organ allograft rejection. I. Delayed-type hypersensitivity and lymphocytotoxicity in heart graft rejection. Transplantation 1983; 36(4): 391–401.

223. Cobbold SP, Jayasuriya A, Nash A et al. Therapy with monoclonal antibodies by elimination of T-cell subsets in vivo. Nature 1984; 312(5994):548–51.

224. Madsen JC, Peugh WN, Wood KJ et al. The effect of anti-L3T4 monoclonal antibody treatment on first-set rejection of murine cardiac allografts. Transplantation 1987; 44(6):849–52.

225. Madsen JC, Superina RA, Wood KJ et al. Immunological unresponsiveness induced by recipient cells transfected with donor MHC genes. Nature 1988; 332:161.

226. Hurme M, Hetherington CM, Chandler PR et al. Cytotoxic T-cell responses to H-Y: mapping of the Ir genes. J Exp Med 1978; 147(3):758–67.

227. Hurme M, Chandler PR, Hetherington CM et al. Cytotoxic T-cell responses to H-Y: correlation with the rejection of syngeneic male skin grafts. J Exp Med 1978; 147(3):768–75.

228. Simpson E, Mobraaten L, Chandler P et al. Cross-reactive cytotoxic responses. H-2 restricted are more specific than anti-H-2 responses. J Exp Med 1978; 148(6):1478–87.

229. Armstrong HE, Bolton EM, McMillan I et al. Prolonged survival of actively enhanced rat renal allografts despite accelerated cellular infiltration and rapid induction of both class I and class II MHC antigens. J Exp Med 1987; 165(3):891–907.

230. Dallman MJ, Wood KJ, Morris PJ. Specific cytotoxic T cells are found in the nonrejected kidneys of blood-transfused rats. J Exp Med 1987; 165(2): 566–71.

231. Walsh CM, Hayashi F, Saffran DC et al. Cell-mediated cytotoxicity results from, but may not be critical for, primary allograft rejection. J Immunol 1996; 156(4):1436–41.

232. Selvaggi G, Ricordi C, Podack ER et al. The role of the perforin and Fas pathways of cytotoxicity in skin graft rejection. Transplantation 1996; 62(12): 1912–15.

233. Schulz M, Schuurman HJ, Joergensen J et al. Acute rejection of vascular heart allografts by perforin-deficient mice. Eur J Immunol 1995; 25(2):474–80.

234. Liew FY, Simpson E. Delayed-type hypersensitivity responses to H-Y: characterization and mapping of Ir genes. Immunogenetics 1980; 11(3):255–66.

235. Chen J, Myllarniemi M, Akyurek LM et al. Identification of differentially expressed genes in rat aortic allograft vasculopathy. Am J Pathol 1996; 149(2):597–611.

236. Paul LC, Saito K, Davidoff A et al. Growth factor transcripts in rat renal transplants. Am J Kidney Dis 1996; 28(3):441–50.

237. Kormendi F, Amend WJ Jr. The importance of eosinophil cells in kidney allograft rejection. Transplantation 1988; 45(3):537–9.

238. Nolan CR, Saenz KP, Thomas CA 3rd et al. Role of the eosinophil in chronic vascular rejection of renal allografts. Am J Kidney Dis 1995; 26(4):634–42.

239. Chan SY, DeBruyne LA, Goodman RE et al. In vivo depletion of CD8+ T cells results in Th2 cytokine production and alternate mechanisms of allograft rejection. Transplantation 1995; 59(8):1155–61.

240. Le Moine A, Surquin M, Demoor FX et al. IL-5 mediates eosinophilic rejection of MHC class II-disparate skin allografts in mice. J Immunol 1999; 163(7):3778–84.

241. Le Moine A, Flamand V, Demoor FX et al. Critical roles for IL-4, IL-5, and eosinophils in chronic skin allograft rejection. J Clin Invest 1999; 103(12): 1659–67.

242. Khanna AK, Cairns VR, Becker CG et al. TGF-beta: a link between immunosuppression, nephrotoxicity, and CsA. Transplant Proc 1998; 30(4):944–5.

243. Khanna A, Cairns V, Hosenpud JD. Tacrolimus induces increased expression of transforming growth factor-beta1 in mammalian lymphoid as well as nonlymphoid cells. Transplantation 1999; 67(4):614–19.

244. Khanna AK, Hosenpud JS, Plummer MS et al. Analysis of transforming growth factor-beta and profibrogenic molecules in a rat cardiac allograft model treated with cyclosporine. Transplantation 2002; 73(10):1543–9.

245. Streilein JW, Takeuchi M, Taylor AW. Immune privilege, T-cell tolerance, and tissue-restricted autoimmunity. Hum Immunol 1997; 52(2):138–43.

246. Streilein JW. Immune privilege as the result of local tissue barriers and immunosuppressive microenvironments. Curr Opin Immunol 1993; 5(3): 428–32.

247. Calne RY, Sells RA, Pena JR et al. Induction of immunological tolerance by porcine liver allografts. Nature 1969; 223(205):472–6.

248. Kamada N, Brons G, Davies HS. Fully allogeneic liver grafting in rats induces a state of systemic

nonreactivity to donor transplantation antigens. Transplantation 1980; 29(5):429–31.

249. Kamada N, Davies HS, Roser B. Reversal of transplantation immunity by liver grafting. Nature 1981; 292(5826):840–2.

250. Doyle HR, Marino IR, Morelli F et al. Assessing risk in liver transplantation. Special reference to the significance of a positive cytotoxic crossmatch. Ann Surg 1996; 224(2):168–77.

251. Kamada N, Wight DG. Antigen-specific immunosuppression induced by liver transplantation in the rat. Transplantation 1984; 38(3):217–21.

252. Farges O, Morris PJ, Dallman MJ. Spontaneous acceptance of liver allografts in the rat. Analysis of the immune response. Transplantation 1994; 57(2):171–7.

253. Farges O, Morris PJ, Dallman MJ. Spontaneous acceptance of rat liver allografts is associated with an early downregulation of intragraft interleukin-4 messenger RNA expression. Hepatology 1995; 21(3):767–75.

254. Niederkorn JY. The immune privilege of corneal grafts. J Leukoc Biol 2003; 74(2):167–71.

255. Niederkorn JY. Immune privilege in the anterior chamber of the eye. Crit Rev Immunol 2002; 22(1):13–46.

256. Lau HT, Yu M, Fontana A et al. Prevention of islet allograft rejection with engineered myoblasts expressing FasL in mice. Science 1996; 273(5271): 109–12.

257. Lau HT, Stoeckert CJ. FasL – too much of a good thing? Transplanted grafts of pancreatic islet cells engineered to express Fas ligand are destroyed not protected by the immune system. Nature Med 1997; 3(7):727–8.

258. Green DR, Flood PM, Gershon RK. Immunoregulatory T-cell pathways. Annu Rev Immunol 1983; 1:439–63.

259. Seddon B, Mason D. Peripheral autoantigen induces regulatory T cells that prevent autoimmunity. J Exp Med 1999; 189(5):877–82.

260. Seddon B, Mason D. Regulatory T cells in the control of autoimmunity: the essential role of transforming growth factor beta and interleukin 4 in the prevention of autoimmune thyroiditis in rats by peripheral CD4(+)CD45RC– cells and CD4(+)CD8(–) thymocytes. J Exp Med 1999; 189(2):279–88.

261. Saoudi A, Seddon B, Fowell D et al. The thymus contains a high frequency of cells that prevent autoimmune diabetes on transfer into prediabetic recipients. J Exp Med 1996; 184(6):2393–8.

262. Asano M, Toda M, Sakaguchi N et al. Autoimmune disease as a consequence of developmental abnormality of a T cell subpopulation. J Exp Med 1996; 184(2):387–96.

This demonstrates that CD4+CD25+ T cells fail to appear in the periphery following day 3 neonatal thymectomy, and that the autoimmune disease associated with day 3 neonatal thymectomy can be prevented by the infusion of such cells. This and other observations from Sakaguchi and colleagues have provoked considerable interest in CD4+CD25+ regulatory T cells. The relevance of these cells to experimental models of transplantation tolerance depends on the precise protocol used as discussed in the text. The significance of these mechanisms to clinically relevant models of transplantation remains to be determined.

263. Sakaguchi S, Sakaguchi N, Asano M et al. Immunologic self-tolerance maintained by activated T cells expressing IL-2 receptor alpha-chains (CD25). Breakdown of a single mechanism of self-tolerance causes various autoimmune diseases. J Immunol 1995; 155(3):1151–64.

264. Asseman C, Mauze S, Leach MW et al. An essential role for interleukin 10 in the function of regulatory T cells that inhibit intestinal inflammation. J Exp Med 1999; 190(7):995–1004.

265. Qin S, Cobbold S, Pope H et al. 'Infectious' transplantation tolerance. Science 1993; 259:974.

266. Davies JD, Leong LY, Mellor A et al. T cell suppression in transplantation tolerance through linked recognition. J Immunol 1996; 156(10):3602–7.

267. Wise MP, Bemelman F, Cobbold SP et al. Linked suppression of skin graft rejection can operate through indirect recognition. J Immunol 1998; 161(11):5813–16.

268. Jonuleit H, Schmitt E, Kakirman H et al. Infectious tolerance: human CD25(+) regulatory T cells convey suppressor activity to conventional CD4(+) T helper cells. J Exp Med 2002; 196(2):255–60.

269. Yin D, Fathman CG. CD4-positive suppressor cells block allotransplant rejection. J Immunol 1995; 154(12):6339–45.

270. Stephens LA, Mason D. CD25 is a marker for CD4+ thymocytes that prevent autoimmune diabetes in rats, but peripheral T cells with this function are found in both CD25+ and CD25– subpopulations. J Immunol 2000; 165(6):3105–10.

271. Kohm AP, Carpentier PA, Anger HA et al. Cutting edge: CD4+CD25+ regulatory T cells suppress antigen-specific autoreactive immune responses and central nervous system inflammation during active experimental autoimmune encephalomyelitis. J Immunol 2002; 169(9):4712–16.

272. Kohm AP, Carpentier PA, Miller SD. Regulation of experimental autoimmune encephalomyelitis (EAE) by CD4+CD25+ regulatory T cells. Novartis Found Symp 2003; 252:45–52; discussion 52–4, 106–14.

273. Mottet C, Uhlig HH, Powrie F. Cutting edge: cure of colitis by CD4+CD25+ regulatory T cells. J Immunol 2003; 170(8):3939–43.

274. Karim M, Kingsley CI, Bushell AR et al. Alloantigen-induced CD25+CD4+ regulatory T cells can develop in vivo from CD25−CD4+ precursors in a thymus-independent process. J Immunol 2004; 172(2):923–8.

275. Kingsley CI, Karim M, Bushell AR et al. CD25+CD4+ regulatory T cells prevent graft rejection: CTLA-4- and IL-10-dependent immunoregulation of allo-responses. J Immunol 2002; 168(3):1080–6.

276. Cobbold SP, Nolan KF, Graca L et al. Regulatory T cells and dendritic cells in transplantation tolerance: molecular markers and mechanisms. Immunol Rev 2003; 196:109–24.

277. Bushell A, Karim M, Kingsley CI et al. Pretransplant blood transfusion without additional immuno-therapy generates CD25+CD4+ regulatory T cells: a potential explanation for the blood-transfusion effect. Transplantation 2003; 76(3):449–55.

278. Lin CY, Graca L, Cobbold SP et al. Dominant transplantation tolerance impairs CD8+ T cell function but not expansion. Nature Immunol 2002; 3(12):1208–13.

279. Sundstedt A, O'Neill EJ, Nicolson KS et al. Role for IL-10 in suppression mediated by peptide-induced regulatory T cells in vivo. J Immunol 2003; 170(3):1240–8.

280. Dieckmann D, Bruett CH, Ploettner H et al. Human CD4(+)CD25(+) regulatory, contact-dependent T cells induce interleukin 10-producing, contact-independent type 1-like regulatory T cells [corrected]. J Exp Med 2002; 196(2):247–53.

281. Levings MK, Sangregorio R, Sartirana C et al. Human CD25+CD4+ T suppressor cell clones produce transforming growth factor beta, but not interleukin 10, and are distinct from type 1 T regulatory cells. J Exp Med 2002; 196(10):1335–46.

282. Piccirillo CA, Letterio JJ, Thornton AM et al. CD4(+)CD25(+) regulatory T cells can mediate suppressor function in the absence of transforming growth factor beta1 production and responsiveness. J Exp Med 2002; 196(2):237–46.

283. Roncarolo MG, Gregori S, Levings M. Type 1 T regulatory cells and their relationship with CD4+CD25+ T regulatory cells. Novartis Found Symp 2003; 252:115–27; discussion 127–31, 203–10.

284. Lombardi G, Sidhu S, Batchelor R et al. Anergic T cells as suppressor cells in vitro. Science 1994; 264(5165):1587–9.

285. Frasca L, Scotta C, Lombardi G et al. Human anergic CD4+ T cells can act as suppressor cells by affecting autologous dendritic cell conditioning and survival. J Immunol 2002; 168(3):1060–8.

286. Mirenda V, Berton I, Read J et al. Modified dendritic cells coexpressing self and allogeneic major histocompatibility complex molecules: an efficient way to induce indirect pathway regulation. J Am Soc Nephrol 2004; 15(4):987–97.

287. Lagaaij EL, Ruigrok MB, van Rood JJ et al. Blood transfusion induced changes in cell-mediated lympholysis: to immunize or not to immunize. J Immunol 1991; 147(10):3348–52.

288. Roelen DL, van Bree S, van Hulst P et al. Regulatory functions of human CD4(+) T cells recognizing allopeptides in the context of self-HLA class II. Hum Immunol 2002; 63(10):902–11.

289. Meier-Kriesche HU, Cibrik DM, Ojo AO et al. Interaction between donor and recipient age in determining the risk of chronic renal allograft failure. J Am Geriatr Soc 2002; 50(1):14–17.

290. McLaren AJ, Jassem W, Gray DW et al. Delayed graft function: risk factors and the relative effects of early function and acute rejection on long-term survival in cadaveric renal transplantation. Clin Transplant 1999; 13(3):266–72.

291. Meier-Kriesche HU, Kaplan B. Cyclosporine microemulsion and tacrolimus are associated with decreased chronic allograft failure and improved long-term graft survival as compared with sandimmune. Am J Transplant 2002; 2(1):100–4.

292. Hornick PI, Mason PD, Baker RJ et al. Significant frequencies of T cells with indirect anti-donor specificity in heart graft recipients with chronic rejection. Circulation 2000; 101(20):2405–10.

293. Martin L, Guignier F, Mousson C et al. Detection of donor-specific anti-HLA antibodies with flow cytometry in eluates and sera from renal transplant recipients with chronic allograft nephropathy. Transplantation 2003; 76(2):395–400.

294. Magro CM, Klinger DM, Adams PW et al. Evidence that humoral allograft rejection in lung transplant patients is not histocompatibility antigen-related. Am J Transplant 2003; 3(10):1264–72.

295. Mandelbrot DA, Furukawa Y, McAdam AJ et al. Expression of B7 molecules in recipient, not donor, mice determines the survival of cardiac allografts. J Immunol 1999; 163(7):3753–7.

296. Ozkaynak E, Gao W, Shemmeri N et al. Importance of ICOS-B7RP-1 costimulation in acute and chronic allograft rejection. Nature Immunol 2001; 2(7):591–6.

297. Salama AD, Yuan X, Nayer A et al. Interaction between ICOS-B7RP1 and B7-CD28 costimulatory pathways in alloimmune responses in vivo. Am J Transplant 2003; 3(4):390–5.

298. Harada H, Salama AD, Sho M et al. The role of the ICOS-B7h T cell costimulatory pathway in transplantation immunity. J Clin Invest 2003; 112(2):234–43.

299. Saito T, Yamasaki S. Negative feedback of T cell activation through inhibitory adapters and costimulatory receptors. Immunol Rev 2003; 192:143–60.

300. Chikuma S, Imboden JB, Bluestone JA. Negative regulation of T cell receptor-lipid raft interaction by cytotoxic T lymphocyte-associated antigen 4. J Exp Med 2003; 197(1):129–35.

301. Ozkaynak E, Wang L, Goodearl A et al. Programmed death-1 targeting can promote allograft survival. J Immunol 2002; 169(11):6546–53.

302. Gao W, Demirci G, Strom TB et al. Stimulating PD-1-negative signals concurrent with blocking CD154 co-stimulation induces long-term islet allograft survival. Transplantation 2003; 76(6):994–9.

303. Yuan X, Dong VM, Coito AJ et al. A novel CD154 monoclonal antibody in acute and chronic rat vascularized cardiac allograft rejection. Transplantation 2002; 73(11):1736–42.

304. Wang J, Guo Z, Dong Y et al. Role of 4-1BB in allograft rejection mediated by CD8+ T cells. Am J Transplant 2003; 3(5):543–51.

305. Yuan X, Salama AD, Dong V et al. The role of the CD134-CD134 ligand costimulatory pathway in alloimmune responses in vivo. J Immunol 2003; 170(6):2949–55.

306. Demirci G, Amanullah F, Kewalaramani R et al. Critical role of OX40 in CD28 and CD154-independent rejection. J Immunol 2004; 172(3):1691–8.

307. Tian L, Guo W, Yuan Z et al. Association of the CD134/CD134L costimulatory pathway with acute rejection of small bowel allograft. Transplantation 2002; 74(1):133–8.

308. Raman VS, Akondy RS, Rath S et al. Ligation of CD27 on B cells in vivo during primary immunization enhances commitment to memory B cell responses. J Immunol 2003; 171(11):5876–81.

309. Hendriks J, Xiao Y, Borst J. CD27 promotes survival of activated T cells and complements CD28 in generation and establishment of the effector T cell pool. J Exp Med 2003; 198(9):1369–80.

310. Rowley TF, Al-Shamkhani A. Stimulation by soluble CD70 promotes strong primary and secondary CD8+ cytotoxic T cell responses in vivo. J Immunol 2004; 172(10):6039–46.

Four

Testing for histocompatibility

Philip A. Dyer, Alison Langton,
Helen Liggett, Karen Wood and
Judith Worthington

INTRODUCTION

The immune system has evolved to specifically recognise and destroy hazardous infective agents such as bacteria and viruses. These same mechanisms function to reject non-self alloimmune tissues, which are an irritant to surgical transplantation. Successful organ transplants occur between monozygotic twins (syngeneic transplants) or between genetically related or unrelated individuals (allogeneic transplants) – but only when the immune system is hindered by effective immunosuppression. The degree of immunosuppression needed, which reflects the frequency and strength of the alloimmune response, will be determined by the immunogenetic disparity between the donor and the recipient. The ability of a recipient to respond to allogeneic tissue will reflect their own immunogenetic constitution – their immune responsiveness. There are two major genetic systems determining human allogenicity, each of which conveys a biological veto or a biological impediment to effective clinical transplantation.

Veto:
- ABO blood group incompatibility.
- Recipient sensitised to donor HLA antigen evidenced by IgG antibody present at the time of transplantation.

Impediment:
- ABO blood group subtype mismatch when recipient has low-titre antibody, e.g. A2 donor to O, B or AB recipient.
- Recipient has been exposed to HLA antigens present in the donor.
- Donor possesses HLA antigen not present in the recipient.

If transplantation should proceed, in the biological veto situation, then usually there will be hyperacute rejection of the transplant.

In the situation of biological impediment, effective clinical transplantation can only be achieved through use of special protocols to remove circulating antibody and to prevent its recurrence or through use of established effective immunosuppression (see Chapter 5).

In this chapter we explain the immunology and genetics of the HLA system in the context of clinical organ transplantation. We will explain current techniques used to identify the extensive HLA polymorphism at the gene (allele) and protein (specificity) levels, and we will detail techniques used to establish recipient allosensitisation. The application of these techniques to attain effective clinical transplantation will be highlighted.

HLA GENETICS

The human leucocyte antigen (HLA) complex is located on the short arm of chromosome 6 at 6p21.3. This region is also known as the major histocompatibility complex (MHC). This collection of highly polymorphic genes codes for HLA molecules, which are cell surface proteins that play a pivotal role in antigen presentation and recognition and hence the survival of transplanted organs and tissues. For the purposes of this chapter the emphasis will be placed on elements of the HLA system that are characterised on a routine basis in the Histocompatibility and Immunogenetics laboratory.

There are two classes of HLA genes that are involved in the immune response to transplanted organs, class I and class II. These classes are structurally and functionally distinct. Class I molecules are involved in the processing and presentation of intracellular peptide to CD8+ T cells. Class II molecules process and present extracellular peptide to CD4+ T cells. This process is described in more detail in Chapter 3 on transplantation immunology.

Potential recipients and donors are tested for HLA class I (HLA-A, HLA-B and HLA-Cw) and HLA class II (HLA-DR, HLA-DQ and in some instances HLA-DP) to facilitate organ allocation (HLA matching), crossmatching and antibody screening. There are two means of determining the HLA type of an individual; by serological methods or DNA polymerase chain reaction (PCR)-based techniques.

HLA NOMENCLATURE

Nomenclature for both accepted and novel HLA alleles is regulated by the WHO Nomenclature Committee for factors of the HLA system.[1] HLA sequences are officially recorded on the IMGT/HLA Sequence Database (www.ebi.ac.uk/imgt), which is updated quarterly and is part of the international Immunogenetics Project (IMGT). HLA genes are highly polymorphic. In February 2005, this database contained sequences for 1179 class I alleles and 725 class II alleles.

Over time, major revisions of HLA nomenclature are necessary due to the ever-increasing numbers of alleles identified. A guide to the most recent

Table 4.1 • HLA nomenclature. Basic overview of the levels of HLA typing performed in the histocompatibility laboratory.

WHO nomenclature	Interpretation
HLA-B	Identification of HLA locus
HLA-B44	HLA antigen defined by serology based technique
HLA-B*44	Asterisk denotes HLA alleles defined by analysis of DNA
HLA-B*44 2-digit resolution	Denotes the allele family Corresponds where possible to the serological group Often termed 'low resolution' Level used for matching in solid organ transplants
HLA-B*4402 4-digit resolution	Allele sequence variation results in amino acid substitutions, coding variation, or non-synonymous changes Level of matching used in haemopoietic stem cell transplantation

nomenclature for HLA antigens and alleles is summarised in **Table 4.1**, where resolution of HLA alleles to the four-digit level is shown. In practice matching beyond this level, even in stem cell transplantation, is impractical. Resolution to eight digits can be carried out and in some instances an alphabetical suffix is used to describe the biological expression of an encoded molecule.

HLA TYPING

Serologically based techniques: complement-dependent cytotoxicity (CDC)

In a CDC test, antisera with specificity for HLA antigens are incubated with peripheral blood lymphocytes in the presence of complement. The antiserum used is usually monoclonal. If the target lymphocytes carry HLA antigen(s) to which the antiserum has specificity the test leads to killing of the target cells. In order to visualise the cell death a cocktail of fluorescent dyes is added to distinguish between live cells (negative test) and dead cells (positive test). CDC serological HLA typing identifies HLA protein polymorphisms as expressed at the cell surface.

Molecular techniques

Molecular techniques for HLA typing of DNA sequence polymorphisms have largely replaced serology since they offer flexibility of resolution, much improved reproducibility and greater accuracy.

The first DNA-based typing techniques identified HLA alleles by analysis of restriction fragment length polymorphisms (RFLPs). This technique relies on polymorphic restriction sites, which are cleaved by enzymes resulting in characteristic electrophoretic patterns from which the HLA type can be deduced. Prior to August 1998, RFLP typing was a requirement in UK law under the Human Organ Transplants Act 1989. Since then RFLP has been superseded by polymerase chain reaction (PCR)-based technologies. The invention of the PCR[2] revolutionised HLA typing techniques by facilitating identification of HLA polymorphisms at the single nucleotide polymorphism (SNP) level.

PRINCIPLE OF THE POLYMERASE CHAIN REACTION

Use of the PCR allows amplification of selected regions of interest within a length of target DNA. The technique involves heat separation of double-stranded DNA, primer annealing and extension resulting in exponential amplification of the template DNA. The essential agent is Taq polymerase, which is a thermostable enzyme that facilitates nucleotide extension from primer pairs, constructing a DNA copy of the template DNA strand. Primers are chemically synthesised oligonucleotides, usually 17–30 nucleotides in length. The primers are designed to flank the region of interest by binding to complementary sequences on the target DNA. Adenine (A) binds to thymine (T) and guanine (G) to cytosine (C) via hydrogen bonds. The PCR mixture contains the target DNA, the primers, the four deoxyribonucleotide triphosphate building blocks (adenine, guanine, cytosine and thymine), Taq polymerase enzyme and reaction buffer.

This process, illustrated in **Fig. 4.1**, is performed in a thermocycler, which creates rapid (millisecond) changes in temperature in a controlled environment.

- Double-stranded DNA is denatured by heating to 90–95°C.
- Cooling to 40–60°C allows the primers to anneal to their complementary sequences on the target DNA.
- Taq polymerase synthesises new strands from the primed sequences using target DNA as template.
- Denaturation, annealing and extension steps are repeated through many cycles and at each cycle new strands can act as templates for the next round of synthesis. This allows exponential increases in product.

PCR-SEQUENCE-SPECIFIC PRIMERS (PCR-SSP)

PCR-SSP is currently the HLA typing system of choice in most histocompatibility and immuno-genetics laboratories. HLA typing of cadaveric donors can be performed in 3 hours using this technique. There are various commercially available PCR-SSP kits in use, such as those manufactured by Dynal Biotech (www.tissue-typing.com), Protrans (www.mediprotrans.de) and Biotest (www.biotest.de). These kits are constantly updated by the manufacturer to incorporate new WHO-recognised alleles. Some laboratories construct in-house SSP trays using their own design primers; however, as more alleles are defined it has become almost impossible for individual laboratories to keep their own primer design up to date.

The underlying concept of PCR-SSP typing of HLA alleles is based on the fact that Taq polymerase lacks 3′ to 5′ exonuclease proofreading activity. Therefore only primers that are matched to the 3′ end of the template will facilitate DNA extension.

To perform HLA typing on one individual, multiple PCRs are performed simultaneously using different combinations of sequence-specific primers. The combinations utilised should allow amplification of all known HLA alleles.

The assignment of alleles is based on the presence or absence of amplified product. To ensure that the absence of a specific product is due to the individual lacking the corresponding sequence and is not simply due to a technical error a control is included

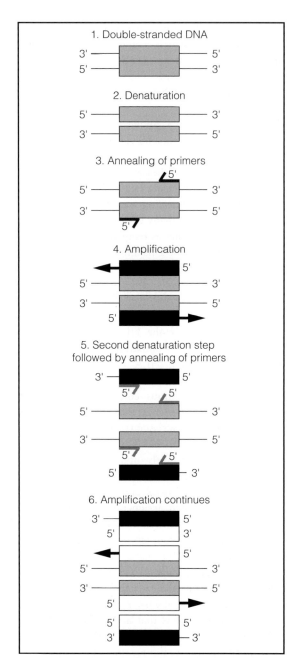

1. Double-stranded DNA

2. Denaturation

3. Annealing of primers

4. Amplification

5. Second denaturation step
followed by annealing of primers

6. Amplification continues

Figure 4.1 • Schematic overview of the polymerase chain reaction (PCR) incorporating denaturation of double-stranded DNA, primer annealing to target DNA sequence and amplification. These three major steps are repeated several times and result in an exponential increase in the target DNA.

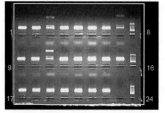

Figure 4.2 • Photograph of a PCR-sequence-specific primer (PCR-SSP) reaction. A control band (DNA) can be seen in each well and specific product bands are visible in wells 3, 8 and 11. By knowing the specific primers in each well the HLA type of an individual can be determined.

in each of the SSP reactions. The control is a gene (or region of a gene) that is constant between all individuals, such as human growth hormone. The PCR-SSP product is visualised by size differences using agarose gel electrophoresis as shown in **Fig. 4.2**. Electrophoresis through agarose relies on the movement of negatively charged DNA (due to the phosphate backbone) towards the anode. Fragments of DNA differentially migrate and thus can be identified according to their size. DNA is visualised on the gel by staining with ethidium bromide, which intercollates between the strands of DNA and fluoresces under ultraviolet light. In **Fig. 4.2**, control bands are visible in each of the SSP reactions and the specific product is visible as a second band in the well. By knowing which wells contain which SSP the HLA type of an individual can be allocated.

PCR-SEQUENCE-SPECIFIC OLIGONUCLEOTIDE PROBES (PCR-SSOP)

PCR-SSOP was the first PCR-based technique used for detecting HLA polymorphisms.[3,4] The technique has advantages over PCR-SSP, in particular a large sample throughput can be achieved; however, the methodology and interpretation of results is complex. PCR-SSOP is not suitable for cadaver donor HLA typing because it takes at least 24 hours to complete.

In PCR-SSOP, generic amplification of the target DNA is performed in a PCR. The amplified DNA is next bound to a solid support membrane. Sequence-specific oligonucleotides (SSO) are used to probe the amplified DNA by hybridisation to complementary regions on the amplified DNA (A to T and G to C). The probes are labelled with a radioactive biotinylated marker for detection. The resulting pattern is used to interpret the HLA type. There are modifications to the basic PCR-SSOP technique, such as reverse dot-blot and PCR oligo-capture assays, but these are not applicable in routine HLA typing.

SEQUENCE-BASED TYPING (SBT)

SBT allows a greater resolution of HLA typing than both PCR-SSP and PCR-SSOP techniques but it is rarely employed for solid organ transplantation as the criteria used for HLA matching usually do not require resolution to the HLA allele level. SBT is mainly used for haemopoietic stem cell transplantation (HSCT) where HLA typing to allele level is necessary due to the risk of graft vs. host disease.

Sequence-based typing involves identification of HLA genes at the nucleotide level, that is, allele level resolution. The technique utilises the elegant way in which DNA is copied by a DNA polymerase enzyme. Bases are incorporated into an extending DNA strand in a PCR through the formation of a phosphodiester bridge between the 3′ hydroxyl group at the growing end of a primer and the 5′ phosphate group of the nucleotide that is being incorporated.[5] In SBT, DNA polymerases incorporate analogues of A, G, T and C that do not have a 3′ hydroxyl group. This results in termination of the strand.[6] The analogues of A, G, T and C are labelled with a fluorescent dye. Detection of the dye then reveals which base is incorporated at each position. In this way the entire sequence can be determined. There are various SBT techniques available from manufacturers such as Applied Biosystems (www.appliedbiosystems.com) and Abbott Diagnostics (www.abbottdiagnostics.com) for HLA typing.

Clinical application of HLA typing

HLA typing and matching are essential prerequisites to renal and stem cell transplantation.

The level of HLA typing employed for solid organ transplantation is generally low to medium resolution (two digits). HLA matching is not employed for heart, liver or lung transplantation; instead other factors such as donor/recipient size compatibility and donor viral exposure status are considered important for allocation. The number of potential recipients for these organs is also less than for renal transplantation, and given the extensive polymorphism of HLA genes, allocation to minimise HLA mismatching is not always practicable. In the case of haemopoietic stem cell transplants (HSCT), medium to high resolution (four digits) HLA typing is performed. The level of matching is increased for HSCT due to the high risk of graft vs. host disease, whereby immunocompetent T cells transferred with the graft attack the recipient's own cells and tissues.

CAUSES OF HLA-SPECIFIC ALLOIMMUNISATION

HLA-specific antibodies can be produced in response to blood transfusions, pregnancy or transplantation.[7–9]

The method of antigen presentation and the dose of the antigen influence the nature of the immune response, which will differ for each of these stimuli.

BLOOD TRANSFUSION

The antigen source in a blood transfusion is the lymphocyte content of the transfused blood.[10] A number of studies have indicated that a low number of transfusions are a minimal risk for sensitisation whilst multiple transfusions are required to cause alloimmunisation.[11,12] These data suggest that one or a few – usually fewer than ten – blood transfusions induce minimal clonal expansion with limited proliferation of T and B cells. This is usually a transient IgM antibody, or IgM antibody followed by IgG antibody production, which is promptly downregulated. Multiple transfusions induce significant clonal expansion where antibody production is more likely and may result in a sustained level of IgG antibody production.[13]

PREGNANCY

HLA-specific antibodies can be produced during pregnancy as a result of stimulation by paternal HLA antigens expressed on the fetus. Stimulation occurs when high levels of antigen enter maternal circulation during the birth of the first child. Subsequent pregnancies may induce a secondary response. Multiparous female patients are at greater risk of sensitisation following blood transfusions, suggesting that a degree of clonal expansion has occurred during pregnancy so that antibodies are more easily induced by subsequent blood transfusions.[14]

PREVIOUS TRANSPLANTATION

An allograft recipient is exposed to those HLA antigens of the donor that were mismatched and consequently may develop antibodies to those antigens. However, transplant recipients are immunosuppressed and the immune response can be immature.

Available evidence suggests that the immune system of all allograft recipients undergoes clonal expansion.

This process develops further if the graft is lost or immunosuppressive therapy is discontinued resulting in detectable donor-specific HLA antibodies in the serum.

DETECTION OF ALLOANTIBODIES

Complement-dependent cytotoxicity

The long-established method used to screen patient sera for HLA-specific antibodies is the CDC assay outlined above. A patient's serum sample is incubated with a panel of lymphocytes of known HLA phenotype. If the test serum contains antibodies specific for HLA molecules on the target, cell death occurs. By using a selected panel of target cells of known HLA phenotype, it is possible to assign specificity to the antibody detected.[15] The CDC assay is also used for recipient/donor crossmatching, which was introduced as an essential pretransplant test in the mid-1960s.[16]

CDC enables the detection and definition of complement-fixing IgG and also IgM antibodies, which may be directed against HLA or non-HLA targets.

Despite its widespread use in antibody screening the CDC assay has a number of inherent problems, not least that non-complement-fixing antibodies, which have been shown to be relevant to graft outcome, cannot be detected.[17] A number of solid-phase laboratory techniques using flow cytometry and enzyme-linked immunosorbent assay (ELISA) are now available for the definition of recipient sensitisation.

Enzyme-linked immunosorbent assays (ELISA)

Several ELISA kits using plate-bound soluble HLA antigens as targets are now commercially available and have a number of advantages over CDC. They detect only HLA-specific antibodies and non-complement-fixing as well as complement-fixing antibodies; they can be semiautomated; and they remove the need for viable target cell panels. The basic principle of ELISA is illustrated in **Fig. 4.3**.

The Quikscreen kit (GTI Inc., www.gtidiagnostics. com) is a solid-phase ELISA-based technique that detects the presence or absence of IgG HLA class I-specific antibodies but does not allow definition of HLA specificities.[18,19] The antigen source is obtained from over 100 platelet donations, which are purified using column chromatography and immobilised directly onto microtitre trays. LATM (One Lambda Inc., www.onelambda.com) is also an ELISA-based screening test, used to detect the presence or absence of HLA class I- and class II-specific antibodies in a single assay. The antigen is purified from either selected Epstein–Barr virus (EBV) transformed cell lines or platelets and bound onto Terasaki trays.[20,21] This assay has the advantage of using only a small volume of serum (10 μl), and its ability to detect both class I- and class II-specific antibodies in the same test.

Quikscreen and LATM are both prescreen tests intended to detect the presence or absence of HLA-specific antibodies; neither is designed to define antibody specificity. ELISA kits are also commercially available for the definition of HLA-specific antibodies. Quik-ID (GTI Inc.) enables the definition of IgG class I HLA-specific antibodies. It uses microtitre trays precoated with a panel of HLA

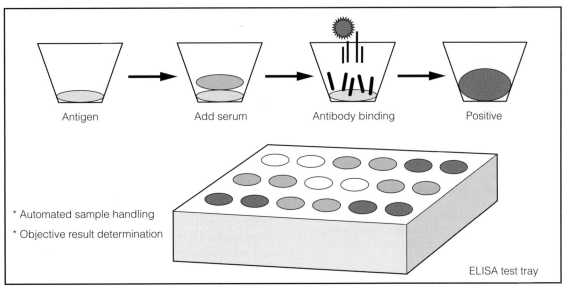

Antigen → Add serum → Antibody binding → Positive

* Automated sample handling

* Objective result determination

ELISA test tray

Figure 4.3 • Schematic representation of the enzyme-linked immunosorbent assay (ELISA). HLA-specific antigen is bound to each well of the ELISA plate. Following the addition of patient serum any HLA-specific antibodies present in the serum will bind to the corresponding target antigen. Binding of the antibody to antigen is detected by using a secondary antibody that causes a colour change in the well. A colour change denotes a positive reaction and hence the presence of HLA-specific antibody.

antigens from platelet donations. In the same manner as CDC the pattern of reactivity can be examined to determine antibody specificity. Class II ID (GTI Inc.) is also designed to define specificity but the antigen source is EBV-transformed cell lines and it detects class II antibodies. The Lambda Antigen Trays (One Lambda Inc.) also feature purified HLA class I and class II antigens attached to a Terasaki-format tray, and are designed for the definition of HLA-specific IgG antibodies.

Flow cytometry assays

Techniques that use a flow cytometer to detect antibody binding have been developed for the identification of IgG antibody binding to lymphocytes.[22] A flow cytometer is a machine in which particles, such as target cells, pass in a fluid phase through a narrow channel at which a laser beam is focused. The particle size and fluorescence are detected by photomultipliers feeding data to a computer. Software is used to interpret the captured data, which is displayed for interpretation.

In detecting antibody binding two pools of equal numbers of ten EBV-transformed lymphoblastoid cell lines are used as targets. Patient sera are screened

against both pools and antibody binding is detected using a fluorescent conjugated antihuman IgG antibody. This technique is not complement dependent and therefore detects antibody subclasses IgG2 and IgG4, which activate complement poorly or not at all. However, a recognised disadvantage of using cell targets is that non-HLA antibodies will also be detected, so further screening products have been developed more recently.

FlowPRA beads ('Flow Panel Reactive Antigen'; One Lambda Inc.) are microparticles coated with purified HLA class I or class II antigen.[23] After incubation of the beads with serum and staining with fluorescence-labelled antihuman IgG antibody, positive sera are detected in the flow cytometer.

A schematic representation of a single FlowPRA bead is illustrated in **Fig. 4.4**. The HLA class I beads are non-fluorescent particles whereas the class II coated beads are internally fluorescent, allowing the FlowPRA class I beads to be separated from the FlowPRA class II beads when tested in the same assay. Consequently it is possible to distinguish HLA class I-specific antibodies from HLA class II-specific antibodies in a single test. In addition to beads used for detecting the presence of antibodies, FlowSpecific (One Lambda Inc.) beads are available

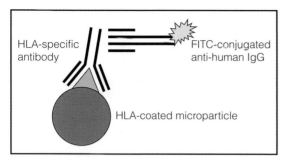

Figure 4.4 • Flow Panel Reactive Antigen (PRA) beads. The bead or microparticle is coated with HLA antigen and is incubated with patient serum. HLA-specific antibody present in the patient serum binds to the corresponding target antigen on the bead. A fluorescently labelled secondary antibody then binds to the antigen/antibody complex. The fluorescently labelled bead is then detected using a flow cytometer.

for the definition of antibody specificity. There are separate tests for the determination of HLA class I and class II specificities. The class I assay involves testing the serum with four pools, each containing eight beads with six antigens per bead. The class II specificity test similarly involves four pools, each of eight beads, but with four antigens per bead. The eight individual bead populations can be distinguished on the basis of their internal fluorescence, and antibody binding is detected by using an FITC-conjugated antihuman IgG. A flow cytometer with several photomultipliers fitted can detect multiple fluorescence spectra.

Luminex technology

Luminex technology uses arrays of antigen-coated microspheres that are coloured with a blend of different intensities of two dyes. After incubation of the test serum with the microspheres any bound antibodies are labelled with a fluorescent anti-human immunoglobulin. The luminex analyser uses a flow cytometer to detect the fluorescence intensity of the antihuman immunoglobulin on each bead. Analysis software determines whether HLA-specific antibody has bound to a specific bead population thus assigning both positivity and HLA specificity.

Tetramers

All the tests discussed to date involve testing sera against antigen sources expressing more than one

HLA antigen. The ultimate aim would be to test serum samples with individually isolated HLA molecules allowing the user to define specificity unequivocally. Individual recombinant HLA antigens have been complexed as tetramers for the detection of HLA/peptide-specific cytotoxic T cells by flow cytometry. Barnardo et al. have already proved the feasibility of using the individual recombinant HLA molecules that make up an HLA tetramer. In their study they found good correlation between CDC-defined specificities and ELISA.[24] Commercial products under development include DynaScreen (Dynal Biotech). This is a solid support antibody screening system in which multiple recombinant HLA molecules are irreversibly bound to a membrane in strips, where each strip is a single HLA allele.

CLINICAL SIGNIFICANCE OF HLA-SPECIFIC ANTIBODIES

The humoral response to an allograft is predominantly an initial IgM response, with low affinity for antigen, followed by a secondary response that is IgG and is of much greater affinity. There have also been reports that IgA may be involved.[25]

The majority of alloantibodies are directed against cell-surface antigens encoded by genes within the MHC at the class I (HLA-A, -B and -Cw) and class II (HLA-DR and -DQ) loci. Such antibodies, if donor specific, cause rapid rejection of vascularised grafts.

Hyperacute rejection (HAR) is apparent within minutes of vascular anastomoses being complete and always within the first 24 hours. Preformed antibodies react with antigens on the vascular endothelial cells of the graft and initiate the complement cascade causing inflammation, blocking the vessels of the graft and causing its death.[26] The introduction of the pretransplant crossmatch has virtually eliminated hyperacute rejection. Acute rejection occurs within a few weeks or months following transplantation. It is caused by the primary response of the recipient to HLA molecules expressed by the transplanted organ. Helper CD4+ T cells stimulate alloreactive B cells to make alloantibody. These antibodies bind to the graft endothelium and initiate rejection in the same way as in hyperacute rejection. Chronic rejection occurs after months or years of good function. There are well-defined pathological changes in the blood vessels, glomeruli and interstitium but the pathogenesis of chronic rejection is less well understood than that of acute rejection.

 A review by McKenna et al. cited more than 23 studies showing that de novo production of donor-specific HLA antibodies is associated with increased acute and chronic rejection and decreased graft survival in kidney, heart, lung, liver and corneal transplants.[27] This was reiterated in a more recent review by Terasaki.[28]

Avoidance of positive crossmatches

The screening of potential transplant recipients for HLA-specific antibodies is an important role of the histocompatibility laboratory. Definition of the HLA specificity of antibodies in patients awaiting renal transplantation avoids not only graft failure but also unnecessary crossmatching as the HLA antigens that must be avoided in a donor can be identified. In addition a comprehensive screening programme reduces the positive crossmatch rate and therefore the unnecessary shipping of organs and prolonged ischaemia times.

Screening strategies

The definition of HLA-specific antibodies in patients awaiting transplantation is time consuming and labour intensive. With the introduction of flow cytometry and ELISA-based techniques the range of technical options available for the laboratory has increased. Flow cytometry and ELISA have generally been considered as alternatives to one another; however, they both have their limitations. Consequently a number of laboratories have devised screening strategies that employ each method in turn to maximise the information obtained whilst limiting the amount of specificity definition work required. The main aim of many of these screening strategies is to screen out antibody-negative sera, which comprise the majority, and focus specificity definition on only those sera known to contain HLA-specific antibodies. By implementing these strategies the workload of the laboratory is reduced whilst improving the level of specificity definition.[29]

Post-transplant monitoring

A number of studies have demonstrated a role for donor HLA-specific antibodies in graft failure and have also illustrated the value of monitoring patients following a transplant.[30] Those patients at risk of humoral rejection by HLA-specific antibody production can be identified and their immunosuppressive therapy can be tailored accordingly.[31] Importantly, by collecting patient samples posttransplant a comprehensive antibody history is available should the graft fail and further transplantation become necessary.

HLAMatchmaker software

HLAMatchmaker is a computer algorithm that identifies donor/recipient HLA compatibility at the molecular level.[32] Amino acid sequence polymorphisms are critical components of immunogenic epitopes and can elicit alloantibody production. The majority of these amino acid sequence polymorphisms reside in the α-helices and β-loops of the HLA protein chain structure – that is, in the sequence positions accessible to alloantibodies. The residues in the strands of the β-pleated sheets of the peptide-binding groove are not considered because they cannot make direct contact with alloantibodies. HLAMatchmaker permits intralocus and interlocus comparisons of polymorphic amino acid sequences of HLA molecules between patients and potential donors to determine the spectrum of non-shared triplets on the mismatched antigens. This software can also be used for highly sensitised patients to identify those antigens that may be mismatched in a transplant but may not elicit a secondary alloresponse, termed 'acceptable mismatches'.

CROSSMATCHING

The complement-dependent cytotoxicity crossmatch (CDC-XM)

This assay follows a protocol similar to that used for cytotoxic antibody screening and is outlined in **Fig. 4.5**. In the CDC-XM, recipient serum is incubated with donor lymphocytes and the subsequent addition of complement results in lysis of

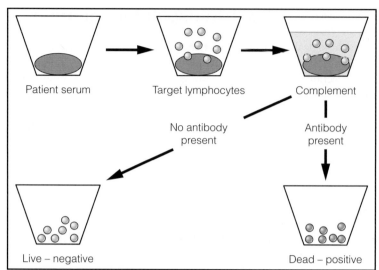

Figure 4.5 • Schematic representation of the complement-dependent cytotoxicity (CDC) assay. Patient serum and target lymphocytes are incubated together and any specific antibodies present in the patient serum will bind to target antigen. Upon addition of complement, target cells that are bound by antibody are lysed. Cell death is visualised and indicates that the patient serum contains antibody. In the case of a crossmatch, cell death is referred to as a 'positive crossmatch' and therefore a contraindication to renal transplantation.

lymphocytes that have been bound by antibody. The mechanism of complement-dependent cytotoxicity is detailed in Chapter 3. Cell viability is visualised by staining the cells and viewing them with a microscope. Cell death indicates a positive crossmatch and is a contraindication to successful renal transplantation. A negative crossmatch means that the renal transplant can proceed. The introduction of the CDC-XM eliminated antibody-mediated hyperacute rejection.

Although the CDC-XM is an essential prerequisite before transplantation there is still debate about the clinical relevance of a positive crossmatch report. The crucial factors in determining clinical relevance are the specificity and immunoglobulin class of the antibody causing the positive results.

 It is accepted that IgG antibodies specific for donor HLA specificities will result in hyperacute rejection. The role of IgM alloantibodies in graft outcome is less clear.

IgM antibodies may be directed against HLA or non-HLA targets. It is now known that IgM antibodies without specificity that react with a patient's own cells in an auto CDC-XM are not clinically relevant and may be an in vitro artefact. The establishment of the presence of such reactivity is important to allow apparently sensitised patients access to transplantation. Other technical problems associated with the CDC-XM include the need for viable target cells, and that only complement-fixing antibodies are detected. Despite its age and simplicity, the CDC-XM is highly effective in the prevention of hyperacute rejection.

The flow cytometry crossmatch (FC-XM)

There is now increasing evidence that more sensitive crossmatch techniques have a role to play in predicting transplant failure. Sensitivity of the crossmatch should equal sensitivity of the screening test used. The first study using a flow cytometer to detect antibody binding in a crossmatch test for renal transplantation showed the technique to be more sensitive than CDC-XM for the detection of donor-specific antibody.[33]

Selected patient sera are crossmatched against donor lymphocytes and incubated at room temperature. The cells are then washed to remove any unbound antigen. Fluorescently tagged antibodies are added in a two-step incubation. Antihuman IgG-FITC in the first step binds with any IgG antibody from the patient sera that may be bound to the donor cells, then CD3-RPE and CD19-RPE separate the lymphocyte population into T and B cells respectively. This three-colour FC-XM is then visualised through the flow cytometer software and a positive crossmatch can be determined by an increase in fluorescence compared with the negative control.[34]

 The association of a positive FC-XM with reduced transplant outcome and the increased sensitivity of this test have now been demonstrated in a number of studies.[35,36]

Many centres have adopted the use of FC-XM for selected cohorts of patients considered to be at high risk, such as repeat transplants, recipients with multiple antibody sensitisation, and in other situations such as transplantation of organs from living donors.

There are few reports on the clinical significance of the FC-XM for non-renal transplants although one study of liver and heart transplants showed that recipients with donor-specific IgG antibodies detected by FC-XM had a poorer prognosis compared with crossmatch-negative recipients.[37]

ELISA crossmatching

ELISA-based assays are increasingly used for antibody screening, and therefore it is logical that they should also be developed for crossmatching. Commercial kits are not yet available because rapid isolation of HLA molecules as targets in the ELISA is technically challenging. The technique would involve purification and capture of donor HLA molecules onto an ELISA tray. These would then be used as targets. Comprehensive studies would be required to establish the role of ELISA crossmatching before it could be widely used in a similar way to research carried out in flow cytometry crossmatching.

PATIENT PROCESS

There now follows a description of the typical patient process seen through the eyes of the histocompatibility and immunogenetics laboratory.

The histocompatibility laboratory HLA types each patient as he or she is referred to the laboratory with a view to going on the transplant list. In addition, HLA-specific antibody screening is performed to identify unacceptable HLA antigens. **Figure 4.6** illustrates the way in which renal patients are investigated in our centre as an example.

Different laboratories may have slightly different procedures but similar investigations will be carried out across the world.

One of the questions most frequently asked by clinicians dealing with solid organ transplantation is how long each laboratory procedure is going to take? An approximate timescale is given in **Box 4.1** to indicate the length of time needed to HLA type a potential organ donor and then to crossmatch the donor with potential renal recipients.

Allocation

The degree of HLA matching required or deemed suitable for successful solid organ transplantation is dependent on the type of organ and the transplant centre at which the transplant is to be performed.

 Evidence-based reviews have demonstrated the effectiveness of HLA matching in improving outcomes, but waiting times may increase as a result.

KIDNEY TRANSPLANTATION

Following evidence-based review and wide discussion with users, a new UK national scheme for the allocation of kidneys from cadaver donors was introduced in mid-1998 with the aim of minimising the degree of HLA mismatching between a donor and the recipient.[38] Patients suitable for kidney transplantation must be identical, or perhaps

Box 4.1 • Approximate timescale for HLA typing of a potential organ donor followed by completion of a crossmatch of donor and potential renal recipient(s) following organ retrieval

0 hours	Lab notified of local donor by transplant coordinator Blood sample sent to the histocompatibility laboratory
After 5 hours	HLA type of donor interpreted UKT run matching programme
After 6 hours	UKT provides shortlist of patients for crossmatch
After organ retrieval	Crossmatch performed
5 hours later	Crossmatch results reported to clinicians

UKT = UK Transplant.

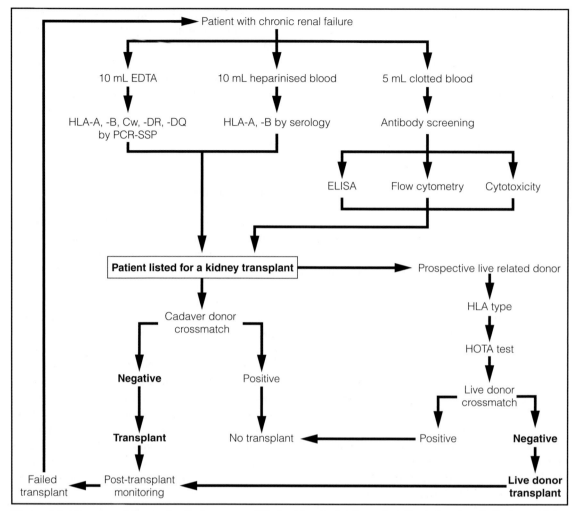

Figure 4.6 • Overview of the renal patient process within the Manchester Transplantation Laboratory. Patients are HLA typed and unacceptable antigens are determined prior to entry onto the renal transplant list. Other histocompatibility laboratories generally follow a similar process.

compatible, for ABO blood group with the donor. They are also HLA typed and screened for the presence of HLA-specific antibodies. These details are entered to local and national 'waiting' lists to which potential donors are matched. Blood group identical recipients can be selected and ranked according to agreed allocation rules. Currently the following rules apply:

- **Tier 1**
  - No HLA-A, -B or -DR mismatch between donor and recipient.
  - Coded as '000'.

- **Tier 2**
  - One mismatch at either HLA-A or -B or at both, but no -DR mismatch.
  - Coded as '100', '010' or '110'.
- **Tier 3**
  - Other degrees of HLA-A, -B, -DR mismatch.
  - Coded appropriately, e.g. '111' up to '222'.

Where there are equal levels of mismatching a points system is used to discriminate. Points are awarded to take account of other factors, most of which have been shown to influence graft outcome:

- Recipient age, favouring younger patients.
- Donor/recipient age differences, minimising age difference.
- Waiting time, favouring long waiters.
- 'Matchability' – favouring those difficult to HLA match.
- HLA sensitisation, favouring highly sensitised patients.
- Centre 'balance of trade' in contributing to organ exchange.

HEART AND LUNG TRANSPLANTATION

Although minimising HLA mismatches has been shown to significantly improve survivals, the irreversible damage caused by prolonged cold storage time discourages exchange of hearts and lungs over large distances simply to minimise HLA mismatches. Recipients in need of a thoracic organ transplant who are sensitised to HLA antigens fare particularly poorly since there is often a prolonged wait for an HLA-compatible, crossmatch-negative donor organ.

LIVER TRANSPLANTATION

 Retrospective reviews of HLA mismatching in liver transplantation have shown little impact on graft survival.

The reason for this remains unclear; however, occurrence of chimerism detected after successful transplantation suggests that tolerance mechanisms may occur in liver transplantation.

CORNEAL TRANSPLANTATION

Corneal transplantation is another area where, in general, the degree of HLA mismatch is not a consideration prior to grafting. The cornea is usually avascular and is therefore considered an 'immunologically privileged' site. However, if a graft bed becomes vascularised as a consequence of primary graft failure, HLA matching has been shown to be beneficial in reducing the risk of rejection in a re-graft.

CONCLUSION

Histocompatibility testing as an effective influence on clinical solid organ transplantation has a mixed reception. The important development of the CDC-XM to prevent hyperacute rejection caused by preformed donor HLA-specific sensitisation by IgG antibodies has saved many thousands of kidneys from immediate failure.

 Avoiding HLA antigen mismatches between the donor and recipient has shown improved survivals at 1 year after transplantation, of between 5 and 10%. However, this effect is dependent on the immunosuppressive regime used.

The clinical value of this phenomenon, as judged by use of HLA matching in allocation of kidneys from deceased donors, varies throughout the world. In North America kidneys are exchanged only if there is no HLA-A, -B and -DR mismatch between the donor and the recipient, whereas in the UK HLA mismatches are minimised at all stages of the allocation algorithm. In countries where there is no exchange system or where there are only a few patients on a waiting list, then avoiding HLA mismatches might not be practicable. The clinical value of the benefit to be gained by allocating kidneys can be measured by the experience of immunosuppressive drugs trials that have taken place since the introduction of ciclosporin in the mid-1980s. Nearly all of these trials, using new drugs or drug combinations, have failed to achieve any improvement in graft survivals at 1 year. This contrasts with the improvement in survival that HLA matching offers. For selection of living kidney donors most centres would include HLA matching as a significant influence when selecting a donor from a group of potential donors. When only one donor is available HLA matching is not a veto to effective transplantation unless there is HLA-specific sensitisation to donor antigens.

Recent advances in effective identification of recipient sensitisation to HLA antigens and definition of the specificity of sensitisation has opened important new approaches to effective allocation of organs for transplantation to avoid antibody-mediated rejection. It remains to be established just what contribution these methods will make to the ongoing attrition in graft loss in the years following stabilisation of graft function. Another possible advantage of the effective definition of recipient sensitisation is a move to transplantation without the need to perform a crossmatch since a sensitisation record will influence organ allocation when unacceptable HLA mismatches are ruled out. It will remain essential that HLA typing of both donor and recipient is performed to facilitate definition of sensitisation. Proceeding to transplantation without performing a crossmatch test should only be considered after careful and expert review of the recipient's sensitisation history and when the kidney cold storage time can be reduced as a result.

The consideration of HLA mismatching in non-renal solid organ transplantation at the time of allocation of donor organs has never been accepted as being of clinical benefit.

 Studies identifying improved survivals when HLA mismatches are minimised (by chance) in heart and lung transplantation have been published, but the picture in liver transplantation is confusing, with studies showing both beneficial and detrimental effects.

In the event, HLA mismatching is not considered as a major factor in non-renal organ allocation except when the recipient is sensitised. In thoracic organ transplantation such patients will often be passed over for a non-sensitised recipient and so will wait much longer with the real possibility of never receiving a transplant.

The true value of histocompatibility testing will reside in supporting clinically effective donor organ allocation systems because of ongoing shortages in donor organ supply and the important need to ensure optimal survival of this rare resource.

Key points

- Mismatching of ABO blood groups is a veto to effective organ transplantation, unless special procedures are used.
- Mismatching of HLA antigens to which a patient is sensitised is a veto to effective organ transplantation, unless special procedures are used.
- The genetics and nomenclature of the HLA system are complex and are defined by a WHO committee.
- Techniques to define HLA types and sensitisation to HLA antigens are precise. Their expert performance and interpretation are vital.
- Application of these techniques to effective transplantation of individual patients requires expert advice and interaction with clinical staff.
- HLA matching, sensitisation and crossmatching are important components of transplant organ allocation.

REFERENCES

1. Marsh SGE, Ekkehard AD, Bodmer WF et al. Nomenclature for factors of the HLA system. Eur J Immunogenet 2002; 29:463–515.

   A WHO Committee report of universally accepted nomenclature.

2. Mullis K, Faloona F. Specific synthesis of DNA in vitro via a polymerase catalysed chain reaction. Methods Enzymol 1987; 155:335.

3. Saika RK, Bugawan TL, Horn GT et al. Analysis of enzymatically amplified β-globin and HLA-DQA DNA with allele specific oligonucleotide probes. Nature 1986; 324:163.

4. Bugawan TL, Horn GT, Long CM. Analysis of HLA-DP allelic sequence polymorphism using the in vitro enzymatic DNA amplification of DP-A and DPB loci. J Immunol 1988; 141:4024.

5. Watson JD, Hopkins NH, Roberts JW et al. Molecular biology of the gene, 4th edn. Menlo Park, CA: Benjamin-Cummings.

6. Sanger F, Nicklen S, Coulson AR. DNA sequencing with chain-terminating inhibitors. Proc Natl Acad Sci USA 1977; 74:5463–7.

7. Opelz G, Graver B, Mickey MR et al. Lymphocytotoxic antibody responses to transfusions in potential kidney transplant recipient. Transplantation 1981; 32:177–83.

8. Nymand G, Heron I, Jensen KG et al. Occurrence of cytotoxic antibodies during pregnancy. Vox Sang 1971; 21:21.

9. Scornick JC, Salomon DR, Lim PB et al. Post-transplant antidonor antibodies and graft rejection. Transplantation 1989; 47:287–90.

10. Martin S, Dyer PA, Harris R. Successful renal transplantation of patients sensitised following deliberate unrelated blood transfusions. Transplantation 1985; 39:256–8.

11. Pfaff WW, Fennell RS, Howard RJ et al. Planned random blood transfusions in preparation for transplantation. Transplantation 1984; 38:701.

12. Reisner EG, Kostyu DD, Phillips G et al. Allo-antibody responses in multiply transfused sickle cell patients. Tissue Antigens 1972; 2:415.

13. Scornick J, Brunson M, Howard R et al. Allo-immunization, memory and the interpretation of crossmatch results for renal transplantation, Transplantation 1992; 54:389–94.

14. Sanfilippo F, Vaughan WK, Bollinger RR et al. Comparative effects of pregnancy, transfusion and prior graft rejection in sensitisation and renal transplant results. Transplantation 1982; 34:360–6.

15. Martin S, Class F. Antibodies and crossmatching for transplantation. In: Dyer PA, Middleton D (eds) Histocompatibility testing – a practical approach. Oxford: IRL Press, 1993; pp. 81–104.

16. Patel R, Terasaki PI. Significance of the positive crossmatch test in kidney transplantation, New Engl J Med 1969: 280:735–9.

   First report of the essential role played by the crossmatch test.

17. Nanni-Costa A, Scolari MP, Lannelli S et al. The presence of posttransplant HLA specific IgG antibodies detected by enzyme-linked immunoabsorbent assay correlates with specific rejection pathologies. Transplantation 1997; 63:167–9.

18. Kao KJ, Scornick JC, Small SJ. Enzyme-linked immunoassay for anti-HLA antibodies – an alternative to panel studies by lymphocytotoxicity. Transplantation 1993; 55:192.

19. Worthington JE, Thomas AA, Dyer PA et al. GTI Quikscreen for the detection of HLA class I specific antibodies. Eur J Immunogenet 1995; 22:110.

20. Wang G, Tarsitani C, Takemura S et al. ELISA assay for the detection of specific antibodies to class I HLA antigens in transplant patients with panel reactive antibodies. Hum Immunol 1996; 49:109.

21. Worthington JE, Sheldon S, Langton A et al. Evaluation of LATM assay for the detection of HLA class I and II specific antibodies. Eur J Immunogenet 1999; 26:69.

22. Harmer AW, Sutton M, Bayne A et al. A highly sensitive rapid screening method for the detection of antibodies directed against HLA Class I and Class II antigens. Transplant Int 1993; 6:277.

23. Pei R, Wang C, Tarsitani C et al. Simultaneous HLA class I and class II antibodies screening with flow cytometry. Hum Immunol 1998; 59:313.

24. Barnardo MC, Harmer AW, Shaw OJ et al. Detection of HLA specific IgG antibodies using recombinant HLA alleles; the MonoLISA assay. Transplantation 2000; 70:531–6.

25. Karuppan SS, Ohlam S, Moller E. The occurrence of cytotoxic and non-complement fixing antibodies in the crossmatch serum of patients with early acute rejection episodes. Transplantation 1992; 54:839–43.

26. Feucht HE, Opelz G. The humoral immune response towards HLA class II determinants in renal transplantation. Kidney Int 1996; 50:1464–75.

27. McKenna RM, Takemoto S, Terasaki PI. Anti HLA antibodies after solid organ transplantation. Transplantation 2000; 69:319–26.

   A seminal report and review.

28. Terasaki PI. Humoral theory of transplantation. Am J Transplant 2003; 3:665–73.

   A synthesis of data supporting an ongoing role for antibody-mediated loss after transplantation.

29. Worthington JE, Langton A, Liggett H et al. A novel strategy for the detection and definition of HLA specific antibodies in patients awaiting renal transplantation. Transplant Int 1998; 11:372–6.

Methodology for efficient detection of pre-transplant sensitisation.

30. Worthington JE, Martin S, Al-Husseini DM et al. Post-transplant production of donor HLA specific antibodies as a predictor of renal transplant outcome. Transplantation 2003: 75;1034–40.

31. Bohmig GA, Regele H. Diagnosis and treatment of antibody-mediated kidney allograft rejection. Transplant Int 2003: 16:773–87.

32. Duquesnoy RJ. HLAMatchmaker: A molecular based algorithm for histocompatibility determination. Description of the algorithm. Hum Immunol 2002: 63:339–52.

33. Garovoy MR, Rheinschmidt MA, Bigos M et al. Flow cytometry analysis: a high technology cross-match technique facilitating transplantation Transplant Proc 1985; 15:1939–44.

34. Robson A, Martin S. T and B cell crossmatching using three-colour flow cytometry. Transplant Immunol 1996; 4:203.

35. Cook DJ, Terasaki PI, Iwaki Y et al. An approach to reducing early kidney transplant failure by flow cytometry crossmatching. Clinical Transplant 1987; 1:253–6.

36. Ogura K, Terasaki PI, Johnson C et al. The significance of a positive flow cytometric crossmatch test in primary kidney transplantation. Transplantation 1993; 56:294–8.

37. Talbot D. Flow cytometric crossmatching in human organ transplantation. Transplant Immunol 1994; 2:138–9.

38. Morris PJ, Johnson RJ, Fuggle SV et al. Analysis of factors that affect outcome of primary cadaveric renal transplantation in the UK. HLA task force of the Kidney Advisory Group of the United Kingdom Transplant Support Service Authority. Lancet 1999; 354:1147–52.

A report that established the current allocation system for deceased donor kidneys in the UK.

Five

Immunosuppression

Neil R. Parrott

INTRODUCTION

I suspect that many of us in transplantation are, like me, bewildered by the variety and combination of immunosuppressive regimens now available to us. For many of us, the burning question would appear to be 'What is the best regimen for my patient?'. This chapter makes no attempt to retrace the extensive review of immunosuppressive drugs that has been undertaken in the two previous editions of this book, but instead aims to answer some of the current outstanding issues. The reader is referred to the corresponding chapter in the earlier editions of this book for 'background reading'.[1,2] Instead of revisiting much of the previous work, it is my intention to ask a few questions that appear to be pertinent to our management of the transplant recipient in the new millennium, and to restrict my review of the published literature largely to those works or studies published since the last edition of this book. I also intend discussing mainly those drugs that currently hold a licence for use in transplantation, and are in 'frequent use'.

At the current time, there are a number of issues that seem to be taxing our thoughts regarding renal transplant immunosuppression:

- What is the current role for the calcineurin inhibitors?

- What can we do to minimise chronic allograft nephropathy?
- Is there a 'gold standard' and what is it?

This chapter aims to focus on these questions and provide evidence to formulate suitable answers.

WHAT IS THE CURRENT ROLE FOR THE CALCINEURIN INHIBITORS?

In renal transplantation

Few would argue that the calcineurin inhibitors (CNIs) have been the mainstay of transplant immunosuppression since the arrival of ciclosporin A over 20 years ago (Sandimmun). However, Sandimmun has been superseded by the micro-emulsion formulation (CSA-ME), and an alternative CNI has now fully established itself in the transplant marketplace. Tacrolimus (Prograf) came into regular use in the UK in 1994, so that transplant physicians have a selection of CNIs from which to choose. Whilst generic forms of ciclosporin are widely available, they are not yet in regular use and therefore will not be discussed further.

However, there is still considerable debate about the relative merits of tacrolimus over ciclosporin.

The US and European 'pivotal studies'[3,4] confirmed that tacrolimus was able to reduce biopsy-confirmed acute rejection, steroid-resistant rejection or the need for 'second-line therapy' treatment with anti-thymocyte globulin (ATG). Neither study demonstrated an increase in 1-year graft or patient survival in patients treated with tacrolimus. However, both studies used the old oil-based formulation of ciclosporin (Sandimmun), and it might be argued that this is an inappropriate comparison for today, given the almost universal use of CSA-ME.

The 5-year follow-up of the phase III US study of tacrolimus has now been published,[5] and makes interesting reading. There are a number of important points in this study. On the intent-to-treat analysis, the 5-year patient and graft survival remained identical in the two groups (79.1% vs. 81.4% and 64.3% vs. 61.6%, tacrolimus vs. ciclosporin respectively). The original study design allowed crossover between groups for treatment failure, and there was a highly significantly greater rate of crossover of patients randomised to the ciclosporin arm than vice versa (27.5% vs. 9.3%, $P < 0.001$). The incidence of treatment failure was significantly lower amongst the patients treated with tacrolimus (43.8% vs. 56.3%, $P = 0.008$). Perhaps even more significant are the 5-year data regarding graft function and other comorbid factors. The median serum creatinine was significantly lower in the tacrolimus arm, and tacrolimus-treated patients had a reduced need for antihypertensives and lipid-lowering agents (Table 5.1).

The later results of the pivotal European study (involving Sandimmun not CSA-ME) have also now been published. This study recruited patients on a 2:1 ratio to tacrolimus or Sandimmun respectively (patients received steroids and azathioprine in addition). The results to 4 years have been analysed[6] and demonstrated that graft survival rates were almost identical at 4 years, with a trend towards lower chronic rejection in the tacrolimus patients. By the time the data were analysed at 5 years for this study,[7] the tacrolimus group had a calculated graft half-life of 15.8 years, vs. 10.8 years for the ciclosporin group, with lower chronic rejection seen in tacrolimus-treated recipients.

As noted above, these two studies might be regarded as obsolete as they compared tacrolimus with the old oil-based formulation of ciclosporin, but there are two prospective, randomised controlled studies addressing the same issue with ciclosporin microemulsion (CSA-ME) that deserve comment. The first is a single-centre, randomised study with 6 years of follow-up, in which patients were randomised to either tacrolimus ($N = 115$) or CSA-ME ($N = 117$) in association with azathioprine and steroids.[8] The study was open label, and was undertaken in Cardiff (Welsh Transplant Research Group). At 6 years, the tacrolimus-treated patients had significantly better graft survival than those receiving CSA-ME (81% vs. 60%, intention-to-treat analysis $P = 0.049$). When crossover for treatment failure was considered, the difference in 6-year graft survival was even more marked (79% vs. 54%, tacrolimus versus CSA-ME respectively, $P = 0.001$). Perhaps more importantly, the renal function at 5 years was significantly better in tacrolimus-treated patients [glomerular filtration rate (GFR) 62 vs. 43 mL/min, tacrolimus vs. CSA-ME respectively,

Table 5.1 • Renal allograft function and cardiovascular risk factors in the 5-year data from the US tacrolimus/ciclosporin study

	Tacrolimus	CSA	P-value
Median serum creatinine (mg/dL)	1.4	1.7	0.0014
Serum Cr >1.5 mg/dL (% patients)	40.4	62.0	0.0017
Mean GFR (±SD)	68.1 ± 31.5	61.1 ± 33.6	<0.0001
Use of antihypertensives (%)	80.9	91.3	0.047
Use of lipid-lowering agents (%)	20.0	58.5	<0.001

CSA, ciclosporin A; Cr, creatinine; GFR, glomerular filtration rate.
Data from ref. 5.

Table 5.2 • Graft survival, renal function and cardiovascular risk factors in the Cardiff randomised study of tacrolimus and CSA-ME

	Tacrolimus	CSA-ME	*P*-value
Graft survival (%)	81	60	0.049
GFR (mL/min)	62	43	0.017
Projected half-life (years)	15	10	not stated
Mean DBP (mmHg)	76	81	0.01
LVM index (g/m)	117	182	0.003
Mean cholesterol (mmol/L)	5.2	6.2	0.007
Hyperglycaemia (%)	16	4	0.002

CSA-ME, ciclosporin A microemulsion; DBP, diastolic blood pressure; LVM index, left ventricular mass index. Data from ref. 8.

$P = 0.017$], and many more patients had what the authors termed 'normal' renal function at 5 years if they had received tacrolimus (**Table 5.2**). The early and late comparisons of serum creatinine in the two groups are summarised in **Fig. 5.1**. These findings are very similar to those reported in the US pivotal study.[5] The authors also examined the effects of treatment on cardiovascular risk factors such as diastolic blood pressure, left ventricular mass and cholesterol, finding that the use of tacrolimus was associated with better cardiovascular risk profiles than CSA-ME.

Although the period of follow-up is significantly shorter (6 months), the European Tacrolimus/ Ciclosporin Study group have reported their findings of a randomised prospective study in 560 patients from 50 centres.[9] Patients received either tacrolimus or CSA-ME with azathioprine and steroids. Biopsy-confirmed acute rejection was reduced in the tacrolimus group (19.6% vs. 37.3%, $P < 0.0001$), graft survival was not statistically different between the groups (94.8% vs. 91.9%, tacrolimus vs. CSA-ME respectively), and renal function was almost identical. As with the other studies cited above, this study also found that cardiovascular risk factors such as hypertension and cholesterol tended to be worse in ciclosporin-treated patients. The incidence of post-transplant diabetes mellitus (PTDM) was higher in the tacrolimus group (8.0% vs. 3.7%, $P = 0.032$), but this difference was diminished and became statistically insignificant if those with pre-existing diabetes were excluded (4.5% vs. 2.0%, tacrolimus vs. CSA-ME respectively).

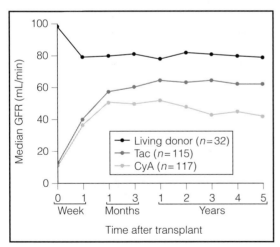

Figure 5.1 • Renal function in a control group of live donor recipients compared with those on tacrolimus or ciclosporin from the Cardiff study. From Jurewicz A. Tacrolimus versus ciclosporin immunosuppression: long term outcome in renal transplantation. Nephrol Dial Transplant 2003; 18(suppl. 1):i7–i11, with permission of Oxford University Press.

In adult renal transplantation:

- Tacrolimus reduces acute and steroid-resistant rejection compared with ciclosporin in renal transplantation.
- Tacrolimus results in better late graft function.

- Tacrolimus results in a better cardiovascular risk profile.

In almost all randomised studies, ciclosporin-treated patients have a greater likelihood of 'treatment failure'.

In paediatric renal transplantation, the use of tacrolimus has been compared with ciclosporin microemulsion (CSA-ME) in a prospective, randomised study in 18 centres from nine European countries. One hundred and three patients received tacrolimus, and 93 received CSA-ME, and data presented are those obtained at their 6-month follow-up. Both groups received azathioprine and corticosteroids.[10] Patient survival was identical, but the incidence of acute rejection was significantly reduced, and calculated GFR was also significantly better in the tacrolimus-treated group. There was a trend towards better graft survival in the tacrolimus group, although this failed to achieve statistical significance (10 grafts lost in tacrolimus group vs. 17 losses in CSA-ME group, $P = 0.06$) (**Table 5.3**).

Liver transplantation

The role of ciclosporin in liver transplantation was discussed in some depth in the second edition of this book. In particular, the prospective randomised trials of ciclosporin (Sandimmun) versus tacrolimus were dealt with in some detail,[11,12] and will not be considered further. However, the pivotal trial comparing CSA-ME with tacrolimus has now been published.[13] The study recruited 606 patients who

had undergone a first orthotopic liver transplant. The authors chose a composite endpoint of combined treatment failure, re-transplantation or death. The study is notable for several reasons. First, it was a very large, prospective, randomised investigator-led study. Second, the study rigorously defined all aspects of immunosuppression to produce what must be regarded as a very statistically sound study. Their results showed a very clear advantage to tacrolimus in liver transplantation. Death or re-transplantation occurred in 19% of the tacrolimus group, and 29% of the CSA-ME group ($P = 0.006$). At the end of year 1, 79% of the patients receiving tacrolimus were alive with their original liver graft, compared with 64% of the CSA-ME patients, and after adjustment for withdrawal for toxicity, 76% and 56% respectively were alive with functioning grafts. The authors concluded that 'data from this trial suggests [sic] that tacrolimus should be the drug of choice in adult liver transplantation'. So far as this author is aware, this recommendation has now been accepted almost universally within liver transplant units in the UK, where tacrolimus is now regarded as the immunosuppressive agent of choice.

Tacrolimus is now regarded as the agent of choice in adult liver transplantation, with superior outcomes in patient and graft survival.

Heart transplantation

In contrast to the numerous studies undertaken in kidney and liver transplantation, the literature is somewhat sparse regarding the comparison of

Table 5.3 • Data from the European randomised study of ciclosporin (CSA-ME) vs. tacrolimus in paediatric renal transplantation

	Tacrolimus	CSA-ME	*P*-value
Acute rejection (%)	36.9	59.1	0.003
Steroid-resistant rejection (%)	7.8	25.8	0.001
Biopsy-confirmed rejection (%)	16.5	39.8	<0.001
Calculated GFR*	62	56	0.03
New-onset diabetes (%)	3.0	2.2	

*GFR, glomerular filtration rate calculated by the Schwartz estimate and expressed as mL/min/1.73 m².
Data from ref. 10.

tacrolimus and ciclosporin in cardiac transplantation. There would appear to be few, if any, major studies comparing the two drugs. None of the studies presents any long-term data, and few are statistically sound studies. The US Multicenter FK506 Study Group examined the outcomes in 16 heart and 15 lung transplant recipients where tacrolimus was used as a rescue therapy, or in cases of intolerance to ciclosporin.[14] The authors concluded that tacrolimus was an effective treatment in this small population, but the study was non-randomised. The Pittsburgh group undertook a study in which 122 patients received tacrolimus, and 121 received ciclosporin. Whilst the groups were large, there was considerable heterogeneity in the use of adjuvant immunosuppressive therapy, the follow-up period in each group differed, and the survival was not different. There was a markedly reduced incidence of rejection in the tacrolimus-treated patients that achieved statistical significance.[15] The European Heart Pilot Study published its own results in a small cohort of patients. Patients were randomised on a 2:1 basis to receive either tacrolimus ($N = 54$) or ciclosporin ($N = 28$). There were no differences in the rates of rejection or graft survival, although it was thought that concomitant use of ATG may have been of benefit in tacrolimus-treated patients.[16] The US study of tacrolimus in heart transplantation was undertaken in six centres, and was prospective, randomised and open label. Patients were randomised to receive either tacrolimus, azathioprine and steroids ($N = 39$) or ciclosporin-based triple therapy ($N = 46$). At the 1-year analysis, there was no difference in the severity or grade of rejection between the groups, but the ciclosporin-treated group developed more new-onset hypertension (71% vs. 48%, $P = 0.05$), and were more likely to receive therapy for raised cholesterol (71% vs. 41%, $P = 0.01$). The authors concluded that tacrolimus therapy was safe and effective in cardiac transplantation.[17] Finally, in a more recent study the Hanover heart transplant group reported their own results with a group of 15 tacrolimus and mycophenolate mofetil (CellCept) (MMF)-treated heart recipients, comparing them to a historical control group of 17 patients receiving ciclosporin–azathioprine. The tacrolimus group had less rejection and lower blood pressure at 3 and 6 months than those treated with ciclosporin.[18]

The published data at present seem insufficient to confirm any major superiority of either immunosuppressant (CSA or tacrolimus) for de novo use in heart transplantation.

Cardiovascular risk profile may be reduced with tacrolimus therapy.

THE CICLOSPORIN C₂ STORY SO FAR

Since the first clinical use of ciclosporin, it has been normal practice to monitor therapy by the use of trough levels taken 12 h post-dose (C_{12} or C_0). However, it has recently been suggested that there is poor correlation between C_0 and the total exposure to the drug as measured by the area under the curve (AUC) in transplant recipients. This has called into question the true value of C_0. In an in-depth investigation of the pharmacokinetics of ciclosporin, the International Neoral Renal Transplantation Study Group has shown a much clearer association between the AUC and the concentration of ciclosporin taken 2 h post-dose (C_2). This group has demonstrated that the C_0 is a very poor correlate of the AUC, and that the most accurate single-point predictor of ciclosporin exposure is the C_2 value.[19] It is a source of great amazement to many of us that after 20 years using the C_0 to monitor ciclosporin therapy we are only now understanding that this has been an entirely inappropriate assay. The poor correlation between AUC and C_0 is shown clearly in **Fig. 5.2**. Based upon their earlier study, Mahalati et al. suggested that a target AUC between hours 0 and 4 (AUC_{0-4}) of between 4400 and 5500 ng/h/mL was associated with less acute rejection, and a minimisation of ciclosporin toxicity.[20] The same group subsequently undertook a prospective study of C_{0-4} in a series of 55 renal transplant recipients.[21] The group targeted the values of 4400–5500 ng/h/mL and showed a very profound correlation between these values and the incidence of acute rejection. In the 22 patients who failed to achieve a level of >4400 ng/h/mL by post-transplant day 3, the incidence of acute rejection was 45%. In very stark contrast, those who achieved C_{0-4} levels >4400 had a rejection rate of just 3% ($P = 0.0002$). The achievement of a 3% rejection rate in a ciclosporin-based regimen at 3 months was previously unheard of. However, for

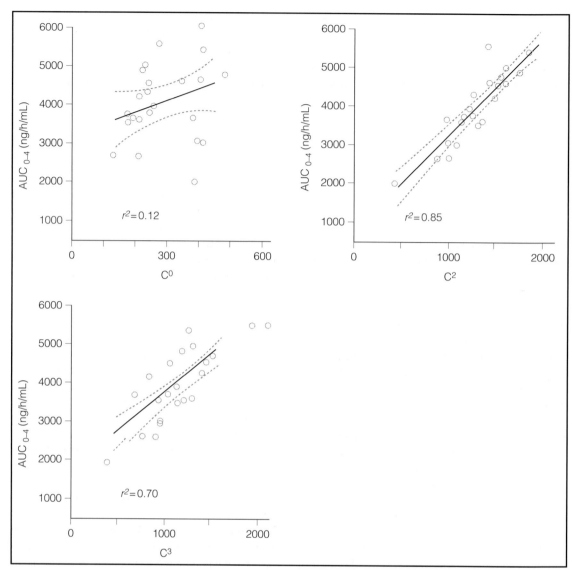

Figure 5.2 • The poor correlation between C_0 (C_{12}) and total ciclosporin exposure (AUC) as demonstrated by the International Neoral Renal Transplantation Study Group. From International Neoral Renal Transplantation Study Group. Cyclosporin microemulsion (Neoral) absorption profiling and sparse-sample predictors during the first three months after renal transplantation. Am J Transplant 2001; 2:148–56, with permission from Blackwell Publishing Ltd.

the majority of clinical transplantation, the routine use of C_{0-4} is clearly impractical, and the Canadian Neoral Renal Transplantation Study Group subsequently undertook a small prospective study of the value of C_2.[22] The association between 'adequate' ciclosporin levels and a rejection-free course was even more marked here. In those who achieved a C_2 level >1.5 µg/mL, there was no acute rejection by the 14th post-transplant day (**Fig. 5.3**). The results

of the first large, prospective, randomised study of C_2 in renal transplantation have now been published.[23] (This is The Monitoring of 2-hour Absorption in Renal Transplantation – MO2ART Study.) The MO2ART study is a 12-month open-label design, with patients' C_2 ciclosporin being targeted to 1.7–1.3 µg/mL for the first 3 months. Patients also received steroids and MMF (89%). After 3 months, patients were randomised to receive

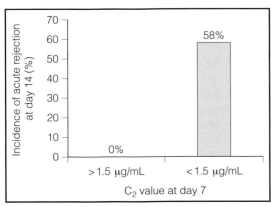

Figure 5.3 • The incidence of acute rejection with C_2 in the Canadian study. From Canadian Neoral Renal Transplantation Study Group. Absorption profiling of cyclosporine microemulsion (Neoral) during the first 2 weeks after renal transplantation. Transplantation 2001; 72:1024–32, with permission.

either 'low' or 'high' C_2 levels. The overall incidence of rejection ($N = 296$) was 11.5%, the incidence in those with immediate graft function was 10.4% ($N = 188$), and in those with delayed graft function was 13.3% ($N = 108$). This study would seem to confirm that at least in the first 3 months, the value of C_2 monitoring is clear, that it is a safe and efficacious method of controlling immunosuppression, and gives acute rejection rates that are still lower than we are used to seeing in renal transplant recipients. Two smaller, single-centre studies in renal transplantation have been undertaken in Riyadh and Toronto. The low incidence of acute rejection has also been confirmed. In each study, a target level of >1.7 µg/mL was mandated, and when achieved, resulted in acute rejection rates of less than 10%.[24,25] Two more recent studies have evaluated the clinical benefits of C_2 monitoring in the stable renal recipient some months after transplantation. In the first Cole et al.[26] assessed the C_2 levels of 175 patients who were 3 or more months out from transplantation. The group compared C_2 with C_0, and found that by C_2 criteria 85 patients had ciclosporin levels above target range (ranges as recommended by the International Consensus document published in 2002 – see ref. 27). Having established that 48% of their maintenance patients had C_2 levels that were above the recommended levels, the group undertook dose reduction on the basis of the C_2 data. In all patients, the renal function remained stable, and in 54% of these, there was a reduction in mean creatinine levels from 153 to 132 µmol/L, with a fall in blood pressure from 135/82 to 131/77. These reductions did not appear to achieve statistical significance. In the second such study Midtvedt et al. examined C_2 and C_0 levels in 1447 renal allograft recipients in Norway, all of whom were greater than 12 months post-transplant.[28] In a series of 203 patients who had C_2 levels of between 700 and 800 µg/L, the mean serum creatinine was 136 µmol/L, but in those with a C_2 of >950 µg/L the serum creatinine was significantly greater (mean 152 µmol/L). The authors found that this difference was statistically signifiant, and concluded that there may be meaningful benefits from the use of C_2 in the maintenance phase of transplantation. A linear regression showed that there was a significant relationship between C_2 and serum creatinine in these patients ($P = 0.03$). However, it must be stressed that these are both observational studies, and need confirmation in other centres and in other study designs.

Is there a national or international consensus on the role of C_2?

The International Consensus statement (CONCERT) on the use of C_2 in both renal and hepatic transplantation is worthy of greater study, and the reader is recommended to read this in detail.[27] However, the thorough review of the published literature in that Consensus comes out with the following recommendations for the renal transplant recipient (these are only very brief summation points):

- There is a strong association between C_2 levels and acute rejection in the de novo renal transplant.
- A C_2 level of 1.5–2.0 µg/mL in the first month is recommended.
- This target should be achieved within the first 3–5 days.
- Lower target C_2 levels should be achieved after the first month (these are shown in **Table 5.4**).
- The data do not yet answer whether the benefits of C_2 extend beyond the first post-transplant year.

Table 5.4 • Comparison of the recommended C_2 levels (all in µg/mL) in the International (CONCERT) Consensus and the recent UK Consensus (see ref. 27)

Time post-transplant (months)	CONCERT (International Consensus)	UK Consensus
<1	1.5–2.0	1.5
2	1.5	1.3
3	1.3	1.1
4–6	1.1	0.9
7–12	0.9	0.7
>12	0.8	0.7

THE UK CONSENSUS ON C_2 MONITORING

In a recent meeting of a number of 'experienced' centres in the UK, a consensus view on the value of C_2 was promulgated. This consensus is, as yet unpublished, but the key findings are presented with the permission of Novartis UK Ltd. The participants agreed the following:

• There was compelling evidence to support the view that C_0 had no clear relationship to AUC and that the best single point to predict this was C_2.
• The formula previously recommended for dosage changes often resulted in significant toxicity in the first few days, and was not to be recommended.
• The dose changes undertaken should be done on the basis of clinical experience, and assessment of biochemical and clinical signs of toxicity.
• The achievement of a target C_2 within 3–5 days was probably too tight, and that achievement of this by day 7 was probably sufficient.
• There was compelling evidence to support the view that the achievement of adequate C_2 levels within the first 7 days was associated with low levels of acute rejection.
• The International Consensus view had suggested C_2 levels that were probably too high (see Table 5.4).

At the present time, it would seem that acceptance of the benefits of C_2 are growing, but are by no means universal. Despite the fact that we've been doing it for 20 years, most would agree that the data support the view that C_0 is a virtually useless measure, that C_2 is certainly a vastly superior method of monitoring ciclosporin therapy, and one that seems to be associated with reduced acute rejection in the early post-transplant phase. However, in this author's view, the two key studies have yet to be undertaken:

1. a prospective, randomised comparison of short- and long-term outcomes of renal transplantation comparing the use of C_0 and C_2; and
2. a comparison by prospective randomised study of tacrolimus and Neoral with the latter therapy monitored by C_2, and tacrolimus monitored by 'traditional' C_0.

The jury may still be out on the C_2 monitoring question, and indeed one wonders if all 'historical' comparisons of ciclosporin using C_0 might even invalidate such past data and comparisons with other immunosuppressive agents.

In renal transplantation:

• Ciclosporin concentration at 2 h post-dose (C_2) is a much more accurate indicator of drug exposure than trough levels.
• C_2 levels of 1500–1700 ng/mL within the first 5–7 days are associated with significantly lower rates of acute rejection.

Further confirmatory prospective studies are indicated in the acute phase.

Promising early data exist to suggest that C_2 might be helpful in the late maintenance phase of renal transplantation, but are insufficient to make strong recommendations for its routine use.

WHAT ABOUT A CALCINEURIN INHIBITOR-FREE REGIMEN?

In the previous edition of this book, the question of a calcineurin inhibitor (CNI)-free regimen was briefly explored. The potential benefits of this approach are immense, and until recently the risks of abandoning our 'gold standard' immunosuppressive agent (ciclosporin or tacrolimus) were also largely unknown.

There are potentially three approaches to a CNI-free regimen:

1. CNI exclusion de novo;
2. planned CNI elimination after a predetermined time period;
3. 'adverse event-driven' CNI elimination.

The majority of cases of 'adverse event-driven' CNI elimination have been in response to chronic allograft nephropathy (CAN), and this indication will be discussed later in this chapter.

Calcineurin-inhibitor exclusion in de novo transplantation

In the first such study of this type, Groth et al. reported the results of a multicentre trial in which 85 first cadaveric renal allograft recipients were randomised to either sirolimus/steroids/azathioprine or ciclosporin/azathioprine/steroids. At 12 months, patient and graft survival were similar in the two groups, but the sirolimus-treated patients had consistently better renal function throughout.[29] Subsequently, Kreis et al. and the European Sirolimus Study Group undertook an open-label, randomised study in renal transplant recipients in 14 centres. Patients were randomised to receive sirolimus, MMF and steroids or therapy with CSA-ME, MMF and steroids. This was a phase II pilot study, and recruited a total of 78 patients.[30] Published data recorded outcomes at 1 year. The two groups were well matched for demographic characteristics, and there were no differences in graft and patient survival. Biopsy-proven rejection was slightly higher in the sirolimus/MMF group, but this did not achieve statistical significance (Table 5.5).

Given that hypercholesterolaemia is a known side effect of sirolimus, it was no surprise that the serum cholesterol was statistically higher in the sirolimus group than the CSA-ME group for the first 6 months, but the magnitude of the effect diminished at 12 months and was not statistically significant at that time. What is most notable in the Kreis study

is the very real improvement in graft function seen in patients who received no CNIs. These data are reproduced in **Fig. 5.4**.

Subsequently, Flechner et al. published their own results from the Cleveland Clinic, in which 61 primary kidney allograft recipients were recruited.[31] All patients received induction therapy with basiliximab, and also MMF 2 g daily and steroids. Thirty patients were randomised to receive ciclosporin, and 31 received sirolimus. Mean follow-up was 18 months. There were no statistical differences between the two groups with respect to patient survival (96.7% vs. 100%, sirolimus vs. CSA respectively), graft survival (96.7% vs. 95.4%, sirolimus vs. CSA respectively) or biopsy-confirmed acute

Table 5.5 • Incidence of rejection, and patient and graft survival in the European phase II study of a sirolimus-based, CNI-free regimen in renal transplantation

	Sirolimus (N = 40)	CSA (N = 38)
Biopsy-proven rejection (%)	27.5	18.4
Graft survival (%)	92.5	89.5
Patient survival (%)	97.5	94.7

Data from ref. 30.

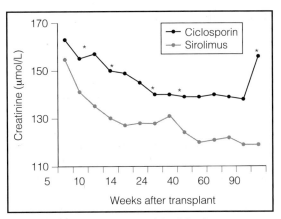

Figure 5.4 • Mean serum creatinine following transplantation in the Kreis study. From Kreis H, Cisterne JM, Land W et al. for the Sirolimus European Renal Transplant Study Group. Sirolimus in association with mycophenolate mofetil induction for the prevention of acute graft rejection in renal allograft recipients. Transplantation 2002; 69:1252–60, with permission.

rejection (6.4% vs. 16.6%, sirolimus vs. CSA). The lower incidence of acute rejection in sirolimus-treated patients (6.4%) in the Flechner study compared with the Kreis study (27.5%) is possibly a consequence of an IL-2 (interleukin 2) receptor blocking agent used by Flechner, and the differing regimens of sirolimus in each study. The Flechner paper also confirmed the fact that renal allograft function was significantly better in patients in the CNI-free protocol (Table 5.6).

In what may be seen as an even greater departure from the accepted wisdom of immunosuppression, Rao et al. reported on a single-centre study using an immunosuppressive regimen that avoided both steroids and CNIs.[32] In a series of 29 primary renal transplant recipients, patients were given Campath-1H, and then sirolimus alone, with doses adjusted to achieve trough levels of 8–12 ng/mL. The study was a non-randomised, single-arm study. Eight patients experienced acute rejection (28%). According to the 12-month data, 21 patients remained on sirolimus monotherapy (82%), with a mean serum creatinine of 1.6 mg/dL in the non-rejectors, and 2.0 mg/dL in those that had rejection ($P = 0.06$). The mean cholesterol and triglyceride levels increased following transplantation, but were not statistically different from baseline, although 60% of patients were started on lipid-lowering therapy in the first 3 months. The study shows that such a regimen is possible and relatively safe, but the serum creatinine levels at 12 months are somewhat higher than one would expect in a CNI-free regimen,

perhaps suggesting underimmunosuppression. There are now a small number of other studies in which the de novo use of CNIs has been avoided. Grimbert et al.[33] randomised 117 low-risk patients to receive either azathioprine and prednisolone ($N = 58$) or triple therapy based upon ciclosporin ($N = 59$). Patients received induction therapy with antithymocyte globulin. The authors presented data after 12 years of follow-up, and showed that the CNI-free group had similar rates of rejection to the ciclosporin-treated patients, and similar 12-year graft survival. In those patients who remained free of rejection, renal allograft function was significantly better at 12 months in the CNI-free group compared with those on ciclosporin (mean creatinine 121 μmol/L vs. 168 μmol/L, $P = 0.006$). This study would seem to be a brave departure from the old philosophy that azathioprine and steroids for maintenance therapy gives inferior results, and would seem to reinforce the growing evidence that CNIs are detrimental in the long term. Stegall et al.[34] reported the results of a small, randomised study in which patients received either tacrolimus MMF/steroids ($N = 40$) or sirolimus/MMF/steroids ($N = 45$). Rejection rates with either regimen were low, 7.5% in the tacrolimus group and 6.7% in the sirolimus group, and renal function was better in the group that did not receive CNIs after 1 month compared with the group that did, but not statistically so. Follow-up was only for 4 months.

The clinical situation in which the avoidance or reduction of CNIs has always been felt to be paramount is in the renal allograft with delayed graft function (DGF). Given the knowledge that CNIs are potentially more damaging in the DGF situation, it is no surprise that studies have attempted to eliminate CNIs altogether or delay their use in this situation. Of the two studies to be cited, neither was randomised, and both were more cohort, observational in type. In the first such study by Hong and Kahan,[35] sirolimus was used with IL-2 receptor blocking antibodies and steroids in the DGF group, and in the second study by Grinyo et al.,[36] MMF was used with thymoglobulin and steroids. Both studies confirmed that there were benefits to CNI avoidance in this situation, but both are 'statistically weak'.

The studies cited above would seem to suggest that there is growing evidence that CNIs can be

Table 5.6 • Creatinine and calculated creatinine clearance (Cockroft–Gault) in patients receiving ciclosporin-based therapy, or sirolimus-based therapy at 6 and 12 months in the Flechner study

	Sirolimus ($N = 31$)	CSA ($N = 30$)	P-value
Creatinine (mg/dL) at:			
6 months	1.29	1.74	0.008
12 months	1.32	1.78	0.004
Calculated creatinine clearance (mL/min) at:			
6 months	77.8	64.1	0.006
12 months	81.1	61.1	0.008

Data from ref. 31.

safely avoided in the de novo renal allograft recipient, but clearly these early results demand more careful, long-term consideration.

Calcineurin inhibitors can be avoided in the de novo renal transplant patient.

Early results are encouraging but long-term follow-up data are required.

Planned CNI elimination

One of the more attractive concepts in current immunosuppression is the idea of planned, early cessation of calcineurin inhibitors, with the aim of introducing a non-nephrotoxic regimen. This may be achieved in one of several ways, but the two most favoured regimens are either (a) the use of sirolimus (Rapamune) to eliminate calcineurin inhibitors; or (b) the use of mycophenolate mofetil (CellCept).

SIROLIMUS AS A 'CNI SUBSTITUTE'

This concept has been explored with considerable success in a number of studies. In one such study, Gonwa et al.[37] recruited patients from 17 centres in the USA and Europe to a prospective, randomised, open-label study. One hundred and ninety-seven patients were randomised to two treatment groups. The first group (group A) received CSA-ME and a fixed dose of sirolimus (2 mg/day), and the second group (group B) received reduced-dose CSA-ME and concentration-controlled doses of sirolimus. All patients received corticosteroids. After 2 months, eligible patients in the second group underwent gradual reduction and cessation of CSA-ME. Follow-up was for 12 months. Patient and graft survival were identical in both groups, and the rates of biopsy-confirmed acute rejection were more-or-less identical at around 20%. Renal function was, however, significantly better in the CSA-ME-elimination arm, and calculated creatinine clearances were higher (**Table 5.7**). Although black recipients have always been known to fare much less well after renal transplantation than non-blacks, this study did show that black recipients in group B (CSA-ME eliminated) had vastly improved renal function compared with black recipients in group A (mean creatinine 2.69 vs. 1.55 mg/dL

Table 5.7 • The effects of CSA elimination on 12-month patient and graft survival, acute rejection and graft function in a sirolimus-based regimen

	Group A* (N = 97)	Group B* (N = 100)	P-value
12-month patient survival (%)	96.9	96.0	
12-month graft survival (%)	92.8	95.0	
Acute rejection (%) (biopsy-confirmed)	18.6	22.0	
Mean creatinine (mg/dL)	1.82	1.38	<0.001
Mean GFR (mL/min) (Nankivell)	57.1	73.5	<0.001

*See text for details of regimens for groups A and B.
Data from ref. 37.

respectively, $P = 0.011$). From this phase II study, the authors concluded that the elimination of CSA resulted in no significant increase in acute rejection, similar graft and patient survival, and much improved renal function.

In a very similar, but phase III study, 525 patients were enrolled into a CSA elimination trial.[38] Four hundred and thirty patients were randomised to either arm. The study design included CSA-ME, steroids and sirolimus for the first 3 months, at which time one group was randomised to remain on a combination of CSA-ME, sirolimus and steroids, and the second group was randomised to have gradual elimination of their CSA, but to remain on sirolimus and steroids (the so-called '310' study). In the CSA-elimination group, sirolimus was targeted to a trough of 20–30 ng/mL, and follow-up was for 12 months. During the prerandomisation phase, the incidence of biopsy-confirmed acute rejection was 13%. At 12 months there were no differences between the groups in terms of patient and graft survival (data not shown here). Once again, there were very significant differences in renal function at 1 year. The patients who remained on a combination of ciclosporin, sirolimus and steroids had a mean calculated GFR of 57 mL/min, and those with ciclosporin elimination had a GFR of 63 mL/min ($P < 0.001$). This pivotal study again demonstrated that the elimination of ciclosporin was a safe and efficacious manoeuvre, but raised some anxiety with respect to the incidence of acute rejection post-randomisation: the incidence of the latter was 4.2% in the CSA triple group and 9.8% in the sirolimus group ($P = 0.035$).

Despite these early anxieties, when the same study was followed to 2 years,[39] there were still no significant differences in patient or graft survival but improvements in renal allograft function continued (**Table 5.8**). High-density lipoprotein (HDL)-cholesterol was significantly higher in the group receiving sirolimus and steroids, but total cholesterol, LDL-cholesterol and triglycerides were not significantly different. Hypertension was reported more frequently in patients who remained on CSA.

Finally, in a very much smaller but similarly designed study to '310', the UK and Ireland Rapamune Study Group recently reported their results in a series of 133 renal recipients.[40] The group reported their own results at 6 months of follow-up. Their findings largely confirmed the results of the two studies above: renal function was significantly improved, with no detriment to patient or graft survival at that timepoint.

It is clear from the three studies above that the use of sirolimus certainly allows the planned, early withdrawal of ciclosporin. This withdrawal may result in a small increase in the incidence of acute rejection, but this would not seem to translate into reduced graft survival after 2 years. Clearly, the 5-year data will be awaited with interest, not least for the graft survival rates in the two groups, but also for evidence of the continued superiority of graft function past the 2-year point.

Planned elimination of CSA with sirolimus is safe and effective.

Planned elimination of CSA with sirolimus results in greatly improved graft function at 2 years, and equal graft survival.

MYCOPHENOLATE MOFETIL AS A 'CNI SUBSTITUTE'

There have been a small number of preliminary studies using this approach in the 'stable' renal allograft recipient, but most such studies have limited follow-up or are non-randomised.[41,42] However, a large, multicentre, randomised study has been published by the Cyclosporine Withdrawal Study Group.[43] One hundred and eighty-seven patients were enrolled from 17 centres, and all were already taking a CSA-based regimen. Those not taking CSA were given MMF for a 3-month 'run-in' period. Patients already taking a CSA/MMF/steroid regimen were randomised directly. Patients randomised to cease CSA had a phased 3-month reduction in their ciclosporin, and the primary efficacy endpoint was renal function 6 months after complete cessation of CSA. Eighty-five patients were randomised in each arm. Interestingly, the analysis of creatinine clearance (as assessed by the Cockroft–Gault formula) showed only a modest trend towards improved renal function in the group who came off CSA, and this did not achieve statistical significance. However, when the data were analysed with respect to the 'per-protocol' patients, there was a statistically significant improvement in renal function (**Table 5.9**).

This study does, however, show that the cessation of CSA is associated with a significant increase in the risks of acute rejection once CSA has been discontinued. In this instance, the rate of acute

Table 5.8 • Two-year follow-up data for the so-called '310' study in which patients underwent planned elimination of CSA after 3 months

	SIR/CSA*	SIR*	*P*-value
Patient survival (%)	94.0	95.3	
Graft survival (%)	91.2	93.5	
Acute rejection (%)	5.1	9.8	
Creatinine (μmol/L)	167	128	<0.001

*SIR, sirolimus; CSA, ciclosporin A; see text for details.
Data from ref. 39.

Table 5.9 • Serum creatinine (μmol/L) in the Cyclosporine Withdrawal Study; per-protocol population. Comparison of renal function at study end

	CSA withdrawal	CSA continuation
Baseline	137	132
End of study	126	136

CSA, ciclosporin A.
Data from ref. 43.

rejection was 10.6% in the group that stopped CSA and 2.4% (P = 0.03) in the group that continued with CSA. Whilst most of the rejection episodes were Banff grade I, some required treatment with mono- or polyclonal antibodies. The CSA-elimination group showed significant reductions in total and HDL-cholesterol but contrary to expectation from previous studies did not demonstrate a benefit in blood pressure control (which was better in the CSA-continuation group). In a similar but smaller study, Schneulle et al. randomised 84 low-risk renal allograft recipients on triple therapy with CSA-ME, MMF and steroids to undergo elimination of either CSA or MMF.[44] The group who ceased CSA remained on MMF and steroids (group A), and those who discontinued MMF remained on CSA and steroids (group B). Randomisation occurred 3 months post-transplantation. Renal function at 6 and 12 months was the primary efficacy endpoint. After 12 months of follow-up, creatinine clearance (72 mL/min vs. 61 mL/min), calculated GFR (73 mL/min vs. 62 mL/min) and serum creatinine (121 µmol/L vs. 138 µmol/L) were all statistically lower in the group on MMF and steroids. There was a trend towards higher rejection following randomisation in the group that discontinued CSA (11.3% vs. 5.0%), but this did not achieve statistical significance. There were also significant falls in systolic and diastolic blood pressure, serum triglycerides and statin usage in the MMF patients. Patient and graft survival at 12 months were identical in each group.

The data from these studies seem to tell us several things, but again, primarily, that it is possible to eliminate CSA at an early stage in a planned and phased way, and that such changes to immuno-suppression should be done in a very slow and controlled manner. There would appear to be benefits in terms of lower cardiovascular risk by the elimination of CSA. The enhanced risk of acute rejection after CSA elimination is very similar in these studies to the findings in the sirolimus-based '310' study (see **Table 5.8** and ref. 38). Finally, one should note that follow-up in these studies is still short, and the influence of CSA elimination on graft survival and renal function after 5 years must be awaited with interest. Thus, compared to the use of sirolimus in this setting, the data on MMF are relatively 'early' and more scant.

'ADVERSE EVENT'-DRIVEN ELIMINATION OF CNIs

The final setting in which one might consider the cessation of CNIs is in the long-term allograft recipient who has developed significant problems with his or her existing regimen of drugs. For some, this might stem from the potentially dysmorphic effects of calcineurin inhibitors, such as ciclosporin-associated gum disease, or hypertrichosis, or the alopecia of tacrolimus. However, for the majority, this is likely to be in the setting of a slow and insidious decline in renal function, with biopsy-proven chronic allograft nephropathy or chronic ciclosporin nephrotoxicity. There are, once again, two current modalities that are open to the clinician – sirolimus and mycophenolate mofetil.

Sirolimus for chronic allograft nephropathy

In an early study from Canada, 20 patients with chronic toxicity secondary to CSA or tacrolimus were switched to therapy with sirolimus.[45] Patients were given fixed-dose sirolimus at 5 mg/day and follow-up was from 7 to 24 months. In this study, mean serum creatinine fell by 17% in the first month after conversion, and 58% of patients had >10% fall in creatinine (mean 22%) after 1 year. In only two cases did the creatinine continue to rise, and in each of these patients the serum creatinine was >285 µmol/L at switch. In a similar uncontrolled, single-centre study, Diekmann et al. converted 22 renal allograft recipients with biopsy-proven nephrotoxicity to sirolimus.[46] Two patients remained stable (9%), 11 patients had improved function (50%), and in 9 cases (41%) renal function continued to deteriorate. A small prospective study was undertaken in Leicester (UK), in which 31 patients with biopsy-proven CAN underwent a 40% reduction in their CSA, with (study group) the addition of sirolimus at 2 mg/day or without the latter (controls). The authors failed to demonstrate any functional or morphological improvement in patients receiving sirolimus but had not eliminated CSA completely, and presumably overlooked the fact that sirolimus may enhance the nephrotoxicity of CSA.[47] In a final study examining the effects of the early use of sirolimus in renal allograft recipients,

40 patients taking a sirolimus/CSA-based regimen were randomised to have continuation or cessation of their CSA.[48] The authors primarily examined renal biopsy samples after 12 months. They concluded that the elimination of CSA resulted in a diminution of the histological indices of chronic rejection after 12 months, but the study was not undertaken in those with 'established' CAN.

All of the above studies are small, mostly uncontrolled, and with short follow-up, and it would appear that there are currently scant good trial data to support the concept that the late addition of sirolimus may reverse established chronic allograft nephropathy.

There are currently no good published trials to support the role of sirolimus in established chronic allograft nephropathy.

Mycophenolate mofetil for chronic allograft nephropathy

Before considering the influence of MMF on established chronic allograft nephropathy, it is worth looking at what evidence might exist regarding the long-term safety of this drug. Ojo et al. looked in some detail at the data of almost 67 000 patients on the US Renal Transplant Scientific Register.[49] The authors used Cox proportional hazard analysis to determine the effect of MMF on chronic allograft failure. The authors came to three important conclusions:

1. MMF reduced the relative risk of chronic allograft failure by 27%.
2. Compared with azathioprine, MMF significantly enhanced 4-year graft survival (85.6% vs. 81.9% respectively).
3. The relative effect of acute rejection on chronic allograft failure had increased over the preceding 10-year period.

In a very similar comparison published in 2003, statistically similar in the methodology used, Meier-Kriesche et al. compared 40 570 patients on azathioprine with 9096 receiving MMF.[50] In this publication, the authors examined the US Renal

Data System (USRDS). To this author it appears that the data are actually from the same, or similar dataset as that used by Ojo et al.[49] However, the conclusions reached are similar and the publication from this large registry seems again to support the contention that the long-term use of MMF is associated with improved late graft function, and some protection against late graft loss.

Outside these analyses of large registries, there are few other studies of the use of MMF in the situation of CAN. In 2001, Weir et al. studied 118 renal recipients with biopsy-proven chronic allograft nephropathy.[51] The study was not randomised, and patients underwent either a 50% reduction in their CSA or tacrolimus trough levels, or they had cessation of their CNI altogether. The authors point out that the decision to either reduce or discontinue CNIs was 'arbitrary'. All patients received MMF in a dose of 2 g/day. One hundred patients had reduction of their CNI (67 on CSA and 33 on tacrolimus), and only 18 had complete cessation. Follow-up was for at least 2 years. In this study, 91.7% of the patients who discontinued their CNI showed significant improvement in their renal function (as measured in a complex way by slopes of decay), improvement was seen in 51.7% of the CSA dose-reduction group and 59.3% of the tacrolimus dose-reduction group. In a small study, McGrath and Shehata randomised 30 patients with biopsy-proven CAN to undergo either conversion to tacrolimus or MMF.[52] All patients started the study on a triple regimen with CSA, azathioprine and steroids. Minimum follow-up was for 6 months. In this study, conversion to tacrolimus had no advantageous effect on renal function, but cessation of CSA and addition of MMF resulted in significant improvement in serum creatinine (creatinine reduced from mean 246 to 188 μmol/L, $P < 0.001$), isotope GFR (increased from mean 26 to 34 mL/min, $P < 0.01$), and also significantly reduced systolic and diastolic blood pressures in the MMF-treated group. Follow-up is again fairly short. Ducloux et al. undertook a non-randomised trial in which 31 patients with CAN were assigned to MMF, and also demonstrated improved renal function, as well as better blood pressure and lipid profiles.[53]

However, what is perhaps the 'pivotal study' to answer this question (and perhaps the only one to date) is the so-called 'Creeping Creatinine Study'.[54]

This was a multicentre, prospective, randomised study in which 73 patients were randomised to cessation of CSA and addition of MMF, or, in the control group, to continue with CSA (N = 70). All had biopsy-confirmed CAN, and follow-up published to date is to 34 weeks. In the MMF group, renal function stabilised or improved in 58% of the patients, compared with 28% in the CSA group (P = 0.002). There were two graft losses in the CSA group, and none in the MMF group, but three patients died in the MMF group from sepsis, liver failure and myocardial infarction. The improvements in renal function appear to be sustained up to 34 weeks in the MMF group, whereas the mean serum creatinine in the CSA group continues to deteriorate (**Fig. 5.5**).

> High-quality controlled trials using MMF as a substitute for calcineurin inhibitors in CAN are few in number, and follow-up is short.
>
> No trials yet have follow-up beyond 2 years.
>
> Despite their statistical shortfalls, most of these trials do demonstrate that cessation of CNIs and substitution of MMF will result in improved allograft function in 60–90% of cases.
>
> Cessation of CNIs is also likely to result in the improvement of cardiovascular risk factors.

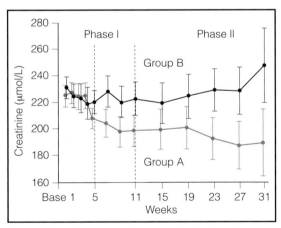

Figure 5.5 • Serum creatinine from the Dudley 'Creeping Creatinine' study. From Dudley CRK, Pohanka E, Riad H et al. Mycophenolate mofetil substitution for cyclosporine A in renal transplant recipients with chronic progressive allograft dysfunction: the creeping creatinine study. Transplantation 2005; 79:466–75, with permission from Lippincott Williams & Wilkins.

IS THERE A 'GOLD STANDARD', AND WHAT IS IT IN RENAL TRANSPLANTATION?

The BTS Consensus Document

In June 2003, the British Transplantation Society undertook the task of producing what it hoped was a consensus document on what might be regarded as the framework for a 'gold standard' in renal transplantation immunosuppression.[55] Space does not permit a full discussion of that document here, but there are a number of key points that deserve emphasising. The final document was produced following a full day's conference attended by key representatives from all the renal transplant units in the UK, as well as representatives from patient groups, UK Transplant and professional groups allied to transplantation. It should be stressed that this does not represent a universal view, but a consensus of the groups represented at that meeting.

Perhaps one of the most important points stressed in the BTS consensus is that there is simply no gold standard, and that in each case 'immunosuppression should be individualised' (Section 1.6), and a comprehensive choice of immunosuppressive agents should always be available to the clinician (Section 1.7). The group agreed unanimously that acute rejection is a predictor of long-term graft survival (Section 2.2), and perhaps even more importantly, that renal function at 1 year 'is an important marker for long-term graft survival' (Section 2.3). In this respect, the consensus document emphasises what has become (perhaps belatedly) a very real issue in renal transplantation – namely that 1-year graft survival is, to some extent, meaningless if one ignores the 'quality of graft survival'. None of us can doubt that to achieve freedom from dialysis after 1 year with a serum creatinine of, say, 250 µmol/L is significantly inferior to the patient who remains free from dialysis with a creatinine of 100 µmol/L. Both might be regarded as successful examples of 1-year graft survival, but can any of us doubt which of the two hypothetical grafts we would rather have?

In terms of baseline immunosuppression, the BTS document has, however, 'sat on the fence' with the following statement:

> *Standard baseline immunosuppression for an intermediate risk patient should consist of the combination of a calcineurin inhibitor, an anti-proliferative agent, oral steroids and an anti-CD25 monoclonal antibody.*

(Ref. 55, Section 5.1)

The statement above is qualified with the term 'intermediate risk patient', and the consensus gives what are very useful guidelines that help to quantify those risk factors that might help the clinician to individualise immunosuppression. The reader is recommended to visit the BTS website for further reading, as the quantified risk factors certainly provide a useful template for optimising and individualising immunosuppression. Whilst the guidelines have recommended the above regimen for what may be regarded as the majority of renal allografts, they have not considered the more controversial concept of de novo exclusion of CNIs (as discussed earlier in this chapter). However, the guidelines have recognised the growing problem of chronic allograft nephropathy with the following statement:

> *In order to minimise calcineurin inhibitor toxicity, allograft dysfunction which is not due to rejection or another identifiable cause may be appropriately treated by reduction and/or withdrawal of calcineurin inhibitor therapy, with or without the addition of an anti-proliferative agent.*

(Ref. 55, Section 4.3)

Although the latter statement recommends the possible use of an antiproliferative agent, the docu-

ment does acknowledge that a TOR inhibitor (target of Rapamycin) may also have a role in this situation, but does not recommend either mycophenolate or sirolimus specifically. The view of this author would be that the data with respect to CNI elimination in favour of steroids and azathioprine are not favourable, and that the incidence of acute rejection following conversion is unacceptably high with this 'old-fashioned' combination. The relative merits of either MMF or sirolimus as a CNI-sparing agent have been discussed earlier in this chapter.

What did NICE have to say?

At the end of 2003, the National Institute for Clinical Excellence (NICE), a regulatory body set up by the Department of Health in the UK, produced what is termed an appraisal entitled 'Immunosuppressive therapy for renal transplantation'.[56] The document is undergoing possible modification in the light of comments received from the transplant profession and pharmaceutical industry. Thus any comments made here must be considered preliminary at this stage.

NICE appraisal is, in some respects, to be viewed in a different light to that for the BTS consensus document. The authors of the BTS document made no effort to analyse the pharmaco-economic impact of any of the regimens that may be used. In contrast, the recommendations from NICE are very much influenced by cost-effectiveness.

The NICE document made the following recommendations:

'1.1 Basiliximab or daclizumab are recommended as options for induction therapy in prophylaxis of acute organ rejection …

1.2 Tacrolimus is recommended as an option when a calcineurin inhibitor is indicated as initial or maintenance immunosuppression … the relative appropriateness should reflect the importance of their different side effect profiles in different patients.

1.3 Mycophenolate mofetil is not recommended in combination with calcineurin inhibitors for the prophylaxis of rejection in renal transplantation … however, it is recommended in cases of severe adverse reactions to calcineurin inhibitors and substitution of an alternative immunosuppressant.

1.4 Sirolimus is not recommended in combination with calcineurin inhibitors for the prophylaxis of rejection in renal transplantation. It is recommended as an option in cases of severe adverse reactions to calcineurin inhibitors **and mycophenolate mofetil** [author's emphasis] necessitating withdrawal of these treatments and substitution of an alternative immunosuppressant.'

There are a number of points worthy of discussion. Firstly the drugs basiliximab and dacluzimab are both CD25-receptor blocking antibodies. They have both been discussed in the previous edition of this book,[2] and have been recommended by both NICE and the BTS consensus document. It would seem that their clinical effectiveness and their cost-effectiveness are in little doubt, and it is likely that we shall see continued growth of their routine use in renal transplantation. The relative cost of the two drugs may also dictate the amount of use each gets in the future. Basiliximab is administered in two × 20-mg doses, with a cost of £1680 (British National Formulary, 48th edn), and daclizumab is typically administered in five doses costing £3600 (British National Formulary, 44th edn).

The second recommendation regarding tacrolimus (recommendation 1.2) clearly recognises that the data show that using tacrolimus is associated with a reduction of the incidence of acute rejection. According to NICE's own pharmaco-economic analysis tacrolimus is indeed a cost-effective treatment. Neither NICE nor the BTS consensus have stated that tacrolimus is the preferred of the two CNIs, although again this author feels that this may be the case (see above).

In very stark contrast to the growing (and now majority practice) in the USA the use of MMF is not supported for de novo treatment but kept in reserve. It is to be hoped that this recommendation will be reviewed to allow tailored immunosuppression. This author certainly believes that the evidence for the routine discontinuation of CNIs after 3–6 months is growing in strength, and it may be that this is the sort of long-term study that might be best pursued in an investigator-led, prospective, randomised trial.

SUMMARY

The use of immunosuppression continues to change and evolve. This chapter has not attempted to address the issues surrounding some of the newer immunosuppressants, such as Myfortic, Certican, Everolimus, FTY720, Campath-1H or FK778, to name but a few. But even for the current spectrum of immunosuppressive drugs, the way that we use them and the combinations that we utilise are continuously changing. There is little doubt that there is a growing emphasis on individualising immunosuppression in a way that reflects the unique combination of every graft and recipient, and their changing clinical circumstances. Finally, the aim of preserving optimum graft function for as long as possible is now gaining considerable impetus. In this respect, the publication by Hariharan et al.[57] has yielded some highly illustrative findings. For this analysis, data were taken from all 256 renal transplant units in the USA, and their data reported to the UNOS (United Network for Organ Sharing) database. The analysis included 105 742 renal transplants undertaken between 1988 and 1998. This paper has a number of very in-depth analyses of renal function and its effect on late graft survival. Perhaps most striking are the values calculated for expected median graft half-life in relation to the serum creatinine at 12 months. Some of these values are reproduced in **Table 5.10**.

Table 5.10 • The calculated graft half-life in relation to serum creatinine after 1 year

1-year creatinine (mg/dL)	Calculated half-life (years)
<1.0	30.7
1.1–1.5	25.8
1.6–2.0	15.4
2.1–2.5	9.0
2.6–3.0	5.8
>3.0	2.8

From Hariharan S, McBride MA, Cherikh WS et al. Post-transplant renal function in the first year predicts long-term kidney transplant survival. Kidney Int 2002; 62:311–18, with permission.

These data emphasise most powerfully that our aim should not be just '1-year graft survival', but that our focus should be on achieving long-term graft survival that will maintain good function and minimise drug-related morbidity. Our current drugs may allow us to do that, and the newer entrants to the clinical field (but not yet licensed) may also help in that aim. The next 3–5 years are likely to see yet further changes in the story of immunosuppression.

• **Key points**

- In renal transplantation, tacrolimus is now a viable and effective alternative to ciclosporin.
- In liver transplantation, tacrolimus is now regarded as the baseline immunosuppressant of choice in many UK centres.
- Tacrolimus has a beneficial effect on cardio-vascular risk profile.
- Monitoring ciclosporin with C_2, and achieving adequate C_2 targets can significantly reduce acute rejection.
- De novo CNI-free protocols have now been validated, but data are still early.
- Cessation of CNIs for chronic allograft neph-ropathy is possible with either mycophenolate or sirolimus.
- CNI elimination protocols may be associated with a slight risk of acute rejection.
- In the majority of studies, the elimination of CNIs is associated with improvement in renal allograft function.

REFERENCES

1. Parrott NR. Immunosuppression: 'The old and the new'. In: Forsythe J (ed.) Transplantation surgery, 1st edn. London: WB Saunders, 1997, 89–121.

2. Parrott NR. Immunosuppression: 'What's new?' In: Forsythe J (ed.) Transplantation surgery, 2nd edn. London: WB Saunders, 2001.

3. Pirsch J, Miller J, Deierhoi M et al. A comparison of Tacrolimus (FK506) and cyclosporine for immunosuppression after cadaveric renal trans-plantation. Transplantation 1997; 63:977–83.

4. Mayer AD, Dmitrewski J, Squifflet JP et al. Multi-centre randomised trial comparing Tacrolimus (FK506) and cyclosporine in the prevention of renal allograft rejection. A report of the European Tacrolimus Multicentre Renal Study group. Transplantation 1997; 64:436–43.

5. Vincenti F, Jensik SC, Filo RS et al. A long-term comparison of Tacrolimus (FK506) and cyclosporine in kidney transplantation: evidence for improved allograft survival at five years. Transplantation 2002; 73:775–82.

   This presents the 5-year follow-up data from the pivotal phase III study comparing ciclosporin with tacrolimus, and shows significant advantages in tacrolimus that are evident at this time interval.

6. Mayer AD for the European Tacrolimus Multi-center Renal Study. Four year follow up of the European Tacrolimus Multicenter Renal Study. Transplant Proc 1999; 31(suppl. 7A):27S–28S.

7. Mayer AD for the European Tacrolimus Multi-center Renal Study Group. Chronic rejection and graft half-life; five year follow-up of the European Tacrolimus Multicenter Renal Study. Transplant Proc 2002; 34:1491–2.

   This is the European counterpart to ref. 5, and demon-strates significant improvement in calculated graft half-life in tacrolimus-treated patients.

8. Jurewicz A. Tacrolimus versus ciclosporin immuno-suppression: long term outcome in renal transplan-tation. Nephrol Dial Transplant 2003; 18(suppl. 1): i7–i11.

   A large, single-centre randomised study with 6 years of follow-up demonstrating superior outcomes in renal recipients treated with tacrolimus.

9. Margreiter R for the European Tacrolimus vs Ciclosporin Microemulsion Renal Transplantation Study group. Efficacy and safety of Tacrolimus compared to ciclosporin microemulsion in renal transplantation: a randomised multicentre study. Lancet 2002; 359:741–6.

   This is the pivotal European multicentre, randomised study comparing ciclosporin microemulsion with tacrolimus.

10. Trompeter R, Filler G, Webb NJA et al. Randomised trial of Tacrolimus versus cyclosporin microemulsion in renal transplantation. Pediatr Nephrol 2002; 17:141–9.

11. Pichlmayr R, Winkler M, Neuhaus P et al. Three year follow up of the European Multicentre Tacrolimus (FK506) Liver Study. Transplant Proc 1997; 29:2499–502.

12. Wiesner RH. Long term comparison of Tacrolimus versus Cyclosporine in liver transplantation. Transplant Proc 1998; 30:1399–400.

13. O'Grady JG, Burroughs A, Hardy P et al. and the UK and Republic of Ireland Liver Transplant Study Group. Tacrolimus versus microemulsified ciclo-sporin in liver transplantation: the TMC randomised controlled trial. Lancet 2002; 360:1119–25.

14. Mentzer RM, Jahania MS, Lasley RD. Tacrolimus as a rescue immunosuppressant after heart and lung transplantation. The US Multicenter FK506 Study Group. Transplantation 1998; 65:109–13.

15. Pham SM, Kormos RL, Hattler BG et al. A prospective trial of Tacrolimus (FK506) in clinical heart transplantation: intermediate term results. J Thorac Cardiovasc Surg 1996; 111:764–72.

16. Reichart B, Meiser B, Vigano M et al. European Multicenter Tacrolimus (FK506) Heart Pilot Group: One year results – European Tacrolimus Heart Study Group. J Heart Lung Transplant 1998; 17:775–81.

17. Taylor DO, Barr ML, Radovancevic B et al. A randomised, multicenter comparison of Tacrolimus and cyclosporine immunosuppressive regimens in cardiac transplantation: decreased hyperlipidaemia and hypertension with Tacrolimus. J Heart Lung Transplant 1999; 18:336–45.

18. Teebken OE, Struber M, Harringer W et al. Primary immunosuppression with Tacrolimus and mycophenolate mofetil versus cyclosporine and azathioprine in heart transplant recipients. Transplant Proc 2002; 34:1265–8.

19. International Neoral Renal Transplantation Study Group. Cyclosporin microemulsion (Neoral) absorption profiling and sparse-sample predictors during the first three months after renal transplantation. Am J Transplant 2001; 2:148–56.

20. Mahalati K, Belitsky P, Sketris I et al. Neoral monitoring by simplified sparse sampling area under the concentration-time curve: its relationship to acute rejection and cyclosporine nephrotoxicity early after kidney transplantation. Transplantation 1999; 68:55–62.

21. Mahalati K, Belitsky P, West K et al. Approaching the therapeutic window for cyclosporine in kidney transplantation: a prospective study. J Am Soc Nephrol 2001; 12:823–33.

22. Canadian Neoral Renal Transplantation Study Group. Absorption profiling of cyclosporine microemulsion (Neoral) during the first 2 weeks after renal transplantation. Transplantation 2001; 72:1024–32.

23. Thervet E, Pfeffer P, Scolari MP et al. Clinical outcomes during the first 3 months posttransplant in renal allograft recipients managed by C2 monitoring of cyclosporine microemulsion. Transplantation 2003; 76:903–8.

24. Keshavamurthy M, Al Ahmadi I, Mohammed Raza S. Single-centre study utilising C2 level as monitoring tool in de novo renal transplant recipients treated with Neoral. Transplant Proc 2001; 33:3112–14.

25. Maham N, Cardella C, Cole E. Optimization of cyclosporine exposure utilising C2 level monitoring in de novo renal transplant recipients. Transplant Proc 2001; 33:3098–9.

26. Cole E, Maham N, Cardella C et al. Clinical benefits of Neoral C2 monitoring in the long-term management of renal transplant recipients. Transplantation 2003; 75:2086–90.

27. Levy G, Thervet E, Lake J et al. on behalf of the Consensus on Neoral C^2 – Expert Review in Renal Transplantation (CONCERT). Patient management by Neoral C^2 monitoring: an international consensus. Transplantation 2002; 73(suppl. 9):S12–18.

    A key early consensus view from the USA on the value of ciclosporin C_2 monitoring.

28. Midtvedt K, Fauchald P, Bergan S et al. C2 monitoring in maintenance renal transplant recipients: is it worthwhile? Transplantation 2003; 76:1236–8.

29. Groth C. Sirolimus (rapamycin)-based therapy in human renal transplantation: similar effects and different toxicity compared with cyclosporine. Transplantation 1999; 67:1036–42.

    The first randomised prospective study using an entirely CNI-free regimen in renal transplantation.

30. Kreis H, Cisterne JM, Land W et al. for the Sirolimus European Renal Transplant Study Group. Sirolimus in association with mycophenolate mofetil induction for the prevention of acute graft rejection in renal allograft recipients. Transplantation 2002; 69:1252–60.

31. Flechner SM, Goldfarb D, Modlin C et al. Kidney transplantation without calcineurin inhibitor drugs: a prospective, randomised trial of Sirolimus versus cyclosporine. Transplantation 2002; 74:1070–6.

32. Rao V, Pirsch JD, Becker BN et al. Sirolimus monotherapy following Campath-1H induction. Transplant Proc 2003; 35(suppl. 3A):128S–30S.

33. Grimbert P, Baron C, Fruchaud G et al. Long-term results of a prospective randomised study comparing two immunosuppressive regimens, one with and one without CsA, in low risk renal transplant recipients. Transplant Int 2002; 15:550–5.

34. Stegall MD, Larson TS, Prieto M et al. Kidney transplantation without calcineurin inhibitors using Sirolimus. Transplant Proc 2003; 35:S125–7.

35. Hong JC, Kahan BD. A calcineurin antagonist-free induction strategy for immunosuppression in cadaveric kidney transplant recipients at risk for delayed graft function. Transplantation 2001; 71:1320–8.

36. Grinyo JM, Gil-vernet S, Cruzado JM et al. Calcineurin inhibitor-free immunosuppression based on antithymocyte globulin and mycophenolate mofetil in cadaveric kidney transplantation: results after 5 years. Transplant Int 2003; 16:820–7.

37. Gonwa T, Hricik DE, Brinker K et al. Improved renal function in Sirolimus-treated renal transplant patients after early cyclosporine elimination. Transplantation 2002; 74:1560–7.

38. Johnson RW, Kreis H, Oberbauer R et al. Sirolimus allows early cyclosporine withdrawal in renal transplantation resulting in improved renal function and lower blood pressure. Transplantation 2001; 72:777–86.

> One of the key early publications looking at the concept of using sirolimus as a ciclosporin substitute.

39. Oberbauer R, Kreis H, Johnson RW et al. Long-term improvement in renal function with Sirolimus after early cyclosporine withdrawal in renal transplant recipients: 2-year results of the Rapamune Maintenance Regimen Study. Transplantation 2003; 76:364–70.

40. Baboolal K for the UK and Ireland Rapamune Study group. A phase III prospective, randomised study to evaluate concentration-controlled Sirolimus (Rapamune) with cyclosporine dose minimisation or elimination at six months in de novo renal allograft recipients. Transplantation 2003; 75:1404–8.

41. Schrama YC, Joles JA, van To et al. Conversion to mycophenolate mofetil in conjunction with stepwise withdrawal of cyclosporine in stable renal transplant recipients. Transplantation 2000; 69:376.

42. Houde I, Isenring P, Boucher D et al. Mycophenolate mofetil, an alternative to cyclosporine A for long-term immunosuppression in kidney transplantation? Transplantation 2000; 70:1251–3.

43. Abramowicz D, Manas D, Lao M et al. Cyclosporine withdrawal from a mycophenolate mofetil-containing immunosuppressive regimen in stable kidney transplant recipients: a randomised, controlled study. Transplantation 2002; 74:1725–34.

44. Schneulle P, Van Der Heide JH, Tegzess A et al. Open randomised trial comparing early withdrawal of either Cyclosporine or Mycophenolate Mofetil in stable renal transplant recipients initially treated with a triple drug regimen. J Am Soc Nephrol 2002; 13:536–43.

45. Dominguez J, Mahalati K, Kiberd B et al. Conversion to Rapamycin immunosuppression in renal transplant recipients: reports of an initial experience. Transplantation 2000; 70:1244–7.

46. Diekmann F, Waiser J, Fritsche L et al. Conversion to Rapamycin in renal allograft recipients with biopsy-proven calcineurin inhibitor-induced nephrotoxicity. Transplant Proc 2001; 33:3234–5.

47. Saunders RN, Bicknell GR, Nicholson ML. The impact of cyclosporine dose reduction with or without the addition of rapamycin on functional, molecular, and histological markers of chronic allograft nephropathy. Transplantation 2003; 75:772–80.

48. Stallone G, Di-Paolo S, Schena A et al. Early withdrawal of cyclosporine A improves 1-year kidney structure and function in Sirolimus-treated patients. Transplantation 2003; 75:998–1003.

49. Ojo A, Meier-Kriesche HU, Hanson JA et al. Mycophenolate mofetil reduces late renal allograft loss independent of acute rejection. Transplantation 2000; 69:2405–9.

> A much-quoted paper that analyses the US renal transplant database of 67 000 patients, and concludes that mycophenolate has an independent effect on long-term allograft function.

50. Meier-Kriesche HU, Steffen BJ, Hochberg AM et al. Mycophenolate mofetil versus azathioprine therapy is associated with a significant protection against long-term renal allograft function deterioration. Transplantation 2003; 75:1341–6.

51. Weir MR, Ward MT, Blahut SA et al. Long-term impact of discontinued or reduced calcineurin inhibitor in patients with chronic allograft nephropathy. Kidney Int 2001; 59:1567–73.

52. McGrath JS, Shehata M. Chronic allograft nephropathy: prospective randomised trial of cyclosporin withdrawal and mycophenolate mofetil or Tacrolimus substitution. Transplant Proc 2001; 33:2193–5.

53. Ducloux D, Motte G, Billerey C et al. Cyclosporin withdrawal with concomitant conversion from azathioprine to mycophenolate mofetil in renal transplant recipients with chronic allograft nephropathy: a 2 year follow-up. Transplant Int 2002; 15:387–92.

54. Dudley CRK on behalf of the MMF 'Creeping Creatinine' Study Group. MMF substitution for CSA is an effective and safe treatment of chronic allograft dysfunction; results of a multi-centre randomised controlled study. Am J Transplant 2002; 2(S3):41.

55. British Transplantation Society. Consensus statement on the use of immunosuppression in renal transplantation. http://www.bts.org.uk

> The BTS standards document that is essential for all readers.

56. National Institute for Clinical Excellence. Appraisal Consultation Document: Immunosuppressive therapy for renal transplantation. www.NICE.org.uk

57. Hariharan S, McBride MA, Cherikh WS et al. Post-transplant renal function in the first year predicts long-term kidney transplant survival. Kidney Int 2002; 62:311–18.

> Very large analysis of the UNOS database, and another often-quoted study, which shows the very powerful influence of graft function at 1 year as a predictor of long-term renal allograft survival.

Six
The donor procedure

Lorna P. Marson

Optimisation of potential donors has become a focus for the transplant community in the face of increasing demand for organs and falling supply. This chapter aims to provide a practical outline of issues surrounding the donor procedure. Areas that will be explored are:

- the concept and physiology of death confirmed by brainstem testing;
- the management of the potential donor.
- criteria for donor selection;
- the surgical technique of organ procurement;
- recent advances in strategies to improve organ donation rates such as non-heart-beating donation and live donation;
- the problems associated with organ injury during procurement, storage and implantation;
- the potential for minimising such damage with advances in organ preservation.

DEATH CONFIRMED BY BRAINSTEM TESTING

The majority of organ donors are patients in intensive care units (ICUs) who have sustained irreversible brain damage for a variety of reasons, including intracerebral haemorrhage, cerebrovascular accident or head injury. The final common pathway is the diagnosis of brainstem death, a concept that has evolved over recent years.

Death is defined as the irreversible loss of capacity for consciousness and the irreversible loss of the capacity to breathe. Neither consciousness nor breathing can be sustained without a functioning brainstem, although understanding of the physiology involved has evolved over the years, with a profound impact on solid organ transplantation.[1] Prior to this, attempts to define death progressed through various stages, involving clinical findings and specific investigations. Initial work focused on the absence of response to electrical stimuli, with negative scalp electroencephalography (EEG) undertaken 18–24 hours following unsuccessful resuscitation resulting in the diagnosis of death.[2] This was followed by the definition of 'coma dépassé', characterised by loss of all reflex and neurological electrical activity.[3] Other investigations that have been adopted in an attempt to define brain death are cerebral angiography, with evidence of cerebral circulatory arrest or 'blocked cerebral circulation';[4] radioisotope techniques, aimed at assessing cerebral blood flow by non-invasive means;[5] computed tomography (CT) and cranial Doppler ultrasound scanning.

The Harvard Committee of 1968 sought to define irreversible coma as a new criterion for death, and listed a number of clinically based criteria, as outlined in **Box 6.1**.[6] The Committee warned of the pitfalls of hypothermia and drug intoxication but

Box 6.1 • Harvard criteria for irreversible coma

1. Unreceptivity and unresponsivity.
2. No movements (observe for 1 hour).
3. Apnoea (3 minutes off ventilator).
4. Absence of elicitable reflexes.
5. 1968: isoelectric EEG of 'great confirmatory value'.

1969: EEG 'not essential'.

Box 6.2 • Minnesota criteria for brainstem death

1. Known but irreparable intracranial lesion.
2. No spontaneous movement.
3. Apnoea (4 minutes).
4. Absent brainstem reflexes.

All findings unchanged for at least 12 hours.

did not specify the context in which the diagnosis of irreversible coma could be made.

The Minnesota criteria emerged when two neurosurgeons challenged contemporary thinking by focusing on the central role played by the brainstem in diagnosis of death. They suggested that irreversible brainstem damage was the point of no return and represented the infratentorial consequences of catastrophic supratentorial events.[7] The novelty of their approach was based on:

1. the requirement for definition of aetiology;
2. the explicit emphasis on the brainstem;
3. the recognition that if the signs of brainstem death were met, the value of an EEG was questionable.

The Minnesota criteria form the basis of the code that has subsequently developed in the UK for the diagnosis of brainstem death, and they are outlined in **Box 6.2**.

The UK code for the diagnosis of brainstem death emphasised the importance of context, stating that strict preconditions must be met before the diagnosis could be made.[8] This forms the basis of current practice in the UK, which involves three steps:

1. preconditions
2. exclusions
3. clinical tests.

Preconditions

The following preconditions must be met before making a diagnosis of brainstem death:

- The patient must be comatose and on a ventilator.

- A positive diagnosis of the underlying cause of coma must have been made.
- The patient must have been ventilated for long enough to determine that irremediable brain damage has been sustained.
- Rigorous efforts to reverse injury must have been made, including surgery where appropriate, optimisation of cerebral perfusion and management of cardiovascular instability.
- In order to ensure that sufficient time passes between onset of injury and diagnosis of brainstem death, there is a suggested interval prior to testing of 6–24 hours from time of last intervention aimed at reversing injury.

Exclusions

The following conditions or treatments delay or prevent a diagnosis of brainstem death from being made:

- Drug or alcohol intoxication requires a delay that is appropriate to the half-life of the drug. For example, 6–8 hours must elapse following alcohol ingestion before confirmation of brainstem death can be undertaken.
- Neuromuscular blocking agents used in many ICUs must also be allowed to clear prior to testing.
- Primary hypothermia, and metabolic and endocrine disturbances are all exclusions.
- It is worth reiterating that coma of unknown aetiology also represents a contraindication to the diagnosis of brainstem death.

Clinical testing

Having established the preconditions and excluded any of the circumstances outlined above, clinical tests must be performed.[9] These demonstrate absent brainstem reflexes and total apnoea. The comment published in the British Medical Journal in 1981 is worthy of note, that 'the doctor is not withdrawing treatment and allowing someone to die, but ceasing to do something useless to someone who is already dead'.[10]

The clinical tests must be performed by two medically qualified personnel who should be senior medics. It is suggested that a period of 2–3 hours should elapse between two sets of tests.

Once brainstem death has been confirmed (**Box 6.3**) the death certificate may be issued; the time of death can be quoted as the time of the first tests.

PHYSIOLOGY OF BRAINSTEM DEATH

Brainstem death is accompanied by significant disturbances in cardiovascular, respiratory and metabolic functions. These occur uniformly in all patients with a dead brainstem, regardless of aetiology.

Box 6.3 • Brainstem death tests

Absent brainstem reflexes

- No papillary response to light.

Potential pitfalls: atropine, topical mydriatic agents.

- Absent corneal reflexes.
- Absent vestibulo-ocular reflexes: caloric tests with 20 mL cold water, with no eye movement within 1 min of completion.
- No motor response to adequate stimulation in cranial nerve distribution.
- No gag reflex or reflex response to bronchial stimulation by suction catheter.

Apnoea testing

- No attempt to breathe despite a P_aCO_2 >6.65 kPa (50 mmHg). Hypoxia must be avoided by preoxygenation with 100% oxygen for 10 minutes.

Potential pitfalls: use of neuromuscular blocking agents and patients with previous respiratory disease such as chronic obstructive pulmonary disease or acute lung pathology.

Cardiovascular disturbances

Raised intracranial pressure results in the Cushing triad of:

1. hypertension: in an attempt to maintain cerebral perfusion pressure;
2. bradycardia: as a result of parasympathetic stimulation and in response to baroreceptor stimulation;
3. alterations in breathing patterns.

Unopposed sympathetic stimulation, or 'autonomic storm', lasts between minutes and hours and results in tachycardia, hypertension, hyperthermia and increased cardiac output. The degree of this stimulation depends on the speed of onset of brainstem death: if it is slow, adrenaline (epinephrine) levels increase 200-fold with resultant ischaemia of 23% of the myocardium; rapid onset results in increased adrenaline levels of 1000-fold with ischaemia of 93% of myocardium.[11]

ASSOCIATED ECG CHANGES

Five distinct changes in the ECG following brainstem death have been described in animal model systems:[12]

1. sinus bradycardia;
2. sinus tachycardia;
3. ventricular ectopics;
4. sinus tachycardia with resulting ischaemia;
5. sinus rhythm with ischaemic changes.

CHANGES IN PERIPHERAL VASCULATURE

There is severe vasoconstriction, with a shift to capacitance vessels, leading to increased venous return to the right heart and increased pulmonary artery pressure. Left ventricular dysfunction leads to elevated left atrial pressure and further increases in pulmonary pressure. This gives rise to capillary wall disruption with fluid leakage and pulmonary oedema.[13]

Following the period of sympathetic stimulation, there is loss of autonomic regulation with resultant hypotension and vasodilation. This is accompanied by reduced myocardial inotropic performance due to severe catecholamine depletion and intrinsic myocardial injury, and results in hypoperfusion to all organs.

Metabolic and hormonal changes

Brainstem death results in a shift from aerobic to anaerobic metabolism, evidenced by a reduction in pyruvate, glucose and palmitate utilisation. The hormonal changes observed following brain death fall into two categories: those associated with the autonomic storm, which represent a transient and massive increase in catecholamines as outlined above; and those associated with hypothalamic–pituitary dysfunction leading to neurogenic diabetes insipidus and a marked decrease in circulating levels of thyroid hormones and cortisol. The development of diabetes insipidus contributes to the hypotension that is almost universally observed, leading to a profound diuresis, with resultant electrolyte imbalance, including hypocalcaemia, hypomagnesaemia and hypophosphataemia. Decreased levels of antidiuretic hormone (ADH; vasopressin) seem to have far-reaching consequences. Patients who develop diabetes insipidus prior to brainstem death are frequently treated with desmopressin, an ADH analogue with minimal pressor activity. However, several investigators have demonstrated improved haemodynamic status in response to arginine vasopressin infusions, with reduction in inotropic requirements in these patients.[14] These findings suggest an intrinsic and crucial contribution of ADH to the maintenance of haemodynamic integrity of the system.

Alterations in thyroid hormone levels following brainstem death have evoked significant interest. Decreased levels of triiodothyronine (T_3) and thyroxine (T_4) have been documented, and some groups have shown that administration of T_3 is associated with increased rates of aerobic metabolism and a reduction in lactate and free fatty acids, products of anaerobic metabolism.[15] Such work has not been universally supported.[16]

Hypothermia is a consistent feature of brainstem death. This is likely to be due to loss of thermal regulation by the central nervous system as well as heat loss by radiation and convection in the critically ill patient. Effects of hypothermia include decreased renal concentrating abilities and a cold diuresis

and a shift of the oxygen dissociation curve to the left, causing decreased oxygen delivery to tissues and local ischaemia. Myocardial consequences of hypothermia include arrhythmias, cardiovascular instability and eventually cardiac arrest.

Coagulopathy is common, with as many as 88% of patients developing disseminated intravascular coagulation after coagulation cascade activation and factor consumption. This occurs secondary to the massive tissue thromboplastin release that accompanies severe neurological injury.

THE MANAGEMENT OF THE DONOR

Following establishment of brainstem death, the goals of patient management alter dramatically from preserving life to optimising the function of specific organs for transplantation.

Strategies for management of potential organ donors

CARDIOVASCULAR SUPPORT

In addition to the cardiovascular disturbances that occur as a consequence of brainstem death (as outlined above), management interventions such as volume depletion and mannitol therapy aimed at minimising intracranial pressure prior to diagnosis of brainstem death may leave the donor hypotensive and inotrope-dependent.

Fluid resuscitation guided by central venous monitoring or even pulmonary artery catheter placement is mandatory. The aims of therapy are to minimise the need for inotropic support but maintain systolic arterial blood pressure greater than 90–100 mmHg. Colloids or crystalloids may be used with the aim of achieving a central venous pressure of 9–12 mmHg. Glucose-containing fluids should be avoided, in order to prevent hyperglycaemia and subsequent osmotic diuresis. Use of a pulmonary artery catheter is indicated for evaluation in thoracic organ donation or where there are coexisting medical conditions in the donor such as valvular disease, cardiomyopathy, severe lung disease or persistent hypotension.

Inotropic support is indicated in hypotension that is resistant to fluid replacement. There has been some debate about the use of inotropes, with inconclusive data regarding the impact of donor pretreatment using vasopressors. A recent study of Registry data has suggested a role for inotropic agents independent of their positive effect on haemodynamic stability, with a reduction in rates of acute rejection in transplants from donors treated with catecholamines.[17] Other centres discourage the use of inotropes due to concerns about catecholamine-induced cardiomyopathy and reduced blood flow to vital organs, possibly resulting in ischaemic injury to the very organs that are intended for transplant.[18] In general, low doses of dopamine (<7.5 µg/kg/min) are used safely, with need for further support guided by invasive monitoring.

RESPIRATORY SUPPORT

The goals for management of the respiratory system are:

1. to ensure adequate oxygen delivery;
2. to maintain acid–base balance;
3. to achieve optimal lung function if these organs are to be transplanted.

The aims of management are to maintain:

1. inspired fraction of oxygen (F_iO_2) at <50%;
2. peak inspiratory pressures of <30 cmH$_2$O with tidal volumes of 15 mL/kg;
3. peak end-expiratory pressures (PEEP) of <5 cmH$_2$O.

Excessive PEEP levels are to be avoided in order to decrease the incidence of barotrauma and maintain venous return to the heart.

MANAGEMENT OF HYPOTHERMIA

Active measures must be taken to prevent heat loss and to rewarm the patient when required. Strategies include use of warm intravenous fluids and ventilating lungs with warmed, humidified air. A temperature of >35°C is the aim.

MANAGEMENT OF METABOLIC AND HORMONAL DISTURBANCES

Treatment of diabetes insipidus requires judicious fluid replacement; hypernatraemia may be aggravated by infusion of large volumes of sodium-containing colloid solutions during resuscitation. Boluses of vasopressin may cause dose-dependent vasoconstriction with potential damage to the organs to be transplanted. Continuous low-dose infusion of the synthetic preparation DDAVP (1-D-amino-8-D-arginine vasopressin) reduces urine output in brainstem-dead donors and is preferred as it has greater potency, less pressor activity and greater duration of action than the natural hormone.[19]

Evidence suggests that certain potential donors may benefit from treatment with a 'hormone replacement package', consisting of T$_3$, cortisol and insulin, which may lead to a reduction in inotrope requirements and improvement in donor status. This may bring about improved transplant survival.[20]

A more recent retrospective study demonstrated improved early graft function following heart transplant with administration of a three-drug hormonal resuscitation treatment in the donor. This included a methylprednisolone bolus and infusions of vasopressin and either triiodothyronine or L-thyroxine.[21]

Defects in coagulation and electrolyte imbalances should be treated with specific replacement therapy, based on frequent laboratory measurements.

CRITERIA FOR DONOR SELECTION

The ideal donor is a young, previously healthy individual who has sustained a fatal injury or suffered a cerebrovascular accident. However, the widening gap between organ demand and supply has led to a relaxation of the criteria for donor selection. The transmission of disease from a donor to a recipient is an undesirable consequence of transplantation and the few absolute contraindications (**Box 6.4**) to organ donation are directed towards preventing such an outcome.

Box 6.4 • Absolute contraindications for organ donation

- Evidence of HIV or active hepatitis B infection
- Presence or history of extracranial malignancy
- Severe systemic sepsis
- Disease of unknown aetiology

History of an intracranial malignancy is not a contraindication for organ donation as the majority of such tumours rarely metastasise outside the central nervous system.

Careful donor selection is required in these cases, as there is evidence that some CNS tumours do spread extracranially in 0.5–2.3% of cases. Risk factors for spread include high-grade tumours, those treated with chemotherapy, and violation of the blood–brain barrier by previous interventions such as craniotomy or shunt formation.[22]

Metastatic disease is commonest in adults with glioblastomas and in children with medulloblastomas, and these groups should thus be excluded as organ donors.[23] The risk of tumour transmission should be weighed against the risk of the patient dying on the waiting list without a transplant. A recent population-based analysis quantified the risk of having a donor with undiagnosed malignancy as 1.3% and the risk of transmission of such malignancy from donor to recipient as 0.2%.[24] Other malignancies that do not preclude organ donation are low-grade skin tumours or cervical carcinoma in situ.

Another major concern is the risk of transmission of infection from the donor into an immunosuppressed recipient. Particularly dangerous infections that precede the terminal illness include active hepatitis B (hepatitis B surface antigen positive), human immunodeficiency virus (HIV), encephalitis of unknown cause, Creutzfeldt–Jakob disease and active tuberculosis. Any evidence of these illnesses in the history or rapid serological tests should classify the potential donor as high risk and may preclude donation.

A more controversial issue relates to patients found to be hepatitis C (HCV) positive. Some groups have suggested that the high risk of HCV transmission means that such donors are unacceptable. However, others are prepared to consider transplanting organs from HCV-positive donors because the slowly progressive nature of the infection means that such infection does not have a major impact on graft or patient survival. Alternatively, HCV-positive organs may be transplanted into HCV-positive recipients. There is concern that a more virulent genotype may be transmitted to the recipient but the evidence for this is weak.

Cytomegalovirus (CMV) can be transmitted to a previously uninfected recipient and may produce a serious primary infection. With the current availability of effective antiviral agents such as ganciclovir and valganciclovir, allocation of an organ from a CMV-positive donor to a CMV-negative recipient is now accepted practice.

The more difficult category of infections to evaluate involves conditions that complicate the terminal care of the donor. Any potential donor with severe systemic sepsis is eliminated from consideration especially if the causative organism is not defined. In contrast, localised infections, such as a chest infection, catheter- or line-related sepsis, even in the presence of positive blood cultures, have not been found to transmit bacterial infections to recipients treated with appropriate antibiotics.

The selection criteria for organ donation depend upon:

- the organ to be transplanted;
- size of recipient waiting list;
- individual circumstances of the potential recipients;
- preferences of transplant centre.

After the diagnosis of brainstem death has been made and consent for organ procurement has been given, a number of baseline investigations should be performed. A blood sample is taken for determination of blood group, tissue type, cytotoxic crossmatch and virology. Where there has been significant transfusion in the donor, a search should be carried out for a pretransfusion sample on which to carry out virology testing. Careful review of the clinical findings coupled with results of routine laboratory and radiological investigations is usually adequate for assessment of the potential donor. A history of intravenous drug abuse and previous therapy with human pituitary growth hormone or other pooled human CNS-derived products are regarded as contraindications to organ donation in most units. Selection criteria for specific organs are outlined in **Box 6.5**.[25]

ORGAN PROCUREMENT TECHNIQUE

Liaison between the donor hospital and the organ procurement teams is provided by the transplant

Kidney

- No evidence of primary renal disease
- No history of longstanding hypertension or diabetes
- Normal urinalysis
- Urine output >0.5 mL/kg/h
- Normal urea and creatinine

Liver

- Age 0–75 years
- History of excessive alcohol consumption may be difficult to assess; inspection of the liver for fatty infiltration is useful

Heart

- Age 0–65 years
- No previous history of heart disease
- Normal electrocardiogram
- Relative contraindications:
  – use of high inotrope doses
  – prolonged hypotension
  – chest trauma
  – prolonged cardiac arrest (>30 min)

Lung

- Age 0–60 years
- No previous history of lung disease
- Normal chest X-ray
- Satisfactory gas exchange ($P_aO_2 > 50$ kPa (370 mmHg) on 100% O_2) with 5 mmHg positive end-expiratory pressure

Pancreas

- Age 10–45 years
- No history of diabetes mellitus
- Relative contraindications:
  – gross obesity
  – peripheral vascular disease
  – ischaemic heart disease

coordinator. Often the procedure occurs at hospitals that are infrequently involved in the process and it is crucial that teams adopt a courteous and considerate approach. Establishment of regional organ procurement teams is helpful in reducing the number of staff attending the procurement operation and in standardising donor management and operative protocols.

Surgical technique for procuring organs from cadaveric donors was first described by Starzl and colleagues.[26] There is considerable variation in tech-

nique and the techniques described are typical of those used. Before starting the procedure, antibiotic prophylaxis is given along with a neuromuscular blocking agent to prevent spinal reflexes.

Procurement of liver and kidneys

PREPARATION

The donor is in the supine position with neck extended and arms by the side. The skin is prepared from the neck to suprapubic region with antiseptic solution. A midline incision is made from xiphisternum to the pubic symphysis and a thorough laparotomy is performed to exclude any concomitant pathology, such as neoplasm and infection. Unexpected lesions should be sent for immediate frozen section.

On completion of the laparotomy the incision is extended upwards towards the root of the neck, to facilitate exposure as shown in **Fig. 6.1**. Following protection of the liver with a large pack, the sternum is divided in the midline. Opening of the pericardium ensures adequate thoracic exposure. The caecum

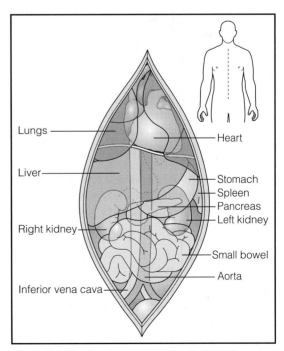

Figure 6.1 • Incision to expose abdominal and thoracic organs.

and right colon are mobilised to expose the aortic bifurcation. The small bowel is lifted superiorly to expose the inferior mesenteric vein, allowing preparation of these two vessels for cannulation.

The liver is mobilised by dividing the right and left triangular ligaments. Careful examination is performed to exclude aberrant hepatic arterial anatomy. Such variations are common: a single hepatic artery arises from the coeliac trunk in about 75% of the population.

The commonest aberrations are:

- accessory right artery arising from the superior mesenteric artery and passing posterior to the portal vein at the porta hepatis;
- accessory left artery arising from the left gastric artery; the accessory left artery then joins the coeliac trunk.

These should be carefully dissected to their origin and included on a common aortic patch.

Dissection at the porta should be carried out as low down as possible. The bile duct is divided and the gallbladder opened and washed out. Finally, the aorta at the level of the diaphragm is isolated. At this stage the thoracic organs are dissected.

PERFUSION

Having ensured that all members of the team are ready for perfusion, the donor is given 20 000 IU heparin intravenously. Perfusion cannulas are inserted and carefully secured into the distal abdominal aorta and inferior mesenteric vein. The ascending aorta is cross-clamped and cold perfusion is started through the aortic and portal cannulas, as shown in **Fig. 6.2**. Approximately 2 litres of organ preservation solution are perfused through each cannula. The inferior vena cava is vented by dividing it in the mediastinum. The abdomen is filled with ice-cold saline to aid surface cooling of the liver and kidneys and removal of the heart and lungs is completed.

REMOVAL OF LIVER

Once the liver is cooled with approximately 1 litre of preservation fluid, the post-perfusion dissection can be performed. The arterial attachments of the liver are divided, with careful dissection back to their origin on the aorta. Care must be taken to

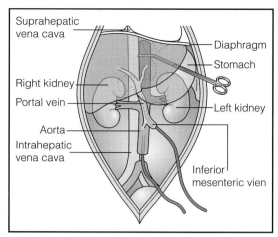

Figure 6.2 • Cannulation of abdominal aorta and inferior mesenteric vein in preparation for perfusion.

preserve the origin of the renal arteries. The suprahepatic inferior vena cava is divided during cardiectomy and the infrahepatic inferior vena cava is divided just above the origin of the renal veins. Finally, the portal vein is divided, preserving maximal length, and the liver is removed and immersed in cold storage solution.

There is some evidence to suggest that perfusion via the portal venous and aortic systems is unnecessary and that perfusion of the liver by the aortic route alone is sufficient.[27]

A prospective randomised study undertaken to examine the effectiveness of aortic-only perfusion for flush-preservation of the liver found that this was as effective as combined aortic and portal perfusion in terms of liver temperature and early graft function.[28]

Back table perfusion of liver

After removal, the portal vein and hepatic artery are flushed with a further 250–500 mL of preservation solution. The bile duct is also flushed and the liver is submerged in cold preservation fluid in a sterile container. Bile is deleterious and should be washed out. Two or three polythene bags are used to pack the liver, which is then stored in ice.

REMOVAL OF KIDNEYS

Simultaneous with the back table work on the liver, the kidneys are excised. The ureters are dissected with as long a length as possible, leaving adequate

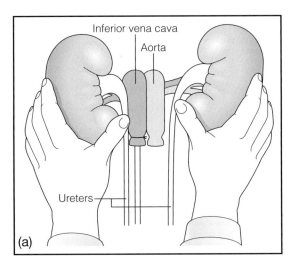

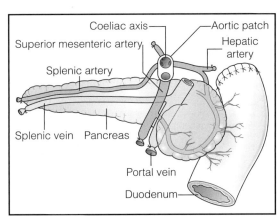

Figure 6.4 • Excision of pancreas with aortic patch.

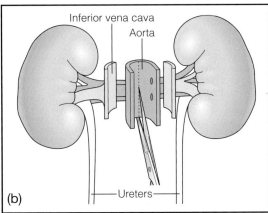

Figure 6.3 • **(a)** En bloc dissection of kidneys.
(b) Separation of kidneys prior to excision.

tissue around them to preserve their blood supply. Care should be taken to preserve the renal arteries on an aortic patch. Once the vascular anatomy of the kidney has been displayed, they can then be separated in situ and removed individually, as shown in **Fig. 6.3**. After having been perfused on the back table with a further 100–200 mL of preservation solution, the kidneys are packed in sterile bags containing cold preservation solution and transported in ice.

Procurement of pancreas

The pancreas is usually retrieved in conjunction with the liver. The blood supply of a pancreatico-duodenal graft is from the coeliac trunk and superior mesenteric artery. Priority is usually given to the liver, so that if there is an aberrant right hepatic artery arising from the superior mesenteric artery close to the aorta, pancreatic transplantation may be more problematic.

In addition to the dissection required for liver retrieval, the duodenum and head of pancreas are mobilised from the right and the spleen and head of pancreas from the left side. The common hepatic artery is dissected proximally to identify the source of the splenic artery. Excision of the pancreas with an aortic patch is shown diagrammatically in **Fig. 6.4**. Overperfusion of the pancreas is undesirable and, after aortic perfusion with 1 litre of preservation fluid, the splenic artery and superior mesenteric arteries are gently occluded and liver and kidney perfusion continued.

After hepatectomy, the duodenum is stapled and divided at the level of the pylorus and third/fourth part. The remaining attachments to the small bowel and transverse colon are divided. The graft is then removed.

BACK TABLE PREPARATION OF THE PANCREAS

Reconstruction of the vascular anatomy is performed at the recipient centre, illustrated in **Fig. 6.5**. The spleen is removed after ligating and dividing the splenic vessels. The distal parts of the splenic artery and superior mesenteric artery are ligated and the proximal ends anastomosed to the internal and external arteries, respectively, of an iliac bifurcation graft obtained from the donor. Thus the common

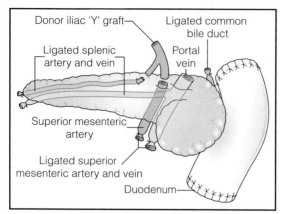

Figure 6.5 • Reconstruction of arterial supply to pancreas graft using donor iliac artery.

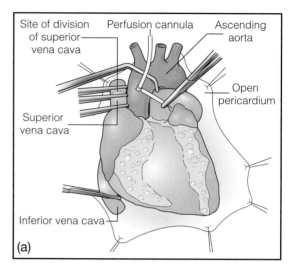

(a)

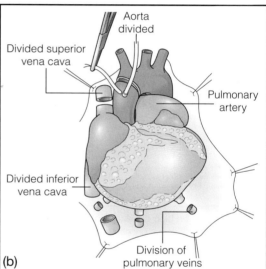

(b)

Figure 6.6 • **(a)** Excision of heart with cannulation of major vessels. **(b)** Division of major vessels prior to excision of heart.

iliac artery becomes the single conduit for supplying blood to the graft. For more detail see Chapter 9.

Heart procurement

After completing the initial dissection of the abdominal organs, the pericardium is opened and the heart examined to confirm its suitability for transplant. The ascending aorta and superior vena cava are mobilised and a perfusion catheter is inserted into the anterior wall of the ascending aorta for the administration of cardioplegia solution. The superior vena cava is then ligated and divided. The ascending aorta is cross-clamped and the cardioplegia solution infused, resulting in cardiac arrest. The left and right heart are emptied via incisions in the left pulmonary veins and inferior vena cava respectively (**Fig. 6.6a**). The heart is excised by dividing all its major vascular attachments (**Fig. 6.6b**).

Procurement of lungs

Preparation of the lungs for procurement is similar to that of the heart with an additional perfusion cannula inserted into the pulmonary artery to perfuse the lungs. After cardioplegia, the left heart is vented via the tip of the atrial appendage rather than via one of the pulmonary veins (**Fig. 6.7**). The lungs are ventilated manually and, just before excision, the endotracheal tube is pulled back and the trachea stapled and divided above the staple line to keep the lungs inflated during storage and transport.

Completion of procurement

On completion of removal of the organs, a portion of spleen and mesenteric lymph nodes is excised for the purpose of tissue typing and crossmatching. In addition, the iliac vessels are excised and preserved for formation of conduits if necessary. Care must be taken to ensure that blood is removed from the body cavity prior to careful closure of the wound with a continuous suture.

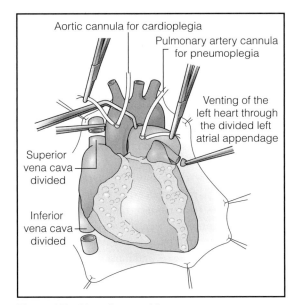

Aortic cannula for cardioplegia

Pulmonary artery cannula for pneumoplegia

Venting of the left heart through the divided left atrial appendage

Superior vena cava divided

Inferior vena cava divided

Figure 6.7 • Heart–lung excision.

Stress associated with organ retrieval

The very nature of the procurement process means that it is associated with tragic death and specific individual circumstances that may be difficult to cope with. Work to date has focused on the impact of this on donor hospital staff. The development of specific liaison nurses between donor hospitals and transplant units has attempted to address this problem. The impact of repeated participation in organ retrievals on individuals within the team has not been addressed and is the subject of ongoing study in the UK. Strategies to manage stress in this group are being investigated in an attempt to minimise staff attrition and to encourage junior surgeons into a career in transplant surgery.

STRATEGIES TO INCREASE ORGAN DONATION

The number of patients on the waiting list for transplantation has increased dramatically over the last two decades and has far outstripped the number of available organs from brainstem-dead donors. Thus, alternative sources of organs have been sought, including 'marginal donors' such as the elderly or diabetics, living donors and donors without a heartbeat.

Marginal donors

The pressure to enlarge the donor pool has prompted the inclusion of cadaveric donors who would previously have been excluded because of advanced age or coexisting illness. The effect of donor age on transplant outcome is controversial, with some studies suggesting an increased risk of organ failure with increasing donor age whilst other groups report good outcomes. Some investigators propose that organs from older cadaveric donors should be allocated to donors at higher risk, defined as those undergoing repeated transplantation, with a high level of sensitisation, older patients, or ones with a poor HLA mismatch (for kidneys).

Recent data suggest that kidneys from donors between the ages of 60 and 74 years can be successfully transplanted provided that less than 15% of glomeruli are shown to be sclerotic on biopsy. An alternative strategy is to transplant two kidneys into a single recipient, thus providing a larger nephron mass.[29,30] Data on the short- and long-term survival of liver transplants from older donors have been encouraging.[31]

Living donation

One potential strategy for overcoming the organ shortage is to develop well-organised living donor programmes for kidney and liver transplants. There is significant expertise in the UK in living donor renal transplantation and it is likely that this will be extended more widely in liver transplantation in the near future. Live donor renal transplantation offers many advantages to the recipient, including the ability to perform the transplant as an elective procedure and reduced incidence of delayed graft function and rejection with improved patient and graft survival figures. But this must be balanced against the risks of donation, including the potential for donor death and serious postoperative complications. The focus of this section will be to investigate different techniques of the donor operation; a more detailed overview of living donation is provided in the previous edition of this book.[32]

Until 1995, living donation was performed exclusively through an open surgical approach, requiring a large incision and resection of the 12th rib, often resulting in significant donor morbidity, including incisional hernia and pneumothorax. With the demonstration of reduced postoperative pain, shorter hospitalisation and quicker recuperation following laparoscopic nephrectomy for disease compared with an open procedure,[33] laparoscopic living donor nephrectomy was introduced into surgical practice in an attempt to reduce morbidity and thus remove a disincentive to organ donation. Laparoscopic nephrectomy now accounts for 31% of live donor procedures in the USA, with 65% of centres offering the procedure.[34] Similar trends have not been seen in the UK, suggesting a greater reluctance to adopt this technique.

There are various techniques of open and laparoscopic donor nephrectomy. Open techniques are performed through either a standard flank incision (which may involve resection of the 12th rib) or an anterior incision, which demands a transperitoneal approach.

Laparoscopically, the operation may be performed via a transperitoneal or extraperitoneal approach. The transperitoneal approach, first adopted by Ratner et al.,[35] is the most commonly used technique. Subsequent developments include the use of a hand-port with certain benefits: it is learnt more quickly by surgeons with less laparoscopic experience and is associated with shorter operating and renal warm ischaemia times.[36,37]

Several studies have investigated the role of laparoscopic donor nephrectomy but there is only one randomised controlled trial comparing hand-assisted laparoscopic and open surgical techniques. The open surgery did not involve rib resection, a factor that has been cited as important in contributing to postoperative pain. The study demonstrated a reduction in analgesia use and hospital stay in the laparoscopic group, with a more rapid return to normal activity, including work, compared with open surgery.[38]

Initial concern regarding increased rate of ureteric complications[39] has not been borne out,[40] but it is worthy of note that there is a learning curve for surgeons developing this technique and that centres

introducing laparoscopic donor nephrectomies may benefit from inviting an experienced guest surgeon to assist in the early stages.

There is wide variation in attitude to living donation across Europe: in Norway approximately 40% of all transplants are from living donors but in France and Germany living donors account for between 2% and 17%. In some centres, introduction of laparoscopic techniques has coincided with increased donor rates,[41,42] but centres performing open surgery claim similarly increased rates of donation.[43] The real impact of laparoscopic surgery on donor rates remains uncertain.

Living donation has been reported for liver, lung, small intestine and pancreas. Living donor liver transplantation is the second most common form of living donor transplant after kidneys. The use of living donors for liver transplantation has been adopted in Japan and the USA,[44,45] but there is not yet an established programme for residents of the UK. Partial hepatectomy is a more hazardous procedure than a unilateral nephrectomy, compounding the ethical and moral dilemma facing the transplant team. Chapter 8 contains a detailed discussion of living donor liver transplantation.

Non-heart-beating donation

During the past decade renewed interest in organ donation after declaration of death by cardiopulmonary criteria has developed because of the potential for increasing the supply of organs for transplantation. Successful long-term results following kidney transplant have led to the development of non-heart-beating donor programmes for use of other organs, including liver, pancreas and lung.

RENAL TRANSPLANTATION

A successful programme of transplantation from donors without a heartbeat could increase the number of kidneys by 30%.[46] By definition a donor without a heartbeat has had a prolonged period of hypotension (lasting several minutes) followed by cardiac arrest before organ procurement. Insufficient perfusion or complete lack of perfusion of such organs was thought to cause irreversible damage, resulting in poor short- and long-term graft survival. There is little doubt that rates of delayed graft function are increased in non-heart-beating donors, caused by acute tubular necrosis, as reported in 50–80% of such transplants.[47]

However, initial concerns about long-term function have not been borne out, with recent case–control studies demonstrating no significant differences in 5-year[48] and 10-year[49] survival of grafts from donors with and without a heartbeat. One finding of concern in a recent study performed by the Leicester group is that at 2 and 5 years, the serum creatinine was significantly higher in the non-heart-beating donor group compared with those with a heartbeat,[48] suggesting that not all of the ischaemic damage is reversible.

Comparison of results of non-heart-beating donation between groups is complicated by lack of clear definition of selection criteria. Kootstra and colleagues described four categories of non-heart-beating donor – the Maastricht categories[50] – shown in **Box 6.6**.

Controlled donations are typically from an ICU and result in short and precisely defined warm ischaemic times as effective cardiopulmonary resuscitation is instituted quickly. Uncontrolled donations, usually from Accident and Emergency departments, arise as a result of sudden and unexpected deaths. By their very nature these tend to have suffered more poorly defined but generally longer warm ischaemic times.[48] The decision to donate must strictly follow and be independent of the decision to withdraw treatment. In these circumstances, organ preservation must be initiated prior to obtaining permission from the family.

Box 6.6 • Maastricht categories

'Uncontrolled' categories
I Patients found dead in the field
II Patients that expire during resuscitation

'Controlled' categories
III Patients with near-fatal head injuries, who are unlikely to become brain dead, and in whom a terminal wean is indicated
IV Patients who suffer a fatal cardiac arrest while brain dead

Ethical issues still constitute one of the main hurdles to wider acceptance of non-heart-beating donation. Definition of the appropriate period of time that should elapse between 'life' and 'death' prior to commencement of the procurement procedure, to eliminate the possibility of spontaneous respiratory effort, is one of the key issues and varies between protocols from 2 minutes (Pittsburgh) to 10 minutes (Maastricht). Development of standardised protocols in this area is important because public concern is likely to have a detrimental effect on all organ donation rates.[51]

Criteria for non-heart-beating donation for kidneys are: age less than 60 years; warm ischaemic time without effective cardiopulmonary resuscitation of less than 40 minutes; and an interval between insertion of aortic balloon and procurement of less than 2 hours. Contraindications are patients with known renal disease, uncontrolled hypertension, complicated diabetes mellitus, systemic sepsis or malignancy.[48]

TECHNIQUE OF RENAL PROCUREMENT FROM NON-HEART-BEATING DONORS

Once the patient is declared dead, external cardiac massage and mechanical ventilation are continued.

In order to minimise the detrimental effects of warm ischaemia, kidneys are cooled to less than 15°C, at which temperature the metabolic rate of the kidney will be 10% of normal. This is achieved by insertion of a double-balloon triple-lumen catheter into the abdominal aorta, as shown in **Fig. 6.8**, to perfuse the kidneys with cold hyperosmolar citrate. This perfusion is continued until the time of retrieval.

Providing consent is obtained within 2 hours of commencement of infusion a midline laparotomy is performed. Outside this time, the procedure is abandoned because of theoretical risk of bacterial translocation from the gut causing contamination and because of prolonged ischaemia. The kidneys are assessed for adequacy of perfusion by macroscopic appearances. Kidneys that appear well perfused are removed and preserved in cold storage.

LIVER TRANSPLANTATION

Historically the first liver transplants were performed using non-heart-beating donors, but function was

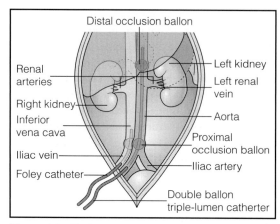

Figure 6.8 • Perfusion of non-heart-beating kidney donor.

less than optimal because of inadequacy of perfusion, immunosuppression and postoperative management. The area has been revisited because of organ shortage, although the number of liver transplants performed from non-heart-beating donors remains relatively small. Between 1993 and 2001, the UNOS database recorded only 191 such liver transplants. Major concerns with the use of such organs centred around reportedly higher rates of primary non-function and hepatic artery thrombosis than with heart-beating donors.[52–54] A more recent retrospective evaluation of outcome following liver transplants from non-heart-beating donors compared with heart-beating donors demonstrated similar rates of graft and patient survival at 1 and 3 years but a significantly higher rate of biliary complications, resulting in multiple interventional procedures, re-transplantation and death.[55] Such complications are likely to be related to ischaemic injury and stricture formation, and the authors urged caution in the use of such grafts.

ORGAN PRESERVATION

Organs for transplantation undergo a variable period of extracorporeal storage during which time they are transferred to the recipient centre and the recipient is prepared for surgery. The principles of organ preservation involve:

- intravascular flushing with chilled preservation fluid;

- hypothermic storage by placing the organ in plastic bags and immersing it in crushed ice in an isolated container until transplantation.

The purpose of organ preservation is to deliver to a recipient a viable graft that will exhibit primary function. Improvements in hypothermic preservation solutions allow extended preservation times, providing important logistic benefits including the institution of HLA-based kidney sharing across geographic boundaries. Static cold storage is an effective means of kidney preservation but increasing cold ischaemic time is associated with non-function of the liver[56] and delayed graft function in renal transplantation.[57] Recent UK Transplant data demonstrate that a cold ischaemic time of greater than 24 hours is associated with a significant delay in graft function in renal transplantation. The liver is less able to tolerate cold ischaemia, with a maximum storage time of 20 hours.

The effect of cold storage on organs

Hypothermic storage at 4°C dramatically reduces, but does not arrest, metabolic activity, by a factor of 1.5–2 for each 10°C fall in temperature. The cellular integrity of the donor organ steadily declines with inhibition of the ATPase-dependent sodium pump. Sodium ions, together with chloride and water, enter the cells causing cellular swelling. Inhibition of calcium–magnesium ATPase activity leads to an influx of calcium and depletion of magnesium in cells.[58] There is a switch from aerobic to anaerobic metabolism, resulting in the accumulation of end-products such as protons, lactate and breakdown products of adenine nucleotides (hypoxanthine). On reperfusion these by-products contribute to the generation of oxygen free radicals, which directly damage tissues and act to induce an acute inflammatory response known as ischaemia–reperfusion injury.[59] There is also direct damage from cold, with physical alterations in cellular membranes and consequent tissue damage.

Organ preservation fluids

To date, the development of preservation fluids has significantly extended cold ischaemic times, particularly for liver transplant, for which cold storage times of 12–18 hours are now possible compared with only 4–8 hours previously. Details regarding components of preservation solutions were given in the previous edition of this book and will not be repeated here.[60] In principle, the chemical composition of preservation fluids is similar to intracellular electrolytes. They all contain impermeants such as sucrose and raffinose, and large anions such as lactobionate or gluconate, which are included to provide osmotic forces and thus limit cell swelling. The other principal constituents are buffers such as citrate, phosphate or bicarbonate, which reduce intracellular acidosis. The preferred flush solution for multiorgan preservation in the majority of centres is University of Wisconsin (UW) solution, and the composition of this is shown in Table 6.1.

The development of solutions such as UW solution has had a major impact on cold storage times, but it is likely that the limits of conventional cold preservation have been reached and further expansion of transplantation will depend on new techniques. This is particularly true in light of the necessity of gaining access to an expanding donor pool to meet the increasing demands for organs, particularly with the use of marginal and non-heart-beating donors.

Table 6.1 • Composition of University of Wisconsin solution

Component	Composition (per litre)
Potassium lactobionate	100 mmol
Sodium phosphate	25 mmol
Magnesium sulphate	5 mmol
Adenosine	5 mmol
Allopurinol	1 mmol
Gluthione	3 mmol
Raffinose	30 mmol
Hydoxethyl starch	50 g
Insulin	100 U
Dexamethasone	8 mg
Potassium	135 mmol
Sodium	35 mmol
Osmolarity	320 mOsm

Organs from such donors are defined according to their risk of dysfunction in the context of current preservation solutions. If significant improvements could be made in preservation, a primary aspect of the risk would be removed, thus rendering such organs more amenable to transplantation.

In addition, current techniques do not allow assessment of organ function until after transplantation has taken place. The inability to assess viability markers during static cold storage is a major limitation in the context of marginal donor organs, particularly in liver and heart transplants. A number of potential strategies for minimising ischaemic injury with alternative techniques of organ preservation are being developed.

Hypothermic perfusion

An alternative to simple cold storage is continuous hypothermic perfusion, which involves a pulsatile pump and oxygenator. It was pioneered in the late 1960s at the University of Wisconsin and was used widely in the USA for storage of kidneys in the 1970s. Unlike simple cold storage, pulsatile machine preservation permits pharmacological manipulation of the perfusate and aids in pretransplant assessment of the graft. Viability markers include the enzyme glutathione S-transferase and measurement of flow/resistance in the circuit. Use of such machine perfusion has been associated with improved early and long-term renal function,[61] but given the short cold ischaemic times used in clinical practice, the cost and logistical problems of machine perfusion have ensured that it has been adopted in only a few centres. More recently, interest has renewed with increased use of marginal and non-heart-beating donors.

Additives to preservation solutions

Novel additives may result in improvements in ischaemia–reperfusion injury or allow longer preservation times. Several compounds are under development with this aim.

The superoxide anion free radical (O^{2-}) has been implicated in the pathogenesis of tissue injury consequent to ischaemia–reperfusion, and the enzyme superoxide dismutase has been used successfully to protect organs from structural damage during reperfusion. This is an enzyme scavenger of free radicals specific for superoxide that has been shown to reduce rates of acute and chronic rejection in a clinical trial, but without an effect on delayed graft function.[62]

Apoptosis, or programmed cell death, has been demonstrated to play a key role in ischaemia–reperfusion injury, with increased levels correlating with increasing cold ischaemic time.[63] Specific inhibitors of apoptosis have been demonstrated to inhibit activation of proapoptotic proteins Bax and p21 in a model of ischaemia–reperfusion injury. Other potentially interesting compounds aimed at limiting ischaemia–reperfusion injury are calcium channel blockers, as calcium accumulation is thought to be a key component of ischaemia–reperfusion injury by effects on mitochondrial function.[64,65]

Perfluorocarbons are hydrocarbon molecules in which hydrogen atoms are replaced by fluorine such that the resulting liquid is able to dissolve 25 times more oxygen than plasma at room temperature. Oxygen release is facilitated by a low oxygen-binding constant thus facilitating oxygen release to tissues. Storage by the two-layer method offers a simple means of supplying oxygen to explanted organs without the necessity for continuous perfusion equipment. Recent studies have utilised perfluorocarbons in the preservation of pancreas grafts using a two-layer method. Pancreas grafts are placed in a chamber containing perfluorocarbon and UW solution. The perfluorocarbon is lipophilic and has a higher density, resulting in separation of the two fluids, with the pancreas graft floating at the interface. Sufficient oxygen is then available from the perfluorocarbon solution to maintain ATP synthesis within the pancreas.[66]

Adoption of this technique by the Edmonton islet transplant group has demonstrated increased islet recovery and improved function from transplanted islets compared with simple UW storage.[67]

Organ modulation during cold ischaemia

The period of cold storage can also be used to modulate the graft in a variety of ways with the aim of altering the immune response or reducing

ischaemia–reperfusion injury. Blockade of potential targets such as the intercellular adhesion molecule-1 (ICAM-1) has been shown to reduce ischaemia–reperfusion injury in clinical trials.[68]

Normothermic perfusion

The problem central to cold storage is the failure to permit normal aerobic metabolism. Machine preservation of the organ at body temperature, normothermic perfusion, allows the maintenance of normal metabolism, thus minimising the accumulation of the substrates for free radical formation on reperfusion and allowing clearance of metabolites.[59] The technique has been applied in several animal models and in human renal transplantation. In the latter study, normothermic perfusion was associated with reduced rates of primary non-function and delayed graft function.[69] A further advantage of normothermic preservation is that of viability assessment. With a functioning organ, it should be possible to define and measure key functional parameters that correlate with post-transplant function.

Other areas of interest in the arena of organ preservation are organ preconditioning, with ischaemia or heat shock, which acts by regulation of apoptosis, and genetic modification of organs during preservation. Genetic transfer offers the possibility of delivering molecules with protective effects, such as adenoviral interleukin 10 (IL-10), Fas ligand and ICAM antisense, to the donor organ with the aim of modulating the graft. Such techniques will be possible only in the context of normothermic machine perfusion.

ORGAN DAMAGE DURING PROCUREMENT

During the course of transplantation, organs may be injured, resulting in delayed graft function or primary non-function, with potential long-term consequences for the graft and the patient. The main donor factors contributing to injury are the process of brain death and haemodynamic instability resulting from hypovolaemia or vasomotor collapse as outlined earlier in the chapter. Several factors associated with organ procurement also contribute to such damage, including cold storage time and implantation.[70]

Sources of injury in the donor

As described previously, the process of brain death triggers massive disruption of control mechanisms, associated with vasomotor collapse and disseminated intravascular coagulation (DIC). DIC occurs commonly following cranial trauma and results in thrombocytopenia and microthrombi in the tissues. Such DIC, coupled with loss of vasomotor control, is likely to result in significant tissue damage in the organs for procurement. The most severe changes are seen in the lungs and heart, rendering them unsuitable for transplantation earlier than other organs.[71]

Injury arising from procurement, preservation and implantation

PROCUREMENT

The process of procurement can give rise to direct vascular or parenchymal injury and to vasospasm. Tension upon or excessive handling of the vessels may contribute to such damage. The technique of 'en bloc' retrieval may reduce such trauma.

ISCHAEMIC TIME

Contributors to total ischaemic time are initial warm ischaemia (the period between clamping of the arterial supply and core cooling), cold ischaemic time (the time for cold storage and transport) and second warm ischaemia time (the time taken to perform the arterial and venous anastomoses prior to reperfusion). Initial warm ischaemia should be minimal in the context of en bloc procurement techniques. Cold ischaemic time will depend on a variety of factors, including distance travelled, organisation of theatres at the recipient centre and time for crossmatching. In the kidney, second warm ischaemia time (SWIT) of 30 minutes or less is associated with excellent initial function rates, whereas a SWIT of 60 minutes or more is more frequently associated with primary graft failure.[72,73] The net effect of such injury is donor endothelial cell damage, which becomes a potential trigger for inflammatory and immunological injury. This is highlighted by evidence from living donor programmes: living donor kidneys with extensive HLA mismatching have excellent graft survival, lacking the injury associated with brain death and prolonged ischaemia.

Pathogenesis of renal ischaemia–reperfusion injury

Although the nature of renal injury associated with brain death is complex, the resulting ischaemic injury is associated with widespread cell injury and decreased activity of the sodium–potassium ATPase pump. This results in an elevated intracellular calcium level, which appears to play a major role in the pathogenesis of cell injury, by inducing nitric oxide synthase and phospholipase A_2.

On return of blood flow to the kidney at reperfusion, further damage occurs. A major event with reperfusion is the interaction of neutrophils with endothelial cells of the organ, giving rise to an inflammatory response, production of preinflammatory cytokines and recruitment of cells of the innate immune system, such as macrophages. Such changes occur not only intraoperatively, with removal of clamps from renal vessels, but also in the donor prior to transplantation, in periods following resuscitation or after release of vasoconstrictive mediators, thus compounding the problem.[74]

Such an inflammatory response promotes immune recognition and makes immunological injury more likely. Immunological injury represents a further insult that can initiate a new injury response and a 'vicious cycle' ensues. Evidence for this in the clinical setting is that initial poor graft function increases the risk of both acute rejection and late graft loss.

SUMMARY

The success of solid organ transplantation has brought with it significant challenges in terms of overwhelming demand and limited organ supply. The importance of optimising management of all potential donors cannot be overestimated. Improvements in donor management, organ preservation and methods aimed at improving donor rates, such as use of marginal donors, live donors and non-heart-beating donors, are all strategies that can be adopted to meet the increasing demand for transplantation.

REFERENCES

1. Pallis C. Brain stem death: evolution of a concept. In: Morris P (ed.) Kidney transplantation, 5th edn. Philadelphia: WB Saunders, 2001:75–88.

2. Jouvet M. Electrosubcorticographic diagnosis of death of the central nervous system during various types of coma. Electroencephalogr Clin Neurophysiol 1959; 11:805.

3. Mollaret P, Goulon M. Le coma dépasse (mémoire preliminaire). Rev Neurol (Paris) 1959; 101:3–5.

4. Bergquist E, Bergstrom K. Angiography in cerebral death. Acta Radiol 1972; 12:283–8.

5. Goodman J, Mishkin F, Dyken M. Determination of brain death by isotope angiography. JAMA 1968; 209:1869.

6. Report of the Ad Hoc Committee of the Harvard Medical School to examine the definition of brain death. A definition of irreversible coma. JAMA 1968; 205:337–40.

7. Mohandas A, Chou S. Brain death: a clinical and pathological study. Neurosurgery 1971; 35:211.

8. Conference of Medical Royal Colleges and their Faculties in the United Kingdom. Diagnosis of brain death. BMJ 1976; 2:1187.

9. Wijdicks E. The diagnosis of brain death. N Engl J Med 2001; 344(16):1215–21.

10. Jennett B, Gleave J, Wilson P. Brain death in three neurosurgical units. BMJ 1981; 282:533.

11. Shivalkar B, Van Loon J, Wieland W et al. Variable effects of explosive or gradual increase of intra-cranial pressure on myocardial structure and function. Circulation 1993; 87(1):230–9.

12. Novitzky D, Wicomb W, Cooper D et al. Electro-cardiographic, haemodynamic and endocrine changes occurring during experimental brain death in the Chacma baboon. J Heart Trans 1984; 4:63.

13. Schroeder R, Kuo P. Organ allocation and donor management. In: Kuo PC, Schoeder R, Johnson L (eds) Clinical management of the transplant patient. London: Arnold, 2001; pp. 201–27.

14. Yoshioka T, Sugimoto H, Uenishi M. Prolonged haemodynamic maintenance by the combined administration of vasopressin and epinephrine in brain death: a clinical study. Neurosurgery 1986; 18:565–7.

15. Novitzky D, Cooper D, Reichart B. Haemodynamic and metabolic responses to hormonal therapy in brain-dead potential organ donors. Transplantation 1987; 43:852–4.

16. Karayalcin K, Umana J, Harrison J et al. Donor thyroid function does not affect outcome in orthotopic liver transplantation. Transplantation 1994; 57(5):669–72.

17. Schnuelle P, Berger S, de Boer J et al. Effects of catecholamine application to brain-dead donors on graft survival in solid organ transplantation. Transplantation 2001; 72:455–63.

18. Walpoth B, Barbalat F, Vitus L. Detrimental effect of endogenous and/or exogenous catecholamine stimulation on ischaemic myocardial tolerance and energetics. Heart Trans 1985; 4:606.

19. Pennefather S, Bullock R, Mantle D et al. Use of low dose arginine vasopressin to support brain-dead organ donors. Transplantation 1995; 59:58–62.

20. Wheeldon D, Potter C, Jonas M et al. Trans-plantation of 'unsuitable' organs. Transplant Proc 1993; 25:3104–5.

21. Rosendale J, Kauffman H, McBride M et al. Hormonal resuscitation yields more transplanted hearts, with improved early function. Transplantation 2003; 75:1336–41.

22. Buell J, Trofe J, Sethuraman G et al. Donors with central nervous system malignancies: are they truly safe? Transplantation 2003; 76(2):340–3.

   This important study from a well-respected surgical oncologist and transplant surgeon highlights the low but real risk of transmission of CNS malignancy from donor to recipient. Specific high-risk categories are stated.

23. Kauffman H, McBride M, Cherikh W et al. Transplant Tumor Registry: donors with central nervous system tumors. Transplantation 2002; 73:579–82.

24. Birkeland S, Storm H. Risk for tumor and other disease transmission by transplantation: a population-based study of unrecognized malignancies and other disease in organ donors. Transplantation 2002; 74:1409–13.

25. Akyol M, Bradley JA. Organ procurement and storage. In: Corson J, Williamson RC (eds) Surgery. London: Mosby, 2001; pp. 6.3.1–6.3.10.

26. Starzl TE, Hakala T, Shaw B. A flexible procedure for multiple cadaveric organ procurement. Surg Gynecol Obstet 1984; 158:223–30.

27. de Ville de Goyet J, Hausleithner V, Malaise J et al. Liver procurement without in situ portal perfusion. Transplantation 1994; 57:1328–32.

28. Chui A, Thompson J, Lam De et al. Cadaveric liver procurement using aortic perfusion only. Aust NZ Surg 1998; 68:275–7.

   This prospective randomised study was undertaken to examine the effectiveness of aortic-only perfusion for flush-preservation of the liver and showed aortic-only perfusion to be as effective as combined aortic and portal perfusion in terms of liver temperature and graft function.

29. Alfrey E, Lee C, Scandling J et al. When should expanded criteria donor kidneys be used for single versus dual kidney transplantation? Transplantation 1997; 64:1142–6.

30. Gridelli B, Remuzzi G. Strategies for making more organs available for transplantation. N Engl J Med 2000; 343(6):404–10.

31. Melendez H, Heaton N. Understanding 'marginal' liver grafts. Transplantation 1999; 68:469–71.

32. Lumsdaine J, Forsythe J, Lear P. Living donation (renal). In: Forsythe J (ed.) Transplantation surgery: current dilemmas, 2nd edn. London: WB Saunders, 2001; pp. 133–154.

33. Clayman R, Kavoussi LR, Soper NJ et al. Laparoscopic nephrectomy: review of the initial 10 cases. J Endourol 1992; 6(2):127.

34. Finelli F, Gongora E, Saaski T et al. A survey: the prevalence of laparoscopic nephrectomy at large US transplant centres. Transplantation 2001; 71:1862–4.

35. Ratner L, Ciseck LJ, Moore RG et al. Laparoscopic live donor nephrectomy. Transplantation 1995; 60(9):1047–9.

This is the first report of laparoscopic live donor nephrectomy, outlining the common transperitoneal approach.

36. Kercher K, Joels C, Matthews B et al. Hand-assisted surgery improves outcomes for laparoscopic nephrectomy. Am Surg 2003; 69(12):1061–6.

37. Lindstrom P, Haggman M, Waldstrom J. Hand-assisted laparoscopic surgery (HALS) for live donor nephrectomy is more time- and cost-effective than standard laparoscopic nephrectomy. Surg Endosc 2002; 16:422–5.

38. Wolf J, Merion R, Leichtman A et al. Randomized controlled trial of hand-assisted laparoscopic versus open surgical live donor nephrectomy. Transplantation 2001; 72:284–90.

This is the only prospective randomised trial comparing outcome following laparoscopic and open techniques for living donor nephrectomy and demonstrates a reduction in analgesia use, shorter hospital stay and earlier return to normal activity in the laparoscopic group.

39. Berends F, den Hoed P, Bonjer H et al. Technical considerations and pitfalls in laparoscopic live donor nephrectomy. Surg Endosc 2002; 16:893–8.

40. Lind M, Hazebroek E, Kirkels W et al. Laparoscopic versus open donor nephrectomy: ureteral complications in recipients. Urology 2004; 63(1):36–9.

41. Sasaki T, Finelli F, Bugarin E et al. Is the laparoscopic donor nephrectomy the new criterion standard? Arch Surg 2000; 135:943–7.

42. Shafizadeh S, McEvoy J, Murray C et al. Laparoscopic donor nephrectomy: impact on an established renal transplant program. Am Surg 2000; 66:1132–5.

43. Barry J. Laparoscopic donor nephrectomy: con. Transplantation 2000; 70:1546–8.

44. Yamaoka Y, Wahhida M, Honda K et al. Liver transplantation using a right lobe graft from a living related donor. Transplantation 1994; 57:1127–8.

45. Brown R, Russo M, Lai M et al. A survey of liver transplantation from living adult donors in the United States. N Engl J Med 2003; 348:818–25.

46. Sanchez-Fructuoso AI, Prats D, Torrente J et al. Renal transplantation from non-heart beating donors: a promising alternative to enlarge the donor pool. J Am Soc Nephrol 2000; 11:350–8.

47. Wijnen R, Booster M, Stubenitsky B et al. Outcome of transplantation from non-heart-beating donor kidneys. Lancet 1995; 345(8957):1067–70.

48. Metcalfe M, Butterworth P, White S et al. A case–control comparison of the results of renal transplantation from heart-beating and non-heart-beating donors. Transplantation 2001; 71:1556–9.

This case–control comparison of renal transplant function following heart-beating and non-heart-beating donation showed no significant difference in overall graft survival between the two groups, despite an increased rate of delayed graft function in the non-heart-beating group.

49. Weber M, Dindo D, Demartines N et al. Kidney transplantation from donors without a heartbeat. N Engl J Med 2002; 347(5):248–55.

50. Kootstra G, Daemen J, Oomen A. Categories of non-heart-beating donors. Transplant Proc 1995; 27:2893.

51. Muiesan P. Can controlled non-heart-beating donors provide a solution to the organ shortage? (Commentary). Transplantation 2003; 75:1627.

52. Casavilla A, Ramirez C, Shapiro R et al. Experience with liver and kidney allografts from non-heart-beating donors. Transplantation 1995; 59:197–203.

53. Gomez M, Garcia-Buitron J, Fernandez-Garcia A et al. Liver transplantation with organs from non-heart-beating donors. Transplant Proc 1997; 29:3478–9.

54. D'Alessandro A, Hoffman R, Knechtle S et al. Liver transplantation from controlled non heart-beating donors. Surgery 2000; 128:579–88.

55. Abt P, Crawford M, Desai N et al. Liver transplantation from controlled non-heart-beating donors: an increased incidence of biliary complications. Transplantation 2003; 75:1659–63.

56. Porte R, Ploeg R, Hansen B et al. Long-term graft survival after liver transplantation in the UW era: late effects of cold ischaemia and primary dysfunction. European Multicentre Study Group. Transplant Int 1998; 11(suppl. 1):164–7.

57. Morris P, Johnson R, Fuggle S et al. Analysis of factors that affect outcome of primary cadaveric renal transplantation in the UK. HLA Task Force of the Kidney Advisory Group of the United Kingdom Support Service Authority. Lancet 1999; 354:1147–52.

58. Macanulty J, Ametani M, Southard J et al. Effect of hypothermia on intracellular Ca^{2+} in rabbit tubules suspended in UW–gluconate preservation solution. Cryobiology 1996; 33:196–204.

59. McLaren AJ, Friend PJ. Trends in organ preservation. Transplant Int 2003; 16:701–8.

60. Attia MS, Prasad KR, Bellamy MC et al. Organ retrieval – fluids and techniques. In: Forsythe J (ed.) Transplantation surgery: current dilemmas, 2nd edn. London: WB Saunders, 2001; pp. 25–64.

61. Polyak M, Arrington B, Stubenbord W et al. The influence of pulsatile preservation on renal transplantation in the 1990s. Transplantation 2000; 69:249–58.

62. Land W, Schneeberger H, Schleibner S et al. The beneficial effect of human recombinant superoxide dismutase on acute and chronic rejection events in recipients of cadaveric renal transplants. Transplantation 1994; 57:211–17.

63. Burns A, Davies D, McLaren AJ et al. Apoptosis in ischaemia/reperfusion injury of human renal allografts. Transplantation 1998; 66:872–6.

64. Ramella-Virieux S, Steghens J, Barbieux A et al. Nifedipine improves recovery function of kidneys preserved in a high-sodium, low-potassium cold-storage solution: study with isolated perfused rat kidney technique. Nephrol Dial Transplant 1997; 12:449–55.

65. Sasaki S, Yasuda K, McCully J et al. Calcium channel blocker enhances lung preservation. J Heart Lung Transplant 1999; 18:127–32.

66. Kuroda Y, Hiraoka K, Tanioka Y et al. Role of adenosine in preservation by the two-layer method of ischaemically damaged canine pancreas. Transplantation 1994; 57:1017–20.

67. Lakey J, Tsujimura T, Shapiro A et al. Preservation of the human pancreas before islet isolation using a two-layer (UW solution-perfluorochemical) cold storage method. Transplantation 2002; 74:1809–11.

68. Haug C, Colvin R, Delmonico F et al. A phase I trial of immunosuppression with anti-ICAM-1 (CD54) mAb in renal allograft recipients. Transplantation 1993; 55:766–72.

69. Valero R, Cabrer C, Oppenheimer F et al. Normothermic recirculation reduces primary graft dysfunction of kidneys obtained from non-heart-beating donors. Transplant Int 2000; 13:303–10.

70. Halloran PF. Renal injury and preservation in transplantation. In: Racusen LC, Solez K, Burdick JF (eds) Kidney transplant rejection. New York: Marcel Dekker, 1998; pp. 149–76.

71. Pratschke J, Wilhelm M, Kusaka M et al. Brain death and its influence on donor organ quality and outcome after transplantation. Transplantation 1999; 67:343–8.

72. Halloran PF, Aprile M, Farewell V. Factors influencing early renal function in cadaver kidney transplants: a case-control study. Transplantation 1988; 45:122–7.

73. Lennard T, Parrott N, Wilson R et al. Primary non-function after renal transplantation: a prospective multifactorial analysis of possible causes in 106 consecutive transplants. Transplant Proc 1988; 20(3):439–41.

74. Land W, Messmer K. The impact of ischaemia/reperfusion injury on specific and non-specific, early and late chronic events after organ transplantation. Early events. Transplant Rev 1996; 10:108–27.

Seven

Renal transplantation in the third millennium

Benjamin E. Hippen and
Robert S. Gaston

INTRODUCTION

At first glance, this assigned topic appears too broad to be addressed in a meaningful fashion. An author might either shy away from the enormity of the subject or choose to trivialise it with irrelevant observations. However, we have chosen to accept the challenge by offering an overview of the current state of renal transplantation, with an eye towards the future. While it reflects our own uniquely American experience, we are hopeful our insights will prove to be of interest elsewhere as well.

Kidney transplantation exploded onto the scene in the second half of the 20th century, the culmination of remarkable advances in surgical technique, pharmacology, and immunological understanding. In a very brief period, the early successes in transplanting identical twins evolved into what is now unquestionably the treatment of choice for most patients with irreversible kidney failure, applied routinely worldwide. In the meantime, liver, heart, small bowel and pancreas transplantation were spawned as offshoots, and immunological discoveries as primitive as histocompatibility antigens and as advanced as lymphocyte trafficking mechanisms were stimulated. Without kidney transplantation, Hitchings and Elion might have applied their enormous intellect to other fields.[1] Jean Borel might have put aside ciclosporin as just another poorly effective antibiotic.[2] In his autobiography, *Surgery*

of the Soul, Nobel laureate Joseph E. Murray mused:

> *There were those who dismissed the [twin transplants] as a one-in-a-million occurrence and not something that would add greatly to the store of medical knowledge. They argued, correctly, that there would be very few identical twins ... so this advance would not benefit the majority of patients with renal failure. But in my view they failed to understand that this was just the first step.*[3,4]

Indeed. Entering the new millennium, we gratefully acknowledge the role of Professor Murray and his contemporaries in successfully surmounting numerous obstacles that impeded the advance of clinical renal transplantation. However, new challenges are emerging that provide equally worthy challenges to current and upcoming generations of transplant professionals.

KIDNEY TRANSPLANTATION: THE TREATMENT OF CHOICE FOR END-STAGE RENAL DISEASE

As recently as a decade ago, it was possible to debate the best treatment option for patients with end-stage renal disease (ESRD). Such innovations as recombinant erythropoietin and biocompatible membranes dramatically reduced the comorbidity associated with chronic haemodialysis. Peritoneal dialysis offered relative freedom from dietary restrictions and thrice-weekly visits to dialysis units. Although the overall mortality rates for those on dialysis appeared stable, given a substantially older patient population, outcomes were clearly improving.[5–8] Transplantation, despite its life-enhancing qualities, was haunted by complications associated with toxic, inadequate immuno-suppression, including rejection, osteonecrosis, opportunistic infections and cancer.[9] Almost half of deceased donor kidneys were lost within 3 years after engraftment (Table 7.1). Rennie's 1978 contention that a kidney transplant was merely a 'temporary respite' from dialysis remained an accurate, if depressing, assessment.[10]

In the last decade, advances in transplantation have increasingly shifted the debate over optimal ESRD treatment from an open question to an established conclusion. After a decade of stagnant graft survival rates, the statistical half-life of allografts began improving in 1988, and, by 1996, had almost doubled, to 13.5 years for deceased donor kidneys and even longer for those from live donors.[11] While still associated with substantial morbidity, new options in maintenance immuno-suppression lessened rejection rates and reliance on corticosteroids, reducing complications after trans-plantation.[12] In the USA, where the Social Security Amendments of 1972 had made payment for ESRD therapy an entitlement for most of the population, transplantation proved substantially less expensive than maintenance dialysis.[13,14] Finally, a new statistical approach has made it possible to compare dialysis outcomes with transplantation outcomes, an analysis previously difficult due to a bias in modality selection. Recent studies have confirmed a survival benefit of transplantation relative to maintenance dialysis for virtually all ages and

Table 7.1 • Evolution in deceased donor transplant outcomes at the University of Alabama at Birmingham, 1968–2003

Years	Immunosuppression	N	Graft survival (%)	
			1-year	3-year
1968–83	Azathioprine Corticosteroids	500	54	42
1984–86	Ciclosporin Corticosteroids	497	65	52
1987–94	ALG/OKT3 Ciclosporin Azathioprine Corticosteroids	1503	78	66
1995–98	OKT3 Ciclosporin/tacrolimus Mycophenolate mofetil Corticosteroids	499	90	81
1998–2003	Daclizumab/ALG Ciclosporin/tacrolimus Mycophenolate mofetil Corticosteroids	749	93	82

ALG, antilymphocyte globulin; OKT3, anti-CD3 antibody.

categories of patients with ESRD.[15] Ironically, longevity on dialysis is now considered a major risk factor for graft loss: those patients transplanted earliest in the course of ESRD experience the best outcomes.[16–18]

Why such a significant change in favour of renal transplantation? More sensitive crossmatch techniques have made donor–recipient compatibility easier to determine.[19] Twenty years ago, the immunosuppressive armamentarium included only polyclonal antilymphocyte globulins (useful for only the short term), azathioprine (relatively ineffective) and large doses of corticosteroids. An improved understanding of the immunobiology of rejection has produced agents with greater specificity and less toxicity.[20] Under current immunosuppressive protocols, fewer than 25% of patients now experience acute rejection, and immunological graft losses are uncommon (at least early after transplantation).[12,21,22] Recent data indicate that quality and stability of renal function (as reflected in the serum creatinine) in the early post-transplant period is a strong predictor of long-term graft survival.[23] Current immunosuppression is associated with unprecedented preservation of renal function.[24] Immunosuppressive complications have become both less common and more manageable. Improved antiviral, antibacterial and antifungal agents have lessened morbidity and mortality due to infections. Moreover, the adoption of prophylactic and pre-emptive approaches to antimicrobial therapies has reduced the incidence of serious infections among transplanted patients, even in the face of more potent immunosuppression.

In a programme whose cost already exceeds all previous projections, Medicare expenditures on ESRD, at $13.8 billion/year in 2000, are estimated to rise to $28 billion/year by 2010, a fact that influences policy-making in the USA.[8,25] Providing care for the average dialysis patient costs Medicare $54 000 annually. Those costs increase to $107 000 in the year a transplant is performed, then decline thereafter to approximately $10 000 per annum. Thus, a graft surviving 2.5–3 years (true in at least 80% of cases) is the most cost-effective way to treat ESRD.[26] Current US statutes mandate transplant evaluation for all ESRD patients.

Dialysis patients, on average, have 20–25% of the life expectancy of healthy, age-matched controls.[8]

While transplant recipients remain at greater risk of cardiovascular and infectious deaths than the general population, transplantation confers a substantial reduction in mortality relative to remaining on dialysis.[27] A recent report indicates that risk of death from common malignancies (lung, breast, colon, etc.) is nearly identical among those on dialysis and those with functioning transplants.[28] While the risk of dying in the perioperative period exceeds that of a wait-listed patient on dialysis, mortality risks decline over time, equalising after about 3 months. After that time, the transplanted patient is less likely to die, and life expectancy with a deceased donor transplant ultimately is about twice that of remaining on dialysis.[15] In the USA, 70% of patients with ESRD are currently undergoing dialysis. However, of those patients living at least 10 years with ESRD, 70% have functioning allografts.[8] Kidney transplantation saves lives, a recently recognised fact that is increasingly understood by patients with ESRD.

Today, the superiority of transplantation over dialysis in improving both the quantity and quality of life is no longer controversial. The challenges facing the next epoch of transplantation are in many ways products of its success, and will be the subject of the remainder of this chapter.

SUPPLY AND DEMAND: MAKING TRANSPLANTATION MORE ACCESSIBLE

Millennial predictions are usually ill-advised, regardless of subject. The best-known millennialists offer dramatic forecasts of the apocalypse to come, often at the expense of facts. Yet, it is difficult to examine the future of renal transplantation without concern, if not alarm, regarding the growing disparity in numbers between available kidneys and patients in need of them. Current successes are diminished by the knowledge that such life-changing therapies will be available to a smaller and smaller fraction of patients who might benefit. The disparity between supply and demand in transplantable kidneys is the single greatest challenge to be faced in the new millennium.

In 2002, 8540 deceased donor kidney transplants and 6230 living donor kidney transplants were

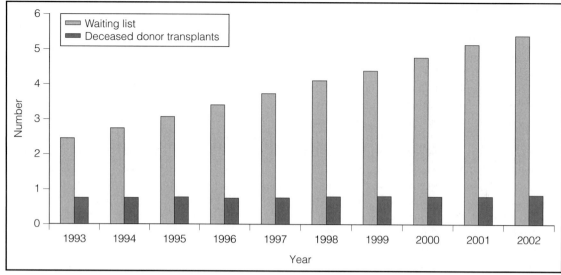

Figure 7.1 • Trends in deceased donor transplantation in the USA, 1993–2002 (actual numbers on *y* axis × 10 000). During this period, the number of patients on the waiting list doubled, while available kidneys increased by approximately 1% per year. From Gaston RS, Alveranga DY, Becker BN et al. Kidney and pancreas transplantation. Am J Transplant 2003; 3(suppl. 4):64–77, with permission from Blackwell Publishing Ltd.

performed in the USA.[29] At present, there are over 56 000 patients in the USA awaiting a renal transplant (**Fig. 7.1**). The US Renal Data System documented a point prevalence of 373 000 patients with ESRD in 2000.[8,30] Approximately a quarter of these have functioning renal transplants, leaving 269 000 prevalent patients on dialysis. Using these proportions as a baseline, approximately 20% of patients with ESRD on dialysis are currently on the waiting list for a renal transplant, and approximately 20% of the patients listed (or 3% of the ESRD population) will be transplanted with a deceased donor kidney on an annual basis. Xue and colleagues projected the number of patients with ESRD in the USA to approach 650 000 by the year 2010, and the transplant waiting list to exceed 100 000 patients.[25] Consider the following extrapolation:

100 000 patients on waiting list × 20% transplanted = 20 000 deceased donor renal transplants annually = 4% of the projected ESRD population.

In short, to **maintain** the current rate of transplanting only 3–4% of the projected ESRD population, annual numbers of deceased donor renal transplants must increase by approximately 220% over the next 7 years. Such numbers, if realised, would severely tax current resources, far exceeding current capacities of transplant centres, surgeons and physicians.[31,32]

Past performance does not always predict future trends, but current data do not portend a dramatic upsurge in the number of deceased donor renal transplants.[33] As seen in **Fig. 7.2**, the sluggish growth in the number of deceased donor kidneys over the past decade contrasts with a dramatic increase in the number of living donors. Indeed, these trends already indicate that, for any individual ESRD patient, the best opportunity for timely transplantation resides in availability of a living donor. By all indications, short-term growth in transplant numbers will remain heavily dependent on living donation. For patients without a living donor, the prospects for transplantation are increasingly grim, with a lengthening waiting period now measured in years.[8]

As noted earlier, extended time waiting on dialysis exacts a toll. Although receipt of a renal transplant, even one of marginal quality,[15,34] confers a significant mortality benefit compared with remaining on dialysis, the progression of cardiovascular morbidity while on dialysis translates into inferior allograft[17] and patient[35] survival. Utilising multivariate analysis, Meier-Kriesche and co-workers demonstrated that any length of time on dialysis results in inferior graft

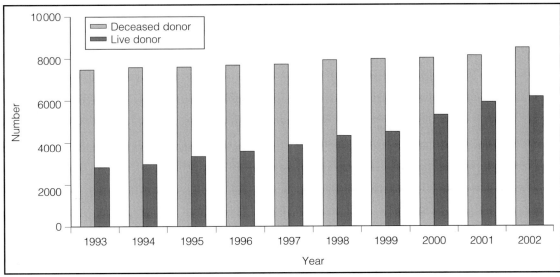

Figure 7.2 • Kidney transplants performed in the USA, 1993–2002, by donor source. In contrast to the sluggish growth in deceased donor transplants, kidneys from living donors almost tripled during the decade. From Gaston RS, Alveranga DY, Becker BN et al. Kidney and pancreas transplantation. Am J Transplant 2003; 3(suppl. 4):64–77, with permission from Blackwell Publishing Ltd.

outcomes when compared with pre-emptive transplantation.[17] Annual mortality on the waiting list is 11% for diabetics, and 6% for non-diabetics,[15,34] meaning that a substantial number of patients will die awaiting transplantation. Currently, a 'low-risk' patient without diabetes who is less than 65 years of age at the time of listing has a greater than 30% chance of death before transplantation.[36]

In the USA the increasing gap between demand and supply is felt disproportionately among minorities, particularly Native and black Americans. The incidence of ESRD among black Americans is four times that of white Americans. This minority group comprises only 13% of the US population, but accounts for 37% of all patients on dialysis. Black Americans receive only 25% of deceased donor kidneys and 14% of kidneys from living donors.[37] In addition, black Americans are likely to suffer a lengthier wait for transplantation than other patients. These numbers reflect the impact of many variables, including later referral for transplant evaluation, a higher frequency of ABO blood types associated with longer waiting times, greater presensitisation, and difficulty matching the donor population.[37]

Recent data indicate that a new class of patients is emerging with claims on the kidney supply. Recipients of extrarenal transplants are developing renal insufficiency with alarming frequency (**Fig. 7.3**).[38] Within 36 months of transplantation, 17% of such patients had a glomerular filtration rate of 29 mL/min or less, and one-third of these had developed ESRD. This new variant of renal insufficiency reflects a combination of pre-existing kidney disease and the nephrotoxicity associated with chronic calcineurin inhibitor (CNI) use. As the number of extrarenal transplants increases, the demand for subsequent (or concurrent) renal transplantation in these patients will further exacerbate the gap between demand and supply.

An outgrowth of these trends is greater attention to the composition and management of the waiting list, factors that are influenced by whatever allocation algorithm is implemented.[39] The purpose of the waiting list is to define patients that are medically suitable for transplantation when an organ becomes available. An allocation system that emphasises HLA matching requires all listed patients to be 'ready' to receive a kidney at any time. In the USA, algorithms are increasingly based on waiting time rather than match grade, requiring only those patients with the longest time on the list to be 'ready' at any given time. Thus, lengthening waiting times require periodic re-evaluation of a

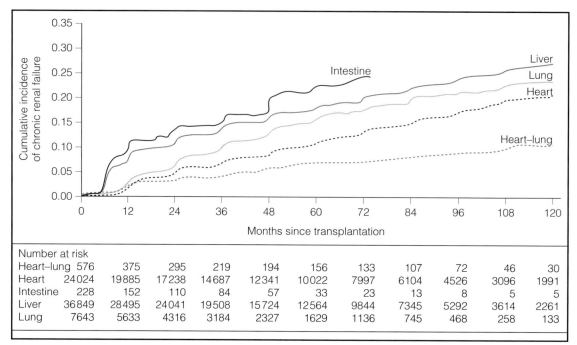

Figure 7.3 • The cumulative incidence of chronic renal failure among 69 321 persons who received non-renal organ transplants in the USA between 1 January 1990 and 31 December 2000. From Ojo AO, Held PJ, Port FK et al. Chronic renal failure after transplantation of a nonrenal organ. N Engl J Med 2003; 349(10):931–40, with permission. Copyright © 2003 Massachusetts Medical Society. All rights reserved.

candidate's status, screening for cardiovascular disease, malignancy and degree of presensitisation. There is no firm evidence as to how often patients awaiting transplantation should be monitored.[40,41] A recent survey of US transplant programmes indicated that 80% regularly re-evaluate patients at high risk for coronary artery disease, although the frequency and method vary widely from centre to centre.[36] Regardless, ensuring that patients on the waiting list remain viable transplant candidates (waiting list management) requires a significant expenditure of time and resources.

Strategies to increase the supply of deceased donor kidneys

Estimating the potential numbers of deceased donors is difficult. From chart reviews, Sheehy and co-workers estimated the annual number of potential brain-dead donors in the USA over a 3-year period (1997–1999) to be between 10 500 and

13 800.[42] During this time, there were 17 000 actual deceased donors in the USA, representing successful 'conversion' (from potential to actual donors) of less than 50%. This gap reflected both failure to enquire about donation and failure to gain consent. Nonetheless, the authors concluded that even dramatic improvement in consent and harvest rates may not meet the rising demand for deceased donor organs.

EXPANDED CRITERIA DONORS

Although something of an anomaly, procurement of kidneys from deceased donors in Spain has been highly effective in addressing the demand for organs[43] (see Chapter 2). A conference convened in Washington to address inadequacies in the USA found that a principal difference between the two systems was utilisation of donors older than 45 years of age.[44] Subsequently, a new category was defined: 'expanded criteria' donors. Previously, a high percentage of these organs were either discarded (18%) or never retrieved. Analysis of these underutilised kidneys documented several

Box 7.1 • Deceased donor variables associated with increased risk of renal allograft failure (relative risk ≥1.7 compared to other donors)

- Age over 60 years
- Age over 50 years, with one of the following characteristics:
  - death from cerebrovascular accident
  - hypertension
  - terminal serum creatinine ≥1.5 mg/dL

From ref. 45.

donor variables as independently associated with increased risk of graft loss (**Box 7.1**).[45,46] Despite a graft failure rate 1.7 times greater than kidneys from more typical donors, Ojo and colleagues demonstrated a substantial survival benefit from marginal donor kidneys, relative to remaining on dialysis (**Fig. 7.4**).[34] Recognising that shorter cold ischaemia time (a modifiable risk factor associated with graft outcome) might improve outcomes further, the United Network for Organ Sharing (UNOS) has implemented a separate allocation list for centres and patients willing to utilise these kidneys. A recent conference recommended that the optimal recipients for these kidneys would be patients with ESRD whose projected wait on the list was longer than their life expectancy on dialysis (e.g. diabetics over age 40 and non-diabetics over age 60).[41] For younger candidates with a longer projected survival on dialysis, acceptance of such an organ might increase risk of earlier-than-expected allograft failure. Another variant on the same theme is the Eurotransplant 'old-for-old' programme. Even the most optimistic projections indicate these new options will yield only a small increase (10–15%) in availability of deceased donor kidneys.

CONSCRIPTION, PRESUMED CONSENT AND MARKET-BASED SOLUTIONS

With substantially more potential donors than retrieved organs, some advocate significant changes in the current strategy of altruistic donation and procurement, and offer no shortage of creative, if morally controversial, suggestions of how to increase numbers. Organ conscription, presumed consent and organ markets are three novel strategies in this regard; reviewing them in depth is beyond the scope of this chapter. However, a few salient points are worth review.

The focal point of the debate over these strategies is the moral propriety of viewing organs as alienable property that can be redistributed by force, presumed consent or after consent and remuneration. Proponents of conscription argue that the demands of distributive justice require confiscation of organs from the dead and distribution to those 'in need', that is, patients on the waiting list. On

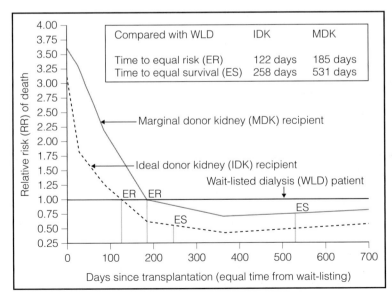

Figure 7.4 • Mortality risks in two groups of deceased donor kidneys, from 'marginal' donors (age over 55 years, MDK, solid line) and from all other donors (ideal donor kidneys, IDK, hatched line), compared with wait-listed dialysis (WLD) patients. There is substantial survival benefit for recipients of kidneys from both donor groups. From Ojo AO, Hanson JA, Meier-Kriesche H et al. Survival in recipients of marginal cadaveric donor kidneys compared with other recipients and wait-listed transplant candidates. J Am Soc Nephrol 2001; 12(3):589–97, with permission.

Compared with WLD	IDK	MDK
Time to equal risk (ER)	122 days	185 days
Time to equal survival (ES)	258 days	531 days

this account, any property rights the dead (or their beneficiaries) might have over organs are over-ridden by the obligations of distributive justice. Mandatory conscription, proponents argue, obviates the need for consent to retrieve, and avoids the charge of financial exploitation. Conscriptionists permit exceptions for religious prohibitions, but rely heavily on the notion that the need for trans-plantable organs outweighs 'irrational' attachments to organs that would otherwise be lost to burial or cremation.[47]

Proponents of presumed consent proceed with similar premises about the rationality of donating organs after death: excepting specific metaphysical/religious beliefs regarding the intact body, it is presumed rational to suppose that most people, were they to reflect on it, would want their organs to go to those in need of them after their death.[48] The right to proceed to donation is presumed unless the individual has 'opted out'.

Thus far, these models appear to have had little impact on availability of deceased donor kidneys for transplantation. In reality, few countries utilise a presumed consent model, and only Austria enforces a presumed consent model so strict as to approach conscription. Although a law enabling presumed consent has existed in Spain since 1979, written permission from the donor's family is nonetheless required in all hospitals prior to retrieval.[49] Further-more, some countries with presumed consent laws, such as France and Italy, retrieve fewer deceased donor kidneys than Spain (in 1999, 16.2 and 13.7 per million for France and Italy respectively, compared with 25.6 per million in Austria and 33.6 per million in Spain).[50]

Market-based approaches to organ procurement operate on the assumption that kidneys are alien-able property that belongs first to the donor, and subsequently to the donor's estate, rather than to the state or society as a whole. Proponents of market-based solutions usually limit their claims to defending the right to sell, rather than the right to purchase organs.[51–53] One example of this is a **monopsony**, wherein only a single buyer (such as the British National Health Service) might be permitted to set the price of and purchase cadaver kidneys. Purchased kidneys would then be distributed in the same fashion as donated cadaver kidneys[51] (see also Chapter 1). Another proposal borrows from the model of a futures market, in which potential donors

would be compensated in advance, based on a con-tractual promise to permit organ harvesting after death.[54] The market value of this promise is based on the likelihood of a successful fulfilment of that promise in the future, the number of other people willing to make such a promise for compensation, and the estimated future need for organs. A futures market has the virtue of obviating the need for a direct 'cash-for-organs' approach from a living donor, with the analogy to a life insurance policy with immediate or deferred benefits. A futures market in organs would ensure, in advance, the consent of the person from whom the organs are to be taken, and enforce compliance through a legally binding contract, rather than leaving the decision to surrogates.

These limited proposals are designed to circum-vent concerns regarding potential abuse of an unregulated organ market, most prominently the exploitation of the poor and disenfranchised. How-ever, proponents vigorously dispute an inevitable connection between organ markets and exploitation. They argue that making altruistic organ donation mandatory unfairly limits the options of both organ vendors and recipients, and that the current system enforces and exploits a societal expectation to donate, recasting the family of the deceased as a barrier to be overcome, rather than the custodian of the deceased person's wishes.[55,56]

Current statutes, at least in the USA, make much of the discussion of organ markets merely theoretical. The National Organ Transplant Act of 1984 prohibits the exchange of any human organ for 'valuable consideration'.[50] Any form of remuner-ation beyond reimbursement for expenses would require substantial legislative changes.

ETHICAL INCENTIVES FOR ORGAN DONATION: A CURIOUS HYBRID

Some who profess moral distaste and operational scepticism regarding unvarnished market-based approaches have proposed so-called 'ethical incen-tives', designed to reward patients and their families who have agreed to organ donation, without under-mining the altruistic nature of the exchange. Rather than cash payments or tax incentives, ethical incen-tives might include reimbursement for funeral expenses, or life insurance for a living donor.[57,58] The premise that poor people are more likely to be exploited in an organ market cuts both ways when applying the same reasoning to ethical incentives: poor people may be more likely to be swayed by such incentives, so the difference may be one of magnitude, not substance.

Notwithstanding the apparent virtues of each of these approaches, it is unclear whether they would substantially increase the number of transplantable organs. Indeed, it is possible that offering incentives, financial or otherwise, to those who might be inclined to act altruistically risks being construed as an offensive devaluation of a gift, resulting in declining availability of organs.[58]

Strategies to increase the supply of living donor kidneys

Living donors fostered the original successes in renal transplantation, have played a key role in its evolution, and have never been more important than today. In non-Western cultures, particularly Japan and Korea, where cadaveric organ procurement systems are either culturally unacceptable or not well developed, living donation has always been the dominant source of transplantable kidneys. A 1999 report from Korea noted that 58% of transplanted kidneys were from living-related donors, 30% from living-unrelated donors and 12% from cadaveric donors.[59] Even in the USA living donors are now more common than deceased donors, and in 2002 they accounted for 45% of transplanted kidneys.[29]

CHANGING RELATIONSHIPS AND MINIMALLY INVASIVE NEPHRECTOMY

Increasing utilisation of live donors reflects the impact of two significant changes. The first is the changing relationship between donors and recipients. As already noted, identical twins were the first successful donor/recipient pairs; technical success equalled immunological success because of genetic identity, even in the absence of effective immunosuppression. Thereafter, with relatively primitive immunosuppressive therapies, HLA similarity between donor and recipient was the key to a successful outcome. However, with the availability of effective antirejection therapies (notably ciclosporin), successful living donor transplantation no longer depended on genetic relationships. The first step beyond the traditional immediate family members was the use of 'emotionally related' donors, such as

long-term friends, distant relatives and spouses.[60] Such transplants are now widely performed in the USA and less so in Western Europe. Moving beyond a documented genetic or emotional relationship between donor and recipient has proven more difficult in terms of defining motivation, and avoiding coercion or exchange of 'valuable consideration'. Nonetheless, a number of programmes in the USA and elsewhere have addressed such situations, typically termed 'non-directed' donation, where donor and recipient may not even know each other.[61,62]

A second major change is the development of laparoscopic or minimally invasive donor nephrectomy.[63] These procedures have been widely adopted in the USA and Europe. Although a debatable issue, reduction in perioperative morbidity and recovery time after surgery is thought to have stimulated some previously reluctant potential donors to participate.[64] A recent multicentre survey confirmed previous reports of low morbidity and mortality (two deaths, one persistent vegetative state out of 10 000 procedures) with the laparoscopic procedure.[65]

There is continuing concern regarding the physical risks undertaken by living kidney donors.[66–68] Current data indicate the perioperative mortality from living donation to be about 0.03%.[65,68] The long-term risk of renal insufficiency in living donors is also controversial, since data on living donors have not been systematically collected. A UNOS study found 56 previous donors on the waiting list for a cadaveric kidney between 1987 and 2002.[67] Of these 56 patients, 36 currently have a functioning allograft, 43 received at least one transplant, and 2 died on the waiting list. Unfortunately, the pool from which these patients were drawn is undetermined, and the incidence of ESRD in previous donors could be anywhere from miniscule to alarming. Alternatively, in data from Sweden, where all outcomes are available via a national database, donors appear to be at less risk for renal problems than the general population.[69,70]

OVERCOMING IMMUNOLOGICAL BARRIERS

Not long ago, ABO incompatibility or a positive T-cell crossmatch were considered contraindications to living donor transplantation. Indeed, as many as 20–30% of willing candidates are excluded from donating to their proposed recipient as a consequence. New approaches enable many previously impossible transplants to occur, with excellent outcomes. The most logistically challenging approach involves paired exchanges, or 'swaps'. A swap programme matches a donor from one family with a compatible recipient in another family, in return for a similar exchange.[59] In some circumstances, a donor pool is employed, with a circle of several donors and recipients paired at the same time. Outcomes for recipients are on a par with those expected from comparably matched controls. List-pairing is a variation on swaps in which an incompatible live donor gives a kidney to the most appropriate recipient on the cadaveric waiting list. In return, the live donor's intended recipient gets the next compatible deceased donor kidney.[71]

Avoiding coercion by offering a donor the opportunity to withdraw consent becomes more complicated in paired and pooled exchange. To avoid the situation of one donor backing out when the exchange donor is undergoing nephrectomy, some centres have arranged simultaneous donor procedures. Confidentiality is sometimes necessary between donor–recipient pairs in order to protect against anger or resentment when complications or graft loss occur.[71]

In overcoming ABO incompatibility, there are significant ethical implications concerning equity of participation. Patients with blood group O can donate to anyone, but transplant candidates with blood group O can only receive a kidney from an O donor. Thus, an O donor might be unlikely to engage in a swap arrangement, since the O donor would have to forgo donating to his or her relative, so-called 'unbalanced' altruism.[72] In a list-pairing arrangement, all O candidates become similarly disadvantaged, even though the net effect is an additional kidney for the 'system'. Such concerns do not apply when a swap is contemplated as a solution for a positive crossmatch. Another concern in list-pairing is trading a known commodity (a living donor kidney) for the uncertainty associated with cadaveric transplantation.

A more immunologically challenging approach to overcoming donor/recipient incompatibility involves transplanting across the ABO barrier and/or a positive T-cell crossmatch. The concept is not new. A successful ABO-incompatible renal transplant was

reported by Starzl et al. in 1964.[73] Plasmapheresis was utilised to treat hyperacute rejection from anti-blood group antibody in 1981.[74] Subsequently, a series of deliberate ABO-incompatible transplants using preoperative plasmapheresis and splenectomy was reported by Alexandre and colleagues in 1985.[75] In this series, all allografts in non-splenectomised patients failed within 5–7 days due to hyperacute rejection, and all patients successfully transplanted demonstrated reduction, but not elimination, of their anti-ABO antibody titre. In a subsequent report of 26 patients with successful ABO-incompatible transplants, the same group reported 88% graft survival at 2 years with related ABO-incompatible donor–recipient pairs.[76] In two recipients, severe antibody-mediated rejection within the first postoperative week was successfully treated with steroids, local radiation therapy and rabbit antilymphocyte globulin, resulting in long-term survival.

Since Alexandre's report, ABO-incompatible renal transplants have become much more common, particularly in Japan, with predictable success. Splenectomy is customarily performed at the time of transplantation. Pretransplant plasmapheresis to remove anti-ABO reactivity is a key part of most protocols, with early administration of potent immunosuppression. It is now generally recognised that the A2 to B or O blood group interaction is quite weak, and such transplants can be performed with little pretransplant manipulation and minimal monitoring.[77] Indeed, defining intensity of anti-ABO responsiveness has proved quite important in predicting who can be successfully desensitised and transplanted. A new twist is substitution of rituximab, an anti-CD20 antibody, for splenectomy in some protocols. Rituximab is a less permanent anti-B-cell intervention with fewer potential long-term consequences for defence against opportunistic infection. The experience at some centres is now quite extensive, with outcomes, both short- and long-term, rivalling those seen with ABO-compatible transplants. Interestingly, after the initial post-transplant period, adaptation appears to occur between graft and host. Despite the return of anti-ABO antibody on allograft vascular endothelium and evidence of complement activation, allograft function remains stable.[78–81]

Surprisingly, transplanting across a positive T-cell crossmatch has proven to be more challenging than

ABO incompatibility. Again, recent advances in immunological testing have allowed rapid identification of recipients likely to respond to desensitisation protocols, with those patients demonstrating less intense antibody reactivity achieving the greatest success.[82,83] Two contrasting approaches to desensitisation have evolved. Some maintain that the anti-idiotype effect of high-dose intravenous immunoglobulin (1 g/kg body weight), followed by potent immunosuppression, is sufficient to allow successful transplantation in suitable individuals.[82,84] Others maintain that aggressive plasma exchange, again with profound immunosuppression, produces more predictable outcomes.[83,85] These protocols may even allow one to simultaneously cross both ABO and major histocompatibility complex (MHC) barriers in the same patient.[86] Both approaches require intense post-transplant surveillance, with early diagnosis and aggressive treatment of antibody-mediated rejection, a common complication.

Though an exciting advance, incompatible transplantation is not yet a viable large-scale solution to the growing demand for transplantation. The financial cost, though clearly greater than with standard donor–recipient pairs, remains substantially less than chronic dialysis. Long-term results are still uncertain. Nonetheless, it appears that ABO incompatibility and/or a positive T-cell crossmatch are increasingly viewed as hurdles to be surmounted rather than a contraindication to transplantation.

EVOLVING IMMUNOSUPPRESSION: MAKING TRANSPLANTATION LESS RISKY

Achieving immunological tolerance of renal allografts remains the elusive grail of organ transplantation. In spite of significant advances in experimental models of tolerance, we are still dependent on effective immunosuppressive drugs to achieve successful clinical outcomes. Fortunately, we now have at our disposal agents that are more effective and less toxic than ever before, with rejection rates in the teens or less, and greater than 90% graft survival after 1 year the norm.[22,87] Unfortunately, patients must still bear the consequences of long-term immunosuppression, including bone disease, cardio-

vascular disease and metabolic disorders such as post-transplant diabetes, as well as the old foes: malignancy and opportunistic infection.[28,88–90]

New classes of immunosuppressant drugs, such as a humanised version of the co-stimulation blocker CTLA4-Ig and modulators of Jak-3 kinase, are under investigation, but demonstrating clinical utility in human trials remains several years away.[91,92] As newer agents are awaited, current developments in clinical immunosuppression are based on maintaining the efficacy of current regimens, with a reduction in toxicity. These 'drug minimisation' protocols typically employ antibody administration – antithymocyte globulin (ATG), anti-CD25 or anti-CD52 monoclonal antibody – in the perioperative period in order to avoid administration or facilitate early withdrawal of a more toxic maintenance agent (usually calcineurin inhibitors or corticosteroids).[93–96]

It is generally accepted that at least some long-term allograft failure is the consequence of calcineurin inhibitor (CNI) nephrotoxicity, making avoidance of these agents (ciclosporin and tacrolimus) attractive. Unfortunately, protocols that exclude CNI use have yielded troubling results, with rejection rates as high as 50%.[97] Attempts to withdraw CNIs as late as 1 year after transplantation have resulted in more rejection than discontinuation of other agents.[98] Few observers, at the current time, believe that CNI therapy will be completely abandoned in the near future.

The introduction of sirolimus has stimulated further interest in CNI-sparing protocols. A recent study of ciclosporin withdrawal in a relatively low-risk cohort of recipients maintained on sirolimus and corticosteroids demonstrated an increased risk of acute rejection, but was generally not accompanied by graft loss, at least in the short term.[99] Concerns regarding an increased propensity for severe hyperlipidaemia have been tempered somewhat by a lack of evidence supporting a subsequent increase in cardiovascular mortality among renal transplant patients.[100,101] Of somewhat greater concern are the observations of impaired surgical wound healing and lymphocele development,[102] as well as an increase in delayed graft function and an unusual form of cast nephropathy when used in combination with tacrolimus.[103] However, the prospect of using sirolimus in place of CNIs, while involving a trade-off in side effects, offers the opportunity to reduce CNI nephrotoxicity as well as the incidence of post-transplant diabetes, a well-known side effect of both ciclosporin and tacrolimus.[104]

A recent randomised, blinded, prospective trial of corticosteroid withdrawal 90 days after transplantation (continuing ciclosporin and mycophenolate) was terminated early due to unacceptably high rejection rates (almost 30%) in the withdrawal cohort.[105] However, it was found that most of the rejection episodes occurred among black American patients, and overall graft survival was not compromised. Armed with new understanding that avoiding corticosteroid use entirely may be safer than withdrawal, as well as a greater appreciation for the importance of patient selection, enthusiasm is again emerging for steroid-free immunosuppression.[97] A pilot study in Canada utilising daclizumab, ciclosporin and mycophenolate mofetil (MMF) documented an acceptably low rejection rate (<25%) and excellent allograft survival after 1 year.[106] Series from some North American centres with similar duration of follow-up are equally intriguing, although widespread application in diverse groups of patients (especially black Americans and those undergoing re-transplantation) cannot yet be advocated.[93,107]

The ultimate drug minimisation protocols seek to induce a state of immunological near-unresponsiveness, so-called 'prope' tolerance.[108] These regimens typically employ aggressive lymphocyte depletion (utilising antithymocyte globulins or an anti-CD52 monoclonal antibody) at the time of transplantation, followed by a single agent (MMF, sirolimus, tacrolimus or ciclosporin). A recent study combining anti-CD52 mAb (Campath 1H) induction with sirolimus monotherapy in 29 patients reported nine episodes of rejection over 2 years.[94] Of interest, five of these cases demonstrated antibody-mediated rejection, and two patients developed a positive T-cell crossmatch, despite having a negative crossmatch prior to transplantation. In another trial utilising single-dose rabbit ATG induction and tacrolimus monotherapy, graft survival appeared quite good, although protocol biopsies appeared to document ongoing immunological injury.[96]

The most significant immunological development of late is greater recognition and understanding of the importance of B-lymphocyte responses and donor-specific antibody in determining graft outcomes. The principal effect of current immunosuppressants is to inhibit cell-mediated rejection, leaving humoral immunity relatively intact. The diagnosis of antibody-mediated rejection (AMR) is not new, but the range of clinical and histological findings implicating antibody-mediated injury has expanded significantly in the last 5 years.[109–113] Immunofluorescent staining for complement fragment C4d has proven to be a reliable marker for antibody-mediated injury, allowing consistent categorisation of clinical events and development of treatment protocols (**Box 7.2**). Such protocols are increasingly standardised, particularly during the early post-transplant period, and most often involve some combination of plasmapheresis, intravenous immune globulin and rituximab.[83,114] Mauiyyedi and colleagues have convincingly demonstrated the importance of donor-specific antibody in chronic allograft nephropathy, although the clinical implications and treatment options remain uncertain.[115] It is clear that future developments in immunosuppressive therapy must address humoral antigraft responses.

Currently, it seems that careful patient selection is of paramount importance in the success or failure of innovative protocols: patients at high risk of rejection will be unlikely to tolerate reduced immunosuppression without adverse consequences.[97] The concept of 'one size fits all' immunosuppressive therapy is no longer viable. The trend towards minimalist immunosuppression for the standard patient provides an interesting contrast with the trend for more intense therapies necessary to prevent antibody-mediated rejection and facilitate transplantation between incompatible pairs. What is required of both approaches are more controlled data over longer periods of time, with better definition of appropriate endpoints by which to evaluate these innovative protocols.[116]

POST-TRANSPLANT MANAGEMENT: MAKING ALLOGRAFTS LAST LONGER

In the new millennium it is no longer acceptable to consider kidney transplantion a 'temporary respite' from dialysis. The majority of patients now achieve

Box 7.2 • Banff '97 diagnostic categories for renal allograft biopsies – updated

1. Normal

2. Antibody-mediated rejection

Rejection due, at least in part, to documented antidonor antibody ('suspicious for' if antibody not demonstrated); may coincide with categories 3, 4 and 5.

Type (grade)

I   ATN-like – C4d+, minimal inflammation.

II   Capillary margination and/or thrombosis, C4d+.

III Arterial – Banff III, C4d+.

3. Borderline changes: 'suspicious' for acute cellular rejection

This category is used when no intimal arteritis is present, but there are foci of mild tubulitis (1–4 mononuclear cells renal tubular cross-section) and at least i1; may coincide with categories 2 and 5.

4. Acute/active cellular rejection

T-cell-mediated rejection; may coincide with categories 2 and 5.

Type (grade)

IA Cases with significant interstitial infiltration (>25% of parenchyma affected) and foci of moderate tubulitis (>4 mononuclear cells/tubular cross-section or group of 10 tubular cells).

IB Cases with significant interstitial infiltration (>25% of parenchyma affected) and foci of severe tubulitis (>10 mononuclear cells/tubular cross-section or group of 10 tubular cells).

IIA Cases with mild to moderate intimal arteritis (Banff IIA).

IIB Cases with severe intimal arteritis comprising >25% of the luminal area (Banff IIB).

III Cases with 'transmural' arteritis and/or arterial fibrinoid change and necrosis of medial smooth muscle cells with accompanying lymphocytic inflammation (Banff III).

5. Chronic/sclerosing allograft nephropathy

Fibrosing changes in the allograft, with or without features of true alloimmune injury to the graft; may coincide with categories 2, 3 and 4.

Grade

I (mild)   Mild interstitial fibrosis and tubular atrophy without (a) or with (b) specific changes suggesting chronic rejection.

II (moderate) Moderate interstitial fibrosis and tubular atrophy (a) or (b).

III (severe)   Severe interstitial fibrosis and tubular atrophy (a) or (b).

6. Other

Changes not considered to be due to rejection; may coincide with categories 2, 3, 4 and 5.

From Racusen LC, Colvin RB, Solez K et al. Antibody-mediated rejection criteria – an addition to the Banff 97 classification of renal allograft rejection. Am J Transplant 2003; 3:708–14 [113], with permission from Blackwell Publishing Ltd.

long-term graft survival, with half-lives for kidneys from deceased donors currently over 13 years and approaching 20 years if the organ is from a live donor. Building on this impressive achievement will require a deeper understanding of the aetiologies of late allograft failure, and strategies for appropriate and effective intervention. Two causes account for over 80% of late graft failures: patient death (with a functioning allograft) and chronic allograft nephropathy.

Of growing importance in providing optimal care for transplant recipients is a potential shortfall in providers experienced in the care of patients with end-stage renal disease and renal allografts. A study commissioned by the American Society of Nephrology to review workforce needs in nephrology estimated that under the current rate of training, the number of new nephrologists being trained equals the attrition due to death and retirement.[32] In other words, **current** training rates are only sufficient to maintain a constant number of practising nephrologists in the USA, not taking into account the increasing prevalence of patients with ESRD. The American Society of Transplantation commissioned a similar study to examine the transplant workforce needs, though it is unclear if the assumptions in the study include the evaluation, listing and follow-up of more than 100 000 patients by 2010. The estimated need by 2007 is an increase of 135 transplant nephrologists, or an additional 75% of the current workforce, and a 25% increase in the number of transplant surgeons.[31] Whether these projections will facilitate sufficient growth in training transplant professionals to meet rapidly expanding needs remains to be determined.

Reducing the impact of chronic kidney disease (CKD) on patient mortality

Early mortality after transplantation is a haunting reminder that chronic kidney disease is also a systemic disease. Despite a more favourable outlook for those with transplants compared with those on dialysis, improving long-term graft survival is tantamount to reducing patient mortality. Patients who die with a functioning allograft most frequently succumb to cardiovascular causes (40–50%), followed by infections and malignancy.[89]

Reducing the impact of infection and malignancy requires more precision in administering immunosuppression, appropriate administration of anti-infective agents (prophylactic, pre-emptive and therapeutic) and effective preventive and screening measures.[117,118] The significant cardiovascular complications associated with kidney transplantation, recognised over three decades ago,[119] have their genesis in chronic kidney disease. Functionally speaking, most renal allograft recipients **are** patients with chronic kidney disease, whose clinical risk is **modulated**, not eliminated, by transplant immunosuppression.

Ironically, the success of renal transplantation entering the third millennium has closed the circle in the treatment of kidney disease. Recent changes in terminology define CKD in a much broader fashion than ever before, with significant implications for patient management as even stage 2 CKD is associated with increased cardiovascular risk compared to the general population (**Table 7.2**).[120] In this context, renal transplantation converts most patients from stage 5 to stage 2 or 3 CKD, with ongoing risk for cardiovascular complications.[89,121] While much of the increased frequency of cardiovascular disease (CVD) after transplantation can be explained by overrepresentation of traditional risk factors (hypertension, hyperlipidaemia) among recipients, other variables (diabetes, older age and cigarette smoking) exert a greater adverse impact than in the general population.[122] Unfortunately, diabetes is more frequent, we are transplanting older patients than ever before, and cigarette smoking remains common among transplanted patients.

It now appears that many of the long-held principles applied to slowing progression of CKD are equally salient in the care of the transplant patient.[123] All potentially modifiable risk factors, including cigarette smoking, hypertension and hyperlipidaemia, should be addressed (**Table 7.3**).[27,118,124] Statins are very effective in reducing low-density lipoprotein (LDL) cholesterol levels. Very high triglyceride levels (>500 mg/dL) require intervention, with fibrates the most commonly utilised agents. In diabetics, glycaemic control must be emphasised. Although preventing immunological insult remains the primary goal of immunosuppressive therapy, it is reasonable to consider the impact of individual agents on CVD risk in formulating protocols.[12]

Table 7.2 • Chronic kidney disease (CKD): a clinical action plan

Stage	Description	GFR (mL/min/1.73 m^2)	Action*
1	Kidney damage with normal or increased GFR	≥90	Diagnosis and treatment, treatment of comorbid conditions, slowing progression, CVD risk reduction
2	Kidney damage with mild decrease in GFR	60–89	Estimating rate of progression
3	Moderate decrease in GFR	30–59	Evaluating and treating complications
4	Severe decrease in GFR	15–29	Preparation for renal replacement therapy
5	Kidney failure	<15 or dialysis	Renal replacement therapy

*Each action plan includes action from the preceding stages.
CVD, cardiovascular disease; GFR, glomerular filtration rate.
From National Kidney Foundation. K/DOQI Clinical practice guidelines for chronic kidney disease: executive summary. Evaluation, classification, and stratification. Am J Kidney Dis 2002; 39(Suppl. 1):S1, with permission. (K/DOQI, Kidney Dialysis Outcome Quality Initiative.)

Table 7.3 • Management goals for metabolic disturbances in chronic kidney disease (CKD) patients before and after transplantation

Parameter	Target
Systemic blood pressure	130/80 mmHg
Glycosylated haemoglobin (A$_1$C)	<7%
LDL cholesterol	<100 mg/dL

Adapted from NCEP and ADA guidelines; see refs 124 and 133.

Of course, diet and exercise are also important components of promoting long-term cardiovascular health.

Reducing the impact of chronic allograft nephropathy (CAN)

It has been generally accepted that the natural history of an allograft is declining function over time in a process termed chronic allograft nephropathy (CAN). The term itself imparts a sense of inevitability that predisposes to therapeutic nihilism. However, recent developments challenge this assumption, giving hope for successful interventions to halt progressive deterioration in graft function. Foremost among these is the observation that with effective immunosuppression, allograft function may remain stable, or even improve, over long periods.[24] In a timely editorial, Halloran challenged the basic terminology and assumptions underlying our approach to CAN.[125] Starting with the premise that the histopathological findings of so-called 'chronic rejection' (namely tubular atrophy, interstitial fibrosis and fibrointimal thickening of arteries) are really the end-product of a wide variety of pathological processes, only by developing greater diagnostic specificity can we hope to spawn effective therapies (**Box 7.3**).

Better diagnostic accuracy will allow identification of specific concomitant pathogenic processes. For example, immunological components of CAN might be subdivided into cellular, humoral and fibrogenic insults, each susceptible to distinct interventions. The identification of C4d deposits in patients with 'chronic' changes indicates that **active** antibody-mediated damage is playing a significant role in a subgroup of patients with CAN.[115,126] Indeed, Lee and colleagues found circulating donor-specific antibody always to precede allograft failure due to CAN.[127] The presence of C4d along with evidence of enhanced chemokine activity may predispose to findings of transplant glomerulopathy.[112,126,128] Finally, application of newer histopathological techniques may allow definition of specific responses, differentiating between immune and non-immune fibrogenesis.[129,130]

It increasingly appears that deterioriation of allograft function is not entirely, and maybe not even

Box 7.3 • Entities responsible for chronic dysfunction in renal allografts

1. Rejection

Allograft injury due to:

(a) T-cell-mediated rejection: tubulitis, endothelialitis, interstitial infiltrate.

(b) Alloantibody-mediated rejection.

2. Allograft nephropathy

Reduced renal function with increased rate of declining function, associated with:

(a) Tubular atrophy, interstitial fibrosis, fibrous intimal thickening of arteries.

(b) Activity of fibrosis and injury.

3. Transplant glomerulopathy

4. Specific diseases

Examples include:

(a) Recurrent or de novo renal disease.

(b) Polyoma-virus nephropathy.

(c) Haemolytic–uraemic syndrome.

(d) Calcineurin inhibitor (CNI) toxicity.

(e) Diabetic nephropathy.

(f) Hypertensive renal disease.

5. Accelerating processes

Factors that may accelerate progression of declining function due to other entities:

(a) Hypertension accelerating other disease.

(b) CNI toxicity accelerating other disease.

(c) Diabetes mellitus.

(d) Proteinuria.

(e) Hyperlipidaemia.

From Halloran PF. Call for revolution: a new approach to describing allograft deterioration. Am J Transplant 2002; 2(3):195–200, with permission from Blackwell Publishing Ltd.

primarily, the result of external insults, but rather reflects the physiological limits of tissue repair following any injury.[131,132] The ability of epithelial cells to undergo repair in response to immunological or non-immunological injury is finite, limited by **senescence**. When such mechanisms are impaired, for whatever reason, atrophy and fibrosis are the result. Thus, the final product in terms of a functioning allograft reflects not only severity of injury, but capacity for repair. The compromised outcomes associated with increased donor age and prolonged preservation time may reflect this interaction.[45,46]

Obviously, our understanding of events and processes influencing allograft function over time remains rather primitive. However, given the immunosuppressive tools currently available, identifying injury and defining the spectrum of responses within the renal graft offer the promise of reducing the adverse impact of CAN on long-term survival.

CONCLUSION

At the beginning of the third millennium, renal transplantation is the beneficiary of unprecedented success, which in turn has generated a host of unforeseen challenges. Dramatic improvement in allograft survival has come on the cusp of an epidemic of chronic kidney disease, with the looming prospect of waiting times approaching a decade for deceased donor kidneys. The expanding chasm between demand and supply has invigorated the search for donors, challenging physicians, philosophers and the general public alike. With successful suppression of T-cell immune responses, attention is now focused on minimising the adverse effects of our intervention, in an effort to reduce the impact of pre-existing comorbidity and enable our patients to survive longer than ever before. As we attempt to overcome previously insurmountable barriers to transplantation, and promote long-term graft survival, we are rediscovering the importance of B-cell responses. The search for mechanisms underlying immunological tolerance remains in the vanguard of research at bench and bedside. Commenting on his original 1954 experience in homotransplantation, Joe Murray noted, 'Our ultimate goal, the glue that bound us, was to help patients. We used every available contemporary form of treatment, but at the same time we also spent a lot of our time and energy in research, trying to find ways to do better'.[4] Some things do not change with time. Even in a new millennium, this must remain our paradigm.

Key points

- The dramatic improvement in outcomes for renal transplantation has made it the renal replacement modality of choice for virtually all patients with end-stage renal disease.
- Renal transplantation, even with marginal kidneys, is cost-effective and cost-efficient compared to dialysis.
- With the plateau of deceased donor transplantation, living-related and living-unrelated donors have become the fastest-growing source of organs.
- Long-term risks to living donors remain uncertain, and should be the subject of prospective study.
- The rapid rate of growth of the waiting list for deceased donor kidneys in the USA entails that the waiting time for a cadaveric organ will soon exceed the lifespan of most incident dialysis patients.
- The disparity between the demand for and supply of available organs has generated unique approaches to allocation, as well as attempts to overcome immunological barriers previously thought to be insurmountable.
- Acute cellular rejection is now of less importance in determining the long-term outcome of renal allografts, and despite recent advances in immunosuppression, allograft half-lives have reached a plateau.
- Efforts to extend the lifespan of renal allografts will focus on control of cardiovascular risk factors, management of the spectrum of conditions associated with chronic kidney disease, and achieving a deeper understanding of the pathophysiology of chronic allograft nephropathy.

REFERENCES

1. Marx JL. The 1988 Nobel Prize for Physiology or Medicine. Science 1988; 242(4878):516–17.

2. Borel JF, Feurer C, Magnee C et al. Effects of the new anti-lymphocytic peptide cyclosporin A in animals. Immunology 1977; 32(6):1017–25.

3. Murray JE. Surgery of the soul: reflections on a curious career. Canton, MA: Boston Medical Library; 2001.

4. Murray JE, Merrill JP, Harrison JH. Renal homo-transplantation in identical twins. 1955. J Am Soc Nephrol 2001; 12(1):201–4.

5. Eknoyan G, Beck GJ, Cheung AK et al. Effect of dialysis dose and membrane flux in maintenance hemodialysis. N Engl J Med 2002; 347(25):2010–19.

6. Meier-Kriesche HU, Ojo AO, Port FK et al. Survival improvement among patients with end-stage renal disease: trends over time for transplant recipients and wait-listed patients. J Am Soc Nephrol 2001; 12(6):1293–6.

   This study demonstrates the improvement in survival for a more contemporary cohort of patients on dialysis, but confirms the comparative survival benefit of renal transplantation.

7. Paniagua R, Amato D, Vonesh E et al. Effects of increased peritoneal clearances on mortality rates in peritoneal dialysis: ADEMEX, a prospective, randomized, controlled trial. J Am Soc Nephrol 2002; 13(5):1307–20.

8. US Renal Data System: Excerpts from the USRDS 2002 Annual Data Report: Atlas of End-Stage Renal Disease in the United States. Am J Kidney Dis 2002; 41(suppl. 2):S1–S260.

   The data reported here have been supplied by the United States Renal Data System (USRDS). The interpretation and reporting of these data are the responsibility of the author(s) and in no way should be seen as an official policy or interpretation of the US Government.

   This document is an accumulation of national data on end-stage renal disease and renal transplantation in the USA.

9. Cameron JL, Whiteside C, Katz J et al. Differences in quality of life across renal replacement therapies: a meta-analytic comparison. Am J Kidney Dis 2000; 35:629–37.

10. Rennie D. Home dialysis and the costs of uremia. N Engl J Med 1978; 298(7):399–400.

11. Hariharan S, Johnson CP, Bresnahan BA et al. Improved graft survival after renal transplantation in the United States, 1988 to 1996. N Engl J Med 2000; 342(9):605–12.

12. Gaston RS. Maintenance immunosuppression in the renal transplant recipient: an overview. Am J Kidney Dis 2001; 38(suppl. 6): S25–S35.

13. Gaston RS. Evolution of Medicare policy involving transplantation and immunosuppressive medications: past developments and future directions. In: Field MJ, Lawrence RL, Zwanziger L (eds) Extending Medicare coverage for preventive and other services. Washington, DC: National Academy Press, 1999; pp. D23–D38.

14. Eggers PW. A quarter century of medicare expenditures for ESRD. Semin Nephrol 2000; 20(6):516–22.

15. Wolfe RA, Ashby VB, Milford EL et al. Comparison of mortality in all patients on dialysis, patients on dialysis awaiting transplantation, and recipients of a first cadaveric transplant. N Engl J Med 1999; 341(23):1725–30.

A seminal study correcting for the selection bias of comparing dialysis patients who are not candidates for transplantation for medical reasons with successful transplant recipients.

16. Meier-Kriesche HU, Port FK, Ojo AO et al. Effect of waiting time on renal transplant outcome. Kidney Int 2000; 58(3):1311–17.

17. Meier-Kriesche HU, Kaplan B. Waiting time on dialysis as the strongest modifiable risk factor for renal transplant outcomes: a paired donor kidney analysis. Transplantation 2002; 74(10):1377–81.

In this study, Meier-Kriesche and colleagues demonstrate a substantial improvement in allograft outcome for pre-emptive transplantation versus transplantation after initiating dialysis, and also confirm that time on dialysis is a risk factor for adverse allograft outcomes.

18. Mange KC, Joffe MM, Feldman HI. Effect of the use or nonuse of long-term dialysis on the subsequent survival of renal transplants from living donors. N Engl J Med 2001; 344(10):726–31.

19. Gaston RS, Shroyer T, Hudson S et al. Renal retransplantation: the role of race, quadruple immunosuppression, and the flow cytometry crossmatch. Transplantation 1994; 57:47–54.

20. Suthanthiran M, Morris RE, Strom TB. Immunosuppressants: cellular and molecular mechanisms of action. Am J Kidney Dis 1996; 28(2):159–72.

21. Vincenti F, Kirkman R, Light S et al. Interleukin-2-receptor blockade with daclizumab to prevent acute rejection in renal transplantation. N Engl J Med 1998; 338:161–5.

22. Margreiter R. Efficacy and safety of tacrolimus compared with ciclosporin microemulsion in renal transplantation: a randomised multicentre study. Lancet 2002; 359:741–6.

23. Hariharan S, McBride MA, Cherikh WS et al. Posttransplant renal function in the first year predicts long-term kidney transplant survival. Kidney Int 2002; 62(1):311–18.

Hariharan et al. show in this study that allograft function in the first year after transplantation, as measured by serum creatinine, predicts long-term outcome independent of other factors, such as rejection.

24. Gourishankar S, Hunsicker LG, Jhangri GS et al. The stability of the glomerular filtration rate after renal transplantation is improving. J Am Soc Nephrol 2003; 14(9):2387–94.

25. Xue JL, Ma JZ, Louis TA et al. Forecast of the number of patients with end-stage renal disease in the United States to the year 2010. J Am Soc Nephrol 2001; 12(12):2753–8.

A harrowing study projecting that the number of patients with ESRD will approach 650 000 by 2010.

26. Field MJ, Lawrence RL, Zwanziger L (eds) Extending Medicare coverage for preventive and other services. Washington, DC: National Academy Press, 2000.

27. Foley RN, Parfrey PS, Sarnak MJ. Clinical epidemiology of cardiovascular disease in chronic renal disease. Am J Kidney Dis 1998; 32(5 suppl. 3): S112–19.

28. Kasiske BL, Snyder JJ, Gilbertson TD. Cancer after kidney transplantatation in the United States. Am J Transplant 2004; 4:905–13.

29. United Network for Organ Sharing. www.unos.org

The UNOS website offers a wide variety of updated donor and recipient data, including a regular update of the waiting list for all transplantable organs.

30. Coresh J, Astor BC, Greene T et al. Prevalence of chronic kidney disease and decreased kidney function in the adult US population: Third National Health and Nutrition Examination Survey. Am J Kidney Dis 2003; 41(1):1–12.

31. Association Research I. Survey of qualified transplant specialists and trainees: Compiled for the American Society of Transplantation, November 2002.

32. Abt Associates I. Estimating workforce and training requirements for nephrologists through the year 2010. J Am Soc Nephrol 1997; 8(suppl. 9)(5):i–xxii.

33. Gaston RS, Alveranga DY, Becker BN et al. Kidney and pancreas transplantation. Am J Transplant 2003; 3(suppl. 4):64–77.

34. Ojo AO, Hanson JA, Meier-Kriesche H et al. Survival in recipients of marginal cadaveric donor kidneys compared with other recipients and wait-listed transplant candidates. J Am Soc Nephrol 2001; 12(3):589–97.

35. Cosio FG, Alamir A, Yim S et al. Patient survival after renal transplantation: I. The impact of dialysis pre-transplant. Kidney Int 1998; 53(3):767–72.

36. Danovitch GM, Hariharan S, Pirsch JD et al. Management of the waiting list for cadaveric kidney transplants: report of a survey and recommendations by the Clinical Practice Guidelines Committee of the American Society of Transplantation. J Am Soc Nephrol 2002; 13(2):528–35.

37. Young CJ, Gaston RS. Renal transplantation in black Americans. N Engl J Med 2000; 343(21):1545–52.

38. Ojo AO, Held PJ, Port FK et al. Chronic renal failure after transplantation of a nonrenal organ. N Engl J Med 2003; 349(10):931–40.

A review of the USRDS database demonstrating that a growing source of patients with ESRD is recipients of nonrenal organs.

39. Danovitch GM, Cecka JM. Allocation of deceased donor kidneys: Past, present, and future. Am J Kidney Dis 2003; 42(5):882–90.

40. Matas AJ, Kasiske B, Miller L. Proposed guidelines for re-evaluation of patients on the waiting list for renal cadaver transplantation. Transplantation 2002; 73(5):811–12.

41. Gaston RS, Danovitch GM, Adams PL et al. The report of a national conference on the wait list for kidney transplantation. Am J Transplant 2003; 3(7):775–85.

42. Sheehy E, Conrad SL, Brigham LE et al. Estimating the number of potential organ donors in the United States. N Engl J Med 2003; 349(7):667–74.

43. Matesanz R. A decade of continuous improvement in cadaveric organ donation: the Spanish model. Nefrologia 2001; 21(suppl. 5):59–67.

44. Rosengard BR, Feng S, Alfrey EJ et al. Report of the Crystal City meeting to maximize the use of organs recovered from the cadaver donor. Am J Transplant 2002; 2(8):701–11.

45. Port FK, Bragg-Gresham JL, Metzger RA et al. Donor characteristics associated with reduced graft survival: an approach to expanding the pool of kidney donors. Transplantation 2002; 74(9):1281–6.

46. Pessione F, Cohen S, Durand D et al. Multivariate analysis of donor risk factors for graft survival in kidney transplantation. Transplantation 2003; 75(3):361–7.

47. Spital A, Erin CA. Conscription of cadaveric organs for transplantation: let's at least talk about it. Am J Kidney Dis 2002; 39(3):611–15.

48. Cohen C. The case for presumed consent to transplant human organs after death. Transplant Proc 1992; 24(5):2168–72.

49. Lopez-Navidad A, Caballero F. Organs for transplantation. N Engl J Med 2000; 343(23):1730–1; author reply 1732.

50. National Organ Transplant Act. Publ L 98-507. 98th Congress (S2048). October 19, 1984. p. Title III-Prohibition of Organ Purchases.

51. Radcliffe-Richards J, Daar AS, Guttman RD et al. The case for allowing kidney sales. Lancet 1998; 351:1950–2.

52. Gill MB, Sade RM. Paying for kidneys: the case against prohibition. Kennedy Institute of Ethics Journal 2002; 12(1):17–45.

53. Kaserman DL, Barnett AH. The US organ procurement system: a prescription for reform. Washington, DC: AEI Press, 2002.

54. Cohen LR. Increasing the supply of transplant organs: the virtue of a futures market. George Washington Law Rev 1989; 58:1–51.

55. Cherry MJ. Is a market in human organs necessarily exploitative? Public Affairs Quarterly October 2000; 14(4):337–60.

56. Radcliffe-Richards J. Nephrarious goings on: kidney sales and moral arguments. J Med Philos 1996; 21:375–416.

A seminal article that challenges several arguments against a limited market in organs.

57. Delmonico FL, Arnold R, Scheper-Hughes N et al. Ethical incentives – not payment – for organ donation. N Engl J Med 2002; 346(25):2002–5.

58. Arnold R, Bartlett S, Bernat J et al. Financial incentives for cadaver organ donation: an ethical reappraisal. Transplantation 2002; 73(8):1361–7.

59. Park K, Moon JI, Kim SI et al. Exchange donor program in kidney transplantation. Transplantation 1999; 67(2):336–8.

60. Terasaki PI, Cecka JM, Gjertson DW et al. High survival rates of kidney transplants from spousal and living unrelated donors. N Engl J Med 1995; 333(6):333–6.

61. Matas AJ, Garvey CA, Jacobs CL et al. Non-directed donation of kidneys from living donors. N Engl J Med 2000; 343(6):433–6.

62. Adams PL, Cohen DJ, Danovitch GM et al. The non-directed live-kidney donor: ethical considerations and practice guidelines: A National Conference Report. Transplantation 2002; 74(4):582–9.

63. Ratner LE, Ciseck LJ, Moore RG et al. Laparoscopic live donor nephrectomy. Transplantation 1995; 60(9):1047–9.

64. Pradel FG, Limcangco MR, Mullins CD et al. Patients' attitudes about living donor transplantation and living donor nephrectomy. Am J Kidney Dis 2003; 41(4):849–58.

65. Matas AJ, Bartlett ST, Leichtman AB et al. Morbidity and mortality after living kidney donation, 1999–2001: survey of United States transplant centers. Am J Transplant 2003; 3(7):830–4.

This article is the source for the widely accepted estimate of the surgical mortality of living kidney donation.

66. Abecassis M, Adams M, Adams P et al. Consensus statement on the live organ donor. JAMA 2000; 284(22):2919–26.

67. Ellison MD, McBride MA, Taranto SE et al. Living kidney donors in need of kidney transplants: a report from the organ procurement and transplantation network. Transplantation 2002; 74(9): 1349–51.

68. Bia MJ, Ramos EL, Danovitch GM et al. Evaluation of living renal donors. The current practice of US transplant centers. Transplantation 1995; 60(4):322–7.

69. Fehrman-Ekholm I, Duner F, Brink B et al. No evidence of accelerated loss of kidney function in living kidney donors: results from a cross-sectional follow-up. Transplantation 2001; 72(3):444–9.

70. Fehrman-Ekholm I, Elinder CG, Stenbeck M et al. Kidney donors live longer. Transplantation 1997; 64(7):976–8.

71. Ross LF, Rubin DT, Siegler M et al. Ethics of a paired-kidney-exchange program. N Engl J Med 1997; 336(24):1752–5.

72. Woodle ES, Ross LF. Paired exchanges should be part of the solution to ABO incompatibility in living donor kidney transplantation. Transplantation 1998; 66(3):406–7.

73. Starzl TE, Marchioro TL, Holmes JH et al. Renal homografts in patients with major donor-recipient blood group incompatibilities. Surgery 1964; 55:195–200.

74. Slapak M, Naik RB, Lee HA. Renal transplant in a patient with major donor-recipient blood group incompatibility: reversal of acute rejection by the use of modified plasmapheresis. Transplantation 1981; 31(1):4–7.

75. Alexandre GPJ, Squifflet JP, DeBruyere M et al. Splenectomy as a prerequisite for successful human ABO-incompatible renal transplantation. Transplant Proc 1985; 17(1):138–43.

76. Alexandre GP, Squifflet JP, De Bruyere M et al. Present experiences in a series of 26 ABO-incompatible living donor renal allografts. Transplant Proc 1987; 19(6):4538–42.

77. Nelson PW, Landreneau MD, Luger AM et al. Ten-year experience in transplantation of A2 kidneys into B and O recipients. Transplantation 1998; 65(2):256–60.

78. Gloor JM, Lager DJ, Moore SB et al. ABO-incompatible kidney transplantation using both A2 and non-A2 living donors. Transplantation 2003; 75(7):971–7.

79. Park WD, Grande JP, Ninova D et al. Accommodation in ABO-incompatible kidney allografts, a novel mechanism of self-protection against antibody-mediated injury. Am J Transplant 2003; 3(8):952–60.

80. Tanabe K, Takahashi K, Sonda K et al. Long-term results of ABO-incompatible living kidney transplantation: a single-center experience. Transplantation 1998; 65(2):224–8.

81. Tyden G, Kumlien G, Fehrman I. Successful ABO-incompatible kidney transplantations without splenectomy using antigen-specific immunoadsorption and rituximab. Transplantation 2003; 76(4):730–1.

82. Glotz D, Antoine C, Julia P et al. Desensitization and subsequent kidney transplantation of patients using intravenous immunoglobulins (IVIg). Am J Transplant 2002; 2:758–60.

83. Schweitzer EJ, Wilson JS, Fernandez-Vina M et al. A high panel-reactive antibody rescue protocol for cross-match-positive live donor kidney transplants. Transplantation 2000; 70:1531–6.

84. Jordan SC. Management of the highly HLA-sensitized patient. A novel role for intravenous gammaglobulin. Am J Transplant 2002; 2:691–2.

85. Sonnenday CJ, Ratner LE, Zachary AA et al. Preemptive therapy with plasmapheresis/intravenous immunoglobulin allows successful live donor renal transplantation in patients with a positive cross-match. Transplant Proc 2002; 34(5):1614–16.

86. Warren DS, Zachary AA, Sonnenday CJ et al. Successful renal transplantation across simultaneous ABO incompatible and positive crossmatch barriers. Am J Transplant 2004; 4:561–8.

87. Suthanthiran M. Acute rejection of renal allografts: mechanistic insights and therapeutic options. Kidney Int 1997; 51(4):1289–304.

88. Miller LW. Cardiovascular toxicities of immunosuppressive agents. Am J Transplant 2002; 2(9):807–18.

89. Ojo AO, Hanson JA, Wolfe RA et al. Long-term survival in renal transplant recipients with graft function. Kidney Int 2000; 57(1):307–13.

90. Weir MR, Fink JC. Risk for posttransplant diabetes mellitus with current immunosuppressive medications. Am J Kidney Dis 1999; 34(1):1–13.

91. Saemann MD, Zeyda M, Diakos C et al. Suppression of early T-cell-receptor-triggered cellular activation by the Janus kinase 3 inhibitor WHI-P-154. Transplantation 2003; 75(11):1864–72.

92. Adams AB, Shirasugi N, Durham MM et al. Calcineurin inhibitor-free CD28 blockade-based protocol protects allogeneic islets in nonhuman primates. Diabetes 2002; 51(2):265–70.

93. Matas AJ, Ramcharan T, Paraskevas S et al. Rapid discontinuation of steroids in living donor kidney transplantation: a pilot study. Am J Transplant 2001; 1(3):278–83.

94. Knechtle SJ, Pirsch JD, H. Fechner J, Jr et al. Campath-1H induction plus rapamycin monotherapy for renal transplantation: results of a pilot study. Am J Transplant 2003; 3(6):722–30.

95. Kirk AD, Hale DA, Mannon RB et al. Results from a human renal allograft tolerance trial evaluating the humanized CD52-specific monoclonal antibody alemtuzumab (CAMPATH-1H). Transplantation 2003; 76(1):120–9.

96. Shapiro R, Jordan ML, Basu A et al. Kidney transplantation under a tolerogenic regimen of recipient pretreatment and low-dose postoperative

immunosuppression with subsequent weaning. Ann Surg 2003; 238(4):520–5; discussion 525–7.

 97. Vincenti F. Immunosuppression minimization: current and future trends in transplant immuno-suppression. J Am Soc Nephrol 2003; 14(7):1940–8.

An important, comprehensive overview of the state of immunosuppression minimisation protocols.

98. Smak Gregoor PJ, de Sevaux RG, Ligtenberg G et al. Withdrawal of cyclosporine or prednisone six months after kidney transplantation in patients on triple drug therapy: a randomized, prospective, multicenter study. J Am Soc Nephrol 2002; 13(5):1365–73.

99. Gonwa TA, Hricik DE, Brinker K et al. Improved renal function in sirolimus-treated renal transplant patients after early cyclosporine elimination. Transplantation 2002; 74(11):1560–7.

100. Blum CB. Effects of sirolimus on lipids in renal allo-graft recipients: an analysis using the Framingham risk model. Am J Transplant 2002; 2(6):551–9.

101. Chueh SC, Kahan BD. Dyslipidemia in renal transplant recipients treated with a sirolimus and cyclosporine-based immunosuppressive regimen: incidence, risk factors, progression, and prognosis. Transplantation 2003; 76(2):375–82.

102. Valente JF, Hricik D, Weigel K et al. Comparison of sirolimus vs. mycophenolate mofetil on surgical complications and wound healing in adult kidney transplantation. Am J Transplant 2003; 3(9): 1128–34.

103. Smith KD, Wrenshall LE, Nicosia RF et al. Delayed graft function and cast nephropathy associated with tacrolimus plus rapamycin use. J Am Soc Nephrol 2003; 14(4):1037–45.

104. Cosio FG, Pesavento TE, Kim S et al. Patient survival after renal transplantation: IV. Impact of post-transplant diabetes. Kidney Int 2002; 62(4):1440–6.

105. Ahsan N, Hricik D, Matas A et al. Prednisone withdrawal in kidney transplant recipients on cyclo-sporine and mycophenolate mofetil – a prospective randomized study. Steroid Withdrawal Study Group. Transplantation 1999; 68(12):1865–74.

106. Cole E, Landsberg D, Russell D et al. A pilot study of steroid-free immunosuppression in the prevention of acute rejection in renal allograft recipients. Transplantation 2001; 72(5):845–50.

107. Hricik DE, Knauss TC, Bodziak KA et al. With-drawal of steroid therapy in African American kidney transplant recipients receiving sirolimus and tacrolimus. Transplantation 2003; 76(6):938–42.

108. Calne R, Friend P, Moffatt S et al. Prope tolerance, perioperative campath 1H, and low-dose cyclo-sporin monotherapy in renal allograft recipients. Lancet 1998; 351(9117):1701–2.

109. Feucht HE, Schneeberger H, Hillebrand G et al. Capillary deposition of C4d complement fragment and early renal graft loss. Kidney Int 1993; 43(6):1333–8.

110. Feucht HE. Complement C4d in graft capillaries – the missing link in the recognition of humoral allo-reactivity. Am J Transplant 2003; 3(6):646–52.

111. Halloran PF, Wadgymar A, Ritchie S et al. The significance of the anti-class I antibody response. I. Clinical and pathologic features of anti-class I-mediated rejection. Transplantation 1990; 49(1): 85–91.

112. Nickeleit V, Zeiler M, Gudat F et al. Detection of the complement degradation product C4d in renal allografts: diagnostic and therapeutic implications. J Am Soc Nephrol 2002; 13(1):242–51.

113. Racusen LC, Colvin RB, Solez K et al. Antibody-mediated rejection criteria – an addition to the Banff 97 classification of renal allograft rejection. Am J Transplant 2003; 3(6):708–14.

114. Montgomery RA, Zachary AA, Racusen LC et al. Plasmapheresis and intravenous immune globulin provides effective rescue therapy for refractory humoral rejection and allows kidneys to be successfully transplanted into cross-match-positive recipients. Transplantation 2000; 70(6):887–95.

115. Mauiyyedi S, Pelle PD, Saidman S et al. Chronic humoral rejection: identification of antibody-mediated chronic renal allograft rejection by C4d deposits in peritubular capillaries. J Am Soc Nephrol 2001; 12(3):574–82.

116. Hariharan S, McBride MA, Cohen EP. Evolution of endpoints for renal transplant outcome. Am J Transplant 2003; 3(8):933–41.

117. Danovitch GM. Guidelines on the firing-line. Am J Transplant 2003; 3(5):514–15.

118. Kiberd B, Keough-Ryan T, Panek R. Cardiovascular disease reduction in the outpatient kidney trans-plant clinic. Am J Transplant 2003; 3(11):1393–9.

119. Rostand SG, Gretes JC, Kirk KA et al. Ischemic heart disease in patients with uremia undergoing maintenance hemodialysis. Kidney Int 1979; 16(5):600–11.

120. Sarnak MJ, Levey AS, Schoolwerth AC et al. Kidney disease as a risk factor for development of cardio-vascular disease: a statement from the American Heart Association Councils on Kidney in Cardio-vascular Disease, High Blood Pressure Research, Clinical Cardiology, and Epidemiology and Pre-vention. Circulation 2003; 108(17):2154–69.

121. Rostand SG. Coronary heart disease in chronic renal insufficiency: some management consider-ations. J Am Soc Nephrol 2000; 11(10):1948–56.

122. Kasiske BL, Chakkera HA, Roel J. Explained and unexplained ischemic heart disease risk after renal

transplantation. J Am Soc Nephrol 2000; 11(9): 1735–43.

123. Kasiske BL, Vazquez MA, Harmon WE et al. Recommendations for the outpatient surveillance of renal transplant recipients. American Society of Transplantation. J Am Soc Nephrol 2000; 11(suppl. 15):S1–86.

124. Third Report of the National Cholesterol Education Program (NCEP) Expert Panel on Detection, Evaluation, and Treatment of High Blood Cholesterol in Adults (Adult Treatment Panel III): final report. Circulation 2002; 106:3143–3421.

125. Halloran PF. Call for revolution: a new approach to describing allograft deterioration. Am J Transplant 2002; 2(3):195–200.

126. Regele H, Bohmig GA, Habicht A et al. Capillary deposition of complement split product C4d in renal allografts is associated with basement membrane injury in peritubular and glomerular capillaries: a contribution of humoral immunity to chronic allograft rejection. J Am Soc Nephrol 2002; 13(9):2371–80.

127. Lee PC, Terasaki PI, Takemoto SK et al. All chronic rejection failures of kidney transplants were preceded by the development of HLA antibodies. Transplantation 2002; 74(8):1192–4.

128. Akalin E, Dikman S, Murphy B et al. Glomerular infiltration by CXCR3+ ICOS+ activated T cells in chronic allograft nephropathy with transplant glomerulopathy. Am J Transplant 2003; 3(9): 1116–20.

129. Badid C, Desmouliere A, Babici D et al. Interstitial expression of alpha-SMA: an early marker of chronic renal allograft dysfunction. Nephrol Dial Transplant 2002; 17(11):1993–8.

130. Grimm PC, Nickerson P, Gough J et al. Computerized image analysis of Sirius Red-stained renal allograft biopsies as a surrogate marker to predict long-term allograft function. J Am Soc Nephrol 2003; 14(6):1662–8.

131. Halloran PF, Melk A, Barth C. Rethinking chronic allograft nephropathy: the concept of accelerated senescence. J Am Soc Nephrol 1999; 10(1):167–81.

  A prescient argument for rethinking the concept of 'chronic rejection'.

132. Gourishankar S, Jhangri GS, Cockfield SM et al. Donor tissue characteristics influence cadaver kidney transplant function and graft survival but not rejection. J Am Soc Nephrol 2003; 14(2):493–9.

133. Standards of medical care for patients with diabetes mellitus. Diabetes Care 2003; 26(suppl. 1):S33–S50.

Eight

Liver transplantation in the third millennium

Olivier Farges

INTRODUCTION

Although the first attempt at liver transplantation, by Thomas Starzl, dates back to 1963, the true development of this procedure only started in 1984 with the availability of an effective immuno-suppressant (ciclosporin). For the first time, acute rejection could be effectively controlled and the 1-year survival was greater than 50%. In these early days, liver transplantation was a formidable procedure, performed by a very limited number of surgeons worldwide, restricted to end-stage patients with a life expectancy measured in weeks, and associated with considerable mortality, morbidity and blood loss. Interestingly, the background of the surgeons who initiated this technique was somewhat different depending on their geographical areas. In Europe, most were surgeons who had significant previous experience with liver surgery. In the USA, on the contrary, most were transplant or vascular surgeons. This difference has had an important impact on how transplant programmes developed, where new techniques were initiated and how technical complications were managed.

Twenty years later, the annual number of liver transplants performed in Europe has increased from 84 to 4274, and liver transplantation has become available in all Western and most Eastern European countries. The procedure is routine in the most active centres, which occasionally have to perform two procedures in a row. Low-risk recipients hardly spend a couple of days in the intensive care unit. The 1-year mortality rate has fallen from 40% in the early 1980s to less than 20% in the late 1990s, and the 5-year survival has increased from 53 to 75%.[1] Immunosuppressive agents are progressively reduced and withdrawn so that most patients with stable graft function are on monotherapy (usually with a calcineurin inhibitor) 6 or 12 months after transplantation. Rejection has become one of the less frequent problems whereas complications related to immunosuppression are responsible for the majority of deaths in patients surviving more than 1 year. Overall, liver transplant recipients enjoy a good quality of life and often return to employment.[2,3] Female recipients are allowed pregnancy and the risk is generally small.[4] This evolution is mainly the result of standardisation of the technique and improved patient selection. These issues will be addressed first in this chapter.

However, whereas the number of potential recipients continues to increase as a result of the success of transplantation, the number of cadaveric donors has only marginally changed over the past 10 years, leading to long waiting times and a significant risk of death on the waiting list. This is probably the main problem facing transplant surgeons at the beginning of the third millennium.

This is particularly true since hepatitis C virus (HCV) infection, which has become the most frequent indication, inevitably recurs within the graft and is sometimes responsible for late graft loss. The second part of this chapter will therefore deal with the management of the waiting list and the means that have been developed to increase the number of grafts.

TECHNIQUES OF LIVER TRANSPLANTATION

Liver transplantation can be performed in different ways depending on where the graft is placed, whether the native liver is retained and whether all the graft or part of it is transplanted. **Orthotopic** and **heterotopic grafts** refer to grafts placed in their usual position or elsewhere (usually the left hypochondrium) respectively. **Auxiliary grafts** refer to grafts that are supposed to only provide part of the liver function with the native liver (or part of it) remaining in place. **Partial grafts** include reduced-size grafts and split grafts. **Reduced-size grafts** are when one part of the liver is retained for transplantation but the other part is discarded. A **split liver** is when the liver is divided into two parts and both are implanted in two different recipients. Domino and living donor transplantation are also techniques used to increase the number of grafts and will be addressed separately later in the chapter. The number of liver transplants performed in Europe with these techniques is shown in **Table 8.1**.

Table 8.1 • Number and types of liver transplants performed in Europe, 1988–June 2003

Liver transplants, overall	51 544
Paediatric transplants (0–15 years)	6137
Orthotopic	51 432
Heterotopic	112
Full-size	44 501
Reduced	2380
Split-liver	2901
Domino	266
Living donor	1286

Data from ref. 1.

The vast majority are orthotopic full-sized graft transplants.

Donor selection

This is addressed in Chapter 6. Liver transplants are only performed between ABO-identical donor–recipients although ABO-compatible grafts are allowed in urgent situations. ABO-incompatible grafts have been successfully used but are associated with decreased survival rates and are therefore no longer allowed in most countries.

 An important consideration is that cold ischaemia time should be kept as short as possible.

Transplant teams are usually informed approximately 4 hours before the retrieval procedure actually starts. Once the donor team has seen the liver and if this is suitable the recipient is brought into the operating room. Preparation of the recipient by the anaesthetists for invasive haemodynamic monitoring takes approximately 1 hour. Removing the recipient's liver lasts 2 to 4 hours. Cold ischaemia time should be less than 12 hours but the shorter the duration, the better the outcome. It is an independent risk factor for post-transplant survival[5] and utilisation of hospital resources.[6] The reduction in cold ischaemia time and better selection of donors have allowed a reduction in graft loss from primary non-function or dysfunction from 4.6% in 1986 to 1.5 % in 2003.[1]

Orthotopic transplantation of full-sized grafts

In the classical technique of liver transplantation, the recipient's liver is removed en bloc with the retrohepatic inferior vena cava, from above the renal veins to below the termination of the hepatic veins. Both ends are anastomosed end-to-end with the corresponding ends of the graft's inferior vena cava, which is also retrieved en bloc. The donor's portal vein is subsequently anastomosed end-to-end with the recipient's portal vein. At that stage, the graft is revascularised. This is frequently associated with a reperfusion syndrome characterised by a decrease in systemic pressure. The magnitude of this syndrome is correlated with graft steatosis and prolonged ischaemia time. The arterial anastomosis is performed subsequently and is rather straightforward as the graft is usually harvested with the coeliac axis. Depending on the surgeon's preference, this arterial graft is either left long or shortened and anastomosed to the recipient's common hepatic artery. It is alternatively anastomosed to the recipient's aorta if the recipient's hepatic artery is thrombosed or injured. Studies have suggested that performing the arterial anastomosis prior to the portal vein anastomosis is associated with a less severe reperfusion syndrome than when the portal vein anastomosis is performed first,[7] although there is no obvious clinical or biological impact.[8] Hence, most surgeons continue to perform the portal vein anastomosis first and start the arterial anastomosis, which is technically more demanding, once the graft is reperfused. The biliary reconstruction is performed last through either a Roux-en-Y anastomosis or a duct-to-duct anastomosis. If a duct-to-duct anastomosis is performed, the routine use of a T-tube is not mandatory as these T-tubes have their own morbidity of approximately 20%.[9] In any case, these tubes should not be removed before 3–4 months post-transplant to avoid biliary leakage.

This technique has evolved mainly for the biliary and caval anastomosis. Most surgeons currently rely on a duct-to-duct anastomosis rather than a Roux-en-Y anastomosis, and this also applies to partial grafts (see below). The former has the advantage over the latter of being quicker, of avoiding an intestinal anastomosis, and of allowing direct access to the bile duct through endoscopic retrograde cholangiopancreatography (ERCP) should this be required to diagnose and treat a leak or stenosis of the anastomosis. Roux-en-Y anastomoses are still performed in patients with primary sclerosing cholangitis, biliary atresia or in case of major disparity between the donor's and recipient's bile duct diameters.

The most significant change is, however, on the caval side. In the initial technique cross-clamping of the inferior vena cava was required as the recipient's inferior vena cava was removed. This would often produce haemodynamic instability, bleeding from the retroperitoneal space and splanchnic congestion, especially in adults. To overcome this problem, surgeons accepted the routine use of veno-venous bypass. Blood is diverted from the inferior vena cava (below the liver) and the portal vein, on the one side, to either the jugular or axillary vein using an external non-oxygenated pump.[10] This technique is fully standardised but requires an additional incision (to access the jugular or axillary vein) and may be associated with specific complications such as thromboembolism or air embolism, hypothermia or haemolysis.

A major breakthrough was the development of the caval preservation technique.[11] The recipient's liver is dissected from the retrohepatic vena cava, which can therefore be left in situ. This allows preservation of the caval flow and avoids the use of an external pump. Besides, a transient end-to-side porto-caval anastomosis may also be constructed to maintain splanchnic flow. Non-randomised studies suggest shorter operating times and fewer requirements for transfused blood with this technique when compared with traditional methods.[12,13] This technique has become the most widely used, at least in France, where a survey found that it accounted for 80% of all transplantations performed between 1991 and 1997.[14] The morbidity rate of this technique is 4%, mainly in bleeding complications or outflow obstruction.[14]

Several studies have reported that the feasibility of caval preservation is 100%.[15] There are nevertheless some situations where this preservation is technically demanding. In particular, this is the case for patients with an enlarged segment 1, encircling the inferior vena cava, such as those with a Budd–Chiari syndrome or cholestatic livers. This difficulty can usually be easily predicted from the recipient's computed tomography (CT) scan. In these patients (approximately 10%), a transient cross-clamping of the inferior vena cava may be indicated to simplify the procedure. As it is usually of short duration, it is better tolerated and does not require an external shunt. In contrast, preservation of the inferior vena cava is much easier in patients with atrophic livers.

Two issues remain controversial. The first is the need for the routine use of a porto-caval shunt during the anhepatic phase. A controlled trial has shown that this shunt was associated with improved haemodynamic status, reduced intraoperative transfusion requirements and preserved renal function during and after liver transplantation.[16] Besides, it takes less than 15 minutes to be created and has no specific morbidity. Nevertheless, many surgeons still use it selectively, in case of congestion of the intestine or poor haemodynamic tolerance.[17] Only in patients with large pre-existing, porto-systemic shunts or collateral circulation is this porto-caval anastomosis not required.

The second evolving issue is how the caval anastomosis should be performed in patients with preservation of their inferior vena cava. The initial method was the piggy-back technique with direct end-to-end anastomosis of the donor's vena cava with the unified stumps of the recipient's hepatic veins[18] (Fig. 8.1). However, several modifications of this technique have been described that differ in the site of the anastomosis on both the donor vena cava (terminal or with a longitudinal extension) and the recipient vena cava (on the common trunk of the left and middle hepatic vein, with or without caval extension, on all three hepatic veins, or on the anterior wall of the inferior vena cava)[19] (Figs 8.1 and 8.2). Whatever method is adopted, experience has shown that a side-biting vascular clamp applied to the front of the recipient cava will allow adequate maintenance of the caval flow during the procedure and thus avoid the need for bypass. The multitude of these methods indicates that the caval anastomosis in recipients with a preserved vena cava is not always straightforward. This is especially the case when the graft is either too small or too large for size. Small for size grafts may have a tendency to slide into the right hypochondrium causing twisting of the caval anastomosis. Large for size grafts may occasionally be very difficult to place as the graft's inferior vena cava may indeed be several centimetres above the level of the recipient's inferior vena cava, and the large size of the graft may prevent adequate visualisation of the anastomosis. This may be overcome by removing the graft's left lateral segment on the back table prior to implantation or by using an interposition venous graft. These large grafts may nevertheless cause anastomotic occlusion by compression. Overall, if there is size disparity between the donor and recipient liver, performing the anastomosis on all three hepatic veins seems to achieve better outflow as it allows a wider anastomosis and avoids positional kinking.[20]

Besides avoiding caval cross-clamping and the use of an external pump, the technique of caval flow preservation has also paved the way for the use of partial grafts (split and living-related grafts) as these grafts do not have a vena cava (see below).

Reduced size grafts

As paediatric donors are rare, size reduction of adult donor grafts was developed in 1984 to allow transplantation of paediatric recipients.[21] This technique consists in removing the right liver or right lobe on the back table as for a conventional hepatectomy. The common bile duct, common hepatic artery, main portal vein and inferior vena cava are retained with the graft (Fig. 8.3). Excellent patient survival of over 90% was obtained with this technique even in children under 1 year of age,[22] and it has therefore been widely adopted internationally resulting in a significant fall in the number of children on waiting lists. However, reduced size grafts have the major disadvantage of discarding the right part of the graft. As this can in fact be used with the technique of split-liver transplantation (see below) most surgeons currently feel that it should only be used in very selected cases where split transplantation cannot be performed. Less than 70 children have been transplanted with this technique in Europe during the past 4 years.

Auxiliary transplantation

In contrast to the previously described technique of liver transplantation, which completely removes the native liver, auxiliary transplantation aims at leaving the native liver (or part of it) in place.

The auxiliary graft was initially used as an alternative to orthotopic whole organ transplantation in patients with end-stage liver disease.[23] The graft was placed heterotopically (usually in the left hypochondrium) and the whole native liver was left in situ. This has almost been abandoned due to the difficulty in achieving optimal outflow of heterotopic grafts combined with the risk of hepatic malignancy developing in the native residual liver of patients grafted for end-stage liver disease with cirrhosis.

Orthotopic auxiliary transplantation has, however, persisted as an option for patients with fulminant liver failure or inborn errors of metabolism. The rationale in patients with fulminant liver failure is

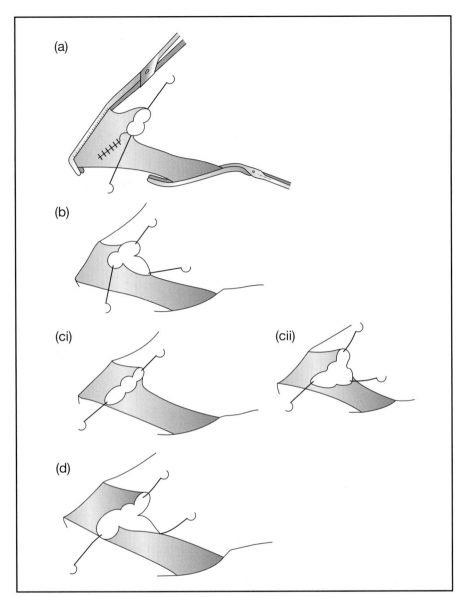

Figure 8.1 • Cavo-caval anastomosis. Caval implantation anastomotic site may vary according to surgeon's choice. In order to decrease the risk of further outflow problems, preference must be given to the largest anastomotic line and to triangulation technique, when possible (**cii** and **d**). **(a)** Trunk of middle and left hepatic veins; **(b)** same as **(a)** with longitudinal split of the vena cava and triangulation; **(ci)** all hepatic veins ostia; **(cii)** same as **(ci)** with triangulation; **(d)** same as **(ci)**, adding vena cava longitudinal split and triangulation technique.

that their liver occasionally regenerates some time after the liver injury has subsided. Auxiliary transplantation aims at providing liver function support during the time period necessary for the liver to regenerate. Once this has occurred, immunosuppression can be stopped and the liver graft undergoes atrophy or can be surgically removed.

Regeneration is mainly observed in patients aged under 40 years transplanted for fulminant liver failure secondary to hepatitis A or B virus or paracetamol overdose. Normal function of the native liver and interruption of the immunosuppressive treatment can be achieved in 65–70% of the 1-year survivors.[24,25]

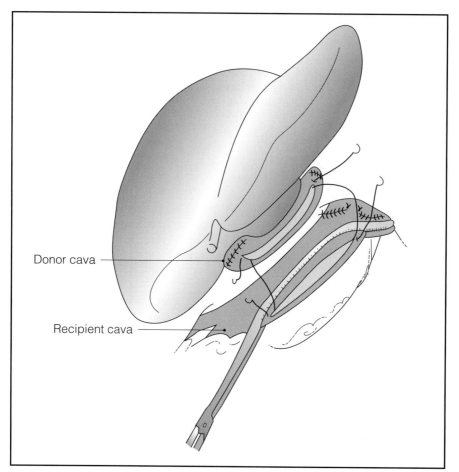

Figure 8.2 • Latero-lateral cavo-cavostomy. The donor and recipient venae cavae are preserved and a large side-to-side anastomosis is performed after suturing both ends of the donor cava. A large clamp is positioned but preserving the recipient caval flow during the procedure.

The technique includes partial hepatectomy of the recipient's liver and transplantation of a partial graft. As the aim, at the initial stage of liver failure, is to provide a sufficient liver mass, the graft is a right liver or a right lobe, which is positioned in place of the previously removed recipient's right liver. The volume and function of both the native liver and graft are monitored postoperatively by CT-scan volumetry and scintigraphy. The procedure is technically more demanding and associated with greater morbidity than whole liver transplantation.[26] The technical complications may, however, be overcome. Besides, the potential for immunosuppression withdrawal is invaluable in young patients.

An additional application of auxiliary grafts is in patients with inborn errors of metabolism caused by a liver defect but not associated with structural liver damage, such as Crigler–Najjar syndrome type 1.[27,28] Good results have been obtained in patients with orthotopically placed auxiliary grafts. However, apart from reducing the risk of losing the patient with acute graft failure with a conventional transplant, there seems limited appeal for this approach in this group of patients since immunosuppression is still required to maintain the graft.

INDICATIONS FOR TRANSPLANTATION AND EVOLUTION

Liver transplantation has specifically been the subject of two Consensus Conferences. The first NIH Consensus Conference held in 1983 in

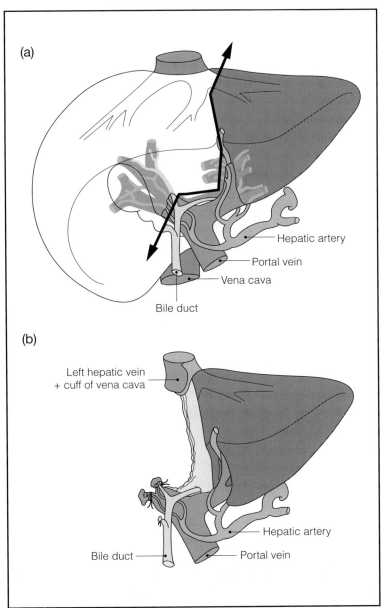

Figure 8.3 • Liver graft reduction technique. **(a)** Section line for preparation of a reduced liver graft using a straight transhilar approach. Right portal vein, hepatic artery and bile duct are electively divided at porta hepatis level. **(b)** Final aspect of the reduced graft.

Bethesda (USA) focused on the clinical usefulness of liver transplantation, justifying its financial cover by the Social Security system and by the Insurance Funds. The second, held in Paris (France) in 1993, aimed at validating the indications due to the growing disparity between need and supply.[29]

The main indications and contraindications in adults agreed at the end of this second conference are listed in **Box 8.1**. As a rule, it was felt that transplantation is indicated when life expectancy is less than 1 year without transplantation and when there are no contraindications. Absolute contraindications were held to be: the presence of extrahepatic organ failure (unless simultaneous transplantation of this organ was performed), uncontrolled immune disease or uncontrolled extrahepatic sepsis. Anticipated poor compliance due to psychiatric disorder was viewed as a relative contraindication.

For most of these chronic liver diseases, mathematical prognosis models have been developed that may help predict the natural history and help decide when transplantation is indicated. The

Box 8.1 • Indications for liver transplantation (LT). Summary of the conclusions of the Consensus Conference held in Paris, 1993

A CLEARLY VALIDATED INDICATIONS	B CONTROVERSIAL INDICATIONS
Primary biliary cirrhosis LT indicated when: • serum bilirubin >100–150 µmol/L, and/or • ascites, and/or • recurring gastrointestinal bleeding, and/or • pruritus resistant to medical treatment, and/or • marked asthenia	**Hepatitis B viral cirrhosis*** Accepted indication if: • no viral replication • routine prophylaxis with anti-HBs immunoglobulin postoperatively
Primary sclerosing cholangitis LT indicated when: • serum bilirubin >100–150 µmol/L, and/or • recurring and poorly controlled cholangitis, and/or • cirrhosis	**Hepatitis C viral cirrhosis*** Accepted indication, although: • HCV infection persists in 75% of the patients • there is no prophylaxis of reinfection
Biliary atresia LT indicated when: • recurrent jaundice after Kasai operation • recurring gastrointestinal bleeding, and/or • recurring and poorly controlled cholangitis • pruritus resistant to medical treatment, and/or • cardiopulmonary complication of cirrhosis • liver failure	**Alcohol cirrhosis*** Accepted indication if: • abstinence of 3–6 months
	Hepatocellular carcinoma Accepted indication if: • the tumour is not too large or multinodular • the tumour is not too small (as these may be resectable without transplantation)
Fulminant or subfulminant liver failure No international standardised criteria; rely on: • factor V or prothrombin time • age • aetiology of liver failure • interval between jaundice and encephalopathy • serum bilirubin	**C NEUROENDOCRINE LIVER METASTASES** **Contraindications** • Liver metastases from colorectal, gastric or breast cancer

*Indication for transplantation in patients with cirrhosis is the deterioration of liver function and/or the occurrence of severe complications such as spontaneous bacterial peritonitis, or recurring bleeding episodes.

progressive deterioration of liver function over time is also an important aspect of selection.

It is important in that respect to be aware that patients with alcoholic cirrhosis may considerably improve their liver function after abstinence and that several months may be required before this becomes evident. Achieving abstinence is therefore crucial, not only to select patients who are less likely to recur after transplantation (see below) but also to assess whether transplantation is indeed necessary.

It is interesting to note that this consensus conference regarded indications for transplant, where the primary disease is likely to recur, as controversial indications. This particularly applied to patients with persistent hepatitis B virus (HBV)-DNA replication or with persistent alcohol consumption. Paradoxically, HCV cirrhosis was not considered as a contraindication despite constant recurrence of HCV infection in the recipient because recurrence was not felt, at that time, to adversely impact outcome. Finally, age was not considered to be a contraindication because several studies had shown it not to impact adversely on survival.

In 1999, 6 years later, the British Society of Gastroenterology also published guidelines on the indications for referral and assessment in adult liver transplantation.[30]

Emphasis was placed on the need for early referral of potential candidates to transplant programmes so as to optimise timing and avoid transplantation being performed when malnutrition or hepatorenal failure have occurred as both significantly increase the risk of the procedure.

Positivity for human immunodeficiency virus (HIV), age above 70 years, portal venous system thrombosis and pulmonary hypertension in the recipient were additional relative contraindications to those already identified in Paris. Most importantly, viral or alcohol cirrhosis was no longer considered as a controversial indication.

Things have indeed evolved over the past 10 years and the main changes will be discussed briefly:

1. Most of the clearly validated indications have become less frequent indications for transplantation.

   (a) Primary biliary cirrhosis (PBC), which initially was the most frequent indication in adults, has become an exceptional indication for liver transplantation except in the few countries where its incidence is high. Most PBC patients have indeed been transplanted in the early period. Besides, treatment with ursodesoxycholic acid has been shown to be very effective in slowing the progression of the disease.[31] Consequently, by the time PBC patients become potential transplant candidates, they may be older than the upper age limit set in most centres. In the year 2000, PBC accounted for only 6% of all liver transplants performed in Europe. The same holds true for primary sclerosing cholangitis (PSC), as its incidence is ten times lower than that of PBC. Hence, the two most validated indications in adults 10 years ago have become relatively rare indications today. Another previously

unrecognised feature of these diseases is that they can recur within the graft although the impact of this recurrence on survival is marginal.[32,33]

   (b) Fulminant liver failure has also become a less frequent indication for liver transplantation than 10 years ago. In 1988, it accounted for 13% of all transplantations performed in Europe but this figure had dropped to 8% by 2001.[34] The most likely explanation is better management of these patients at the initial stage of liver failure, use of N-acetylcysteine and reduction in the incidence of HBV infection.

2. The proportion of transplantations performed for viral hepatitis has, in contrast, increased considerably. In the USA, for example, HBV or HCV cirrhosis accounted for 60% of all transplantations performed in 2002 as compared with 12% in 1991.

   (a) HBV-DNA replication prior to transplantation, which was the main limitation to the transplantation of HBV-cirrhotic patients, can now be stopped with the most recent antiviral treatments in up to 90% of patients.

Post-transplant prevention of viral recurrence within the graft relies on the administration of hepatitis B immunoglobulin and lamivudine.

The major concern is the development of lamivudine resistance due to mutations in the YMDD motif of the HBV-DNA polymerase gene. New drugs such as adefovir dipivoxil and entecavir have been demonstrated to be effective against both wild-type and lamivudine-resistant mutants. Survival of patients transplanted for an HBV and an HBV-HDV (hepatitis D virus) coinfection is 70% and 85% at 5 years and 65% and 85% at 10 years.

   (b) In contrast, HCV recurrence within the graft is a rising and unforeseen problem. HCV recurrence, although recognised as potentially resulting in severe liver damage, was initially thought to have a relatively slow progression and not to impact on survival significantly.[35] However, recent studies have reported a much higher and quicker rate of severe graft damage than previously thought.[36]

 HCV recurrence is now recognised as having a significant impact on the survival of both patients and grafts.

Following transplantation, HCV infection recurs in all patients who are HCV RNA-positive at the time of transplantation and viral load is considerably higher than prior to transplantation.[37] The rate of progression of fibrosis is 3–6 times faster in transplant recipients than in naive patients, and it is estimated that 30% of recipients develop cirrhosis by the end of the fifth postoperative year. Once cirrhosis is established, decompensation occurs in 42% after 1 year as compared with 3% per year in non-transplant patients. The 5-year survival rate in HCV-positive recipients is 10% less than in HCV-negative recipients.[38,39] Furthermore, survival curves continue to decline after the fifth postoperative year at a much faster rate than for other cirrhosis, with a 10-year survival of only 55%. Only patients transplanted for a malignancy have a lower survival.

The rate of fibrosis progression appears to be highly dependent on the date of transplantation.[40] Median time interval to the detection of cirrhosis has shortened from more than 10 years in patients transplanted in the late 1980s to around 3 years in patients transplanted in the late 1990s. Some of the risk factors for recurrence have been identified recently and include the use of organs from older donors (as the donor pool has been extended in recent years to such donors),[41] prolonged ischaemia time, heavy induction immunosuppression and treatment for acute rejection.[42] The impact of the use of reduced rather than whole grafts (through splitting or living-related liver transplantation) is uncertain. As the trend

for severe recurrence has emerged only recently, it may be feared that the 55% 10-year survival reported in the European Liver Transplant Registry for the period 1988–2000 may be an overestimate. Furthermore, as HCV disease accounts for at least 40% of liver transplantations and as re-transplantation for HCV recurrence is not contraindicated (although controversial in some countries), there is even concern that HCV disease alone may overwhelm the system. Hence the great interest in the development of antiviral treatments.[43]

Antiviral treatment in patients on the waiting list can induce a sustained response in 20% but many patients do not meet inclusion criteria and serious adverse events occur frequently. Post-transplant combination therapy with interferon and ribavirin also achieves a sustained virological response rate of 20%.[44] Ribavirin is, however, poorly tolerated in transplant recipients and, overall, almost two-thirds of the patients require dose adjustment. Higher response rates are expected with utilising pegylated interferon,[45] although it is less efficacious than in immunocompetent patients. Infusions of high-titre HCV antibody in the peri- and postoperative period are currently under study as prophylaxis against re-emergence.

3. Relative contraindications have been more clearly defined.

(a) Hepatocellular carcinoma (HCC) initially accounted for 30% of liver transplant procedures but currently accounts for less than 15%. This is related to a radical change in the selection criteria. In the early 1980s, liver transplantation was performed in patients whose tumour could not be resected due to the severity of their cirrhosis or size of their tumour. Survival following transplantation of patients with large tumours was, however, very low due to a prohibitive recurrence rate.

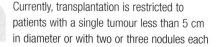 Currently, transplantation is restricted to patients with a single tumour less than 5 cm in diameter or with two or three nodules each

less than 3 cm, provided there is neither vascular invasion, lymph node metastases, nor extrahepatic disease (the so-called Milan criteria).[46]

Provided these criteria are fulfilled, the 5-year survival is 70%, comparable to that of patients transplanted without a malignancy.

(b) HIV infection is no longer considered as a formal contraindication to transplantation[47] (provided CD4 levels are above 400/mm^3) and trials are under way in different countries to assess the efficacy of transplantation in this setting. As a matter of fact, incidence of HIV positivity amongst HBV- or HCV-cirrhotic patients is high. Preliminary results indicate that these patients should be transplanted at a somewhat earlier stage than HIV-negative patients and that the management of antiviral treatment requires adaptation.

It is of course difficult to predict how these indications will evolve over the next decade. There is, in particular, considerable variation in the proportion of each indication between countries, a likely reflection of the epidemiology of diseases and in particular HCV infection. One approach is to consider the prevalence of some liver diseases, and figures are given for the USA in **Table 8.2**. Although HCV infection is currently a growing problem, the age of cirrhosis decompensation or HCC development (the two most frequent indications for trans-

Table 8.2 • Prevalence of some liver diseases in the USA

NAFLD	2/10
Alcohol abuse	8/100
HBsAg or anti-HBc Ab	5/100
Anti-HCV	2/100
NASH	2/100
Haemochromatosis	2–5/1000
Primary biliary cirrhosis	3/10 000
Wilson disease	3/100 000

NAFLD, non-alcoholic fatty liver disease; NASH, non-alcoholic steato-hepatitis.

plantation) is increasing. It currently peaks above 70 years old and this will certainly be a limitation in the access to transplantation. Non-alcoholic fatty liver disease (NAFLD) and non-alcoholic steato-hepatitis (NASH), a spectrum of histopathological changes in the liver correlated with obesity and type 2 diabetes, seem in contrast to emerge as rising causes of cirrhosis or as additional risk factors for fibrosis progression in patients with alcohol or viral injuries.

THE WAITING LIST

As for other organs, most notably the kidney, there is an obvious discrepancy between the number of transplant candidates and the number of grafts available. Increasing waiting time and mortality rates on the waiting list are evidence for this. Most importantly, the number of candidates continues to increase whereas the number of cadaveric grafts is stable. During the year 2000 in the USA, the number of candidates increased by 17% whereas there was no increase in the number of cadaver grafts. It is likely that the number of cadaveric donors will even decrease in the future.

These figures require, however, some comments:

- The mortality rates on most waiting lists range between 5 and 10%. However, these figures are difficult to interpret as they do not take into account patients who are removed from the list because they become too sick.
- The discrepancy between the numbers of donors and recipients is highly variable from one country to another. **Table 8.3** for example shows that although there is a shortage in the UK and France, this is considerably less than in the USA. Part of this discrepancy can be explained by a much earlier listing of potential transplant candidates in the USA compared with other countries (see below).
- The number of transplant candidates refers to those actually listed, not all potential transplant candidates, some of whom are not listed. Prevention of access to the waiting list may be financial, cultural or medical. In Virginia for example, Medicare did not recognise liver transplantation as a standard therapy for adult patients until 3 years ago. There is also a perception that the well-educated portions of

Table 8.3 • Comparison between the number of liver transplants performed (first figure) and the number of patients still on the waiting list at the end of the year (second figure)

Year	USA	UK	France
1993	3440/2902	533/98	653/371
1995	3933/5529	668/138	646/304
1998	4516/11 579	665/201	693/238
2001	5188/18 047	675/158	803/404
2002	5330/16 974	706/163	882/458
2003	5671/na	627/239	na

Data available from www.unos.org (USA), www.uktransplant.org.uk (United Kingdom), www.efg.sante.fr (France).

our societies access healthcare systems earlier and more frequently than individuals from less favoured communities. Finally, attitudes of physicians or transplant centres towards liver transplantation are not homogeneous. There remain, for example, concerns in some transplant units about the appropriateness of offering scarce livers to those with alcoholic liver disease or those who use illegal drugs. Moreover, considerable variations exist between and within countries regarding access to medical care.

- Such discrepancies are not homogeneous. Paediatric recipients, for example, are relatively spared. This is somewhat paradoxical as children were initially limited in their access to liver grafts due to the preponderance of adult donor grafts. There is, however, a cultural tradition to favour children, and measures have been implemented in most countries to speed up their access to the list. In France, for example, all donors less than 30 years old are offered to paediatric recipients as a priority.
- There are also highly variable waiting times between regions or centres within the same country. This seems particularly true in countries where the number of transplant programmes is high or the number of transplantations performed in each programme is highly variable. In that respect, the UK, where only seven, albeit very active,

programmes are running appears to be an exception.

- Finally, and probably most importantly, the number of cadaveric grafts is only a small fraction of the number of cadaveric donors. This is best evidenced by the highly variable number of donors per million inhabitants in various countries. This figure ranges between 15 (in most European countries and Canada) and 35 in Spain.

As a rule, the number of transplantations performed has not increased markedly over time except in the USA (**Table 8.3**). The increase observed in France in 2001 is mainly related to the development of living-relative liver transplantations.

Several approaches have been used to decrease the disparity between the number of transplant candidates and grafts, such as optimising allocation, increasing the number of cadaveric grafts, and use of living-related liver transplantation.

OPTIMISING ALLOCATION OF GRAFTS

The principles of allocation are not unique to transplantation and parallels have even been made with what happened during the sinking of the Titanic.[48] Situations vary greatly between countries due to the difference in the burden of liver disease, methods of delivering and paying for healthcare services, amount of resources put into healthcare and rates of organ donation. An important aspect is also that the views of medical practitioners and policy-makers may be different from that of the public. The former are very likely to place emphasis on medical outcome. The latter places a very high value on considerations other than outcomes, particularly that of giving everyone a chance at receiving scarce resources.[49] Studies to date have shown that, all things equal, the public prefers that life-saving procedures such as transplantation be given to the young over the old, to those not responsible for their illness over those whose illness is self-inflicted, and to primary transplantations over re-transplantations.

Several systems have been implemented worldwide to optimise graft allocation and reduce mortality rates on the waiting list. All consist of prioritising high-risk recipients.[50] This applies particularly to patients with acute liver failure, which includes fulminant liver failure, primary graft non-function or post-transplantation hepatic artery thrombosis and acute decompensation of Wilson's disease. The main difference for the other recipients is whether the allocation of the graft is patient- or centre-orientated. Below are three examples on how these systems work.

US models

In the USA, the earliest system of liver allocation employed the 'sickest first' principle, with some priority also given to the time spent on the waiting list. Patients in an intensive care unit (ICU) received first priority, followed by patients requiring continuous hospitalisation, and lastly patients who were being cared for at home. However, the drawbacks of this method were that the criteria for grading these patients were not standardised and that patients were listed years before they actually needed a transplant merely to accrue waiting time. Because the waiting list and waiting times were growing, this system was changed in 1997, when minimal criteria for placement on the waiting list were introduced.[51] Disease severity was graded using the Child–Turcotte–Pugh (CTP) scoring system, initially devised to predict outcomes after portal decompression. The minimal criterion was that patients be CTP class B. In addition, a separate status 1 category was created for patients with fulminant hepatic failure, primary non-function of a liver transplant or hepatic artery thrombosis diagnosed within 7 days of transplantation, as well as patients with acute decompensated Wilson's disease. Patients with chronic liver disease were grouped into status 2A (CTP score $\geqslant$ 10 and less than 7 days predicted survival), status 2B (CTP score = 10 or CTP score = 7–9 with major complications of portal hypertension) and status 3 (CTP score = 7–9), in order of diminishing priority. Unfortunately, the minimal criteria adopted in 1997 also proved too broad and inexact to control placement on the list. This also failed to reduce waiting times.

The most recently implemented system therefore gives less priority to the waiting time and removes subjective elements in the evaluation of the severity of the liver disease. It is based on the Mayo End-stage Liver Disease Model (later renamed Model for End-stage Liver Disease, or MELD), which had initially been designed to predict mortality after transjugular intrahepatic portosystemic shunt (TIPS). This model was tested in various groups of patients with end-stage liver disease, including transplant candidates, and underwent some modifications including the withdrawal of variables referring to the complications of portal hypertension and cause of cirrhosis before being implemented for the national waiting list at the end of March 2002.

$$MELD\ score\ =\ 0.957 \times \log N\ (LN)\ (creatinine)\ +$$
$$0.378 \times LN\ (bilirubin)\ +$$
$$1.12 \times LN\ [International$$
$$Normalized\ Ratio\ (INR)]\ +\ 0.643$$

Patients with hepatocellular carcinoma (HCC) are somewhat prioritised on this list. In fact, according to UNOS data, wait-list times for a liver transplant can approach or exceed 2 years for 45% of the listed patients. This greatly disfavoured HCC patients, whose indication for transplantation depends more on the tumour stage than on the severity of their liver disease. During this waiting time, the tumour could evolve to a point when liver transplantation was becoming contraindicated. This occurred in up to 50% of the patients after 1 year on the waiting list.[52] The goal for prioritising HCC patients is to equate the risk of tumour progression beyond the transplantation criteria with the risk of death in non-HCC patients with chronic liver disease on the waiting list over the same period of time. HCC patients were therefore assigned 24 points when their tumour was less than 2 cm (stage 1) and 29 points if they had a single tumour 2–5 cm or two or three nodules all less than 3 cm (stage 2). This arbitrary scoring assignment was downgraded in April 2003 after it was found that HCC patients were being preferentially transplanted compared with others having equal MELD scores on the waiting list (20 points for stage 1 and 24 points for stage 2). More changes were made in April 2004 when it was further uncovered that 30% of stage 1 patients in fact had no tumours on their liver explants. Patients with stage 1 tumours therefore no longer receive priority while stage 2 patients continue to receive 24 points.

These changes show how complicated it is to define the rules for a national waiting list. Besides, the 'sickest first' principle has the inherent drawback of compromising the overall efficiency of transplantation as the survival is lower in the sickest patients. Finally, this system gives little flexibility to the attribution of non-optimal grafts (see below).

The UK model

In the UK, compared with the USA, liver transplantation is more tightly regulated, performed in fewer centres and associated with shorter waiting lists and times. The centrally funded body, UK Transplant, maintains the waiting list nationally. Super-urgent patients (fulminant liver failure, emergency re-transplantation or total absence of liver function) are given national priority. If there is no super-urgent recipient, grafts are allocated to the transplant unit in whose area the donor is located. The transplant unit selects the recipient judged the most suitable for the given donor. If no recipient is suitable or if the graft is judged unusable, it is offered, in sequence, to the other units, in turn. This system offers considerable flexibility. There is in addition little pressure to list patients at a too early stage, which may explain the much reduced waiting list. Agreement of the centres to give priority to very urgent patients (such as those with fulminant hepatic failure) further removed these concerns.

The fundamental principles that govern liver transplantation in the UK were laid down in Edinburgh in 1998, and may be summarised as follows:

1. Donor livers are a national resource that is limited. Guidelines drawn up to indicate the selection criteria for transplantation should be publicised and agreed by all those involved in transplantation (including patients and lay members) and followed by all the designated centres in the UK.
2. Livers should be allocated to give a maximum outcome in preference to allowing every potential recipient to have a chance to receive an available organ; i.e. utility prevails over equity. The main criteria for selection of patients should be based on the quality of life and anticipated life expectancy set out in the guidelines, and patients should be offered transplantation if there is a more than 50% probability of the patient being alive 5 years

after transplantation with a quality of life acceptable to the patient.
3. Selection of the recipients is the responsibility of the transplant unit as physicians taking care of the waiting list are the best placed to select the ideal recipient of a given donor.

The French model

In France, graft allocation is also centre- rather than patient-orientated. The advantage of this system is that each centre coordinates its waiting list and there is therefore little pressure to list patients prematurely. It also affords greater flexibility in the use of marginal or split livers depending on the clinical condition of the recipient. There nevertheless also exists the concept of super-emergencies and adult emergencies. The former include fulminant liver failures and graft failures within 7 days of transplantation. The latter patients have priority over all the others at the national level and the mean waiting time is less than 2 days. These include adult patients with acute decompensation of a chronic liver disease, provided agreement is given by external experts. Such patients have a priority at the regional level. Finally, there also exists a local priority. Grafts retrieved within a hospital are offered first to the corresponding transplant unit provided there are no regional or national priorities. If no recipient is available, the graft is offered to the other units of the region, in turn. Interestingly, transplant centres that are approached through this process go to the end of the list whether or not they accept the graft. This is a direct but effective way to increase the use of available grafts.

INCREASING THE NUMBER OF CADAVERIC GRAFTS

Four methods have been used to increase the number of cadaveric grafts: (1) the use of cadaveric donors previously considered as unsuitable for donation; (2) transplanting more than one recipient with one graft, through splitting or domino transplantation; (3) developing living-related liver transplantation; and (4) improving the identification of cadaveric donors. Xenotransplantation and the use of stem cell technology will not be addressed in the present chapter.

Use of marginal donors

Marginal grafts include those from older donors, those with steatotic grafts or evidence of current or prior viral hepatitis – anti-HCV or anti-hepatitis B core (HBc) antibodies – and non-heart-beating donors. These marginal grafts, as a rule, were initially used for urgent recipients in whom transplantation could not be delayed. Results were clearly unsatisfactory, leading to the conclusion that high-risk recipients should be given optimal grafts and that marginal grafts would best suit recipients with preserved liver function and nutritional status who nevertheless could not wait too long for their transplant.

 Marginal grafts best suit recipients with preserved liver function and nutritional status who nevertheless cannot wait long for their transplant.

The ideal example of such a situation is a child grade A or B patient with hepatocellular carcinoma. The policy for optimal allocation of these marginal livers to individual patients may therefore not be the same as those for the standard liver from a heart-beating donor. Hence, centre-orientated allocation systems are more effective than patient-orientated ones. Another issue is whether recipients should be informed about this policy and what degree of information or veto should be given to the patient.

NON-HEART-BEATING DONORS

Another area of renewed interest is the use of non-heart-beating donors (NHBDs). These include haemodynamically stable individuals who are extubated in the operating room or intensive care unit following a decision by the patient's next of kin to withdraw care and provide consent for organ donation (controlled NHBD). In contrast, uncontrolled NHBD refers to those patients who sustain cessation of cardiopulmonary function prior to arriving at hospital, within the emergency department or as hospital inpatients. A recent North American survey shows that the number of NHBDs (predominantly controlled) is increasing but still

accounts for only 1% of all liver transplantations although there are estimates that it could increase to up to 20%. In recipients of these grafts, the risk of graft failure is increased by 30% and the survival curves decrease by 10%. Nevertheless, this technique appears to be a promising option provided donors are less than 60 years old, donor warm ischaemic time is less than 30 minutes, cold ischaemia time is less than 8 hours and recipients are in relatively good general condition.[61]

OLDER DONORS

Although there is no clear definition of an older donor, it was usually considered that these were associated with an increased risk for the recipient as a result of delayed graft function, arterial complications (due to arteriosclerosis of the graft's arteries) and transmission of occult tumours. There is, however, growing evidence that even donors older than 70 years may be used safely provided there are no additional risk factors.[53] These in particular include steatosis (which should be ruled out by a liver biopsy) and a long cold ischaemia time.[54] As a matter of fact, the age of the donor population has increased considerably over the past 10 years. In 1990, the proportion of donors more than 60 years was less than 1% whereas it is currently close to 20% in Europe.

STEATOTIC GRAFTS

There is a clear link between steatosis in the donor liver and graft dysfunction after transplantation,[55,56] which, in itself, has been shown to have a detrimental effect on eventual graft outcome. Steatosis is induced by several factors, including obesity, alcohol consumption and type 2 diabetes, making it a common histological finding in the normal population. In the cadaveric donor population, the prevalence of steatosis ranges between 15 and 30%.[57] Impaired liver function tests or the presence of a hyperechoic liver at ultrasound may raise suspicion but both lack sensitivity. Macroscopically, steatotic livers have a greasy consistency, yellow discoloration and rounded edges. However, these are relatively subjective and in one series, 66% of steatotic livers were described as 'normal' on macroscopic appearance.[58] When steatosis is suspected, histological evaluation of the donor liver is performed before transplantation. The percentage area of hepatic parenchyma involved with steatosis is evaluated on a frozen-section biopsy specimen. Both microvesicular steatosis (i.e. fat vacuoles smaller than the nuclear diameter) and macrovesicular steatosis (i.e. fat vacuoles larger than the nuclear diameter) are usually taken into account, although graft dysfunction has been shown to correlate best with macrovesicular steatosis.[59] Mild, moderate and severe steatosis are defined as being <30%, 30–60% or >60% respectively.

Most surgeons consider severe steatosis as an absolute contraindication to the use of the liver for transplantation, and use grafts with moderate steatosis only if other risk factors such as prolonged preservation time and poor condition of the recipient are not present.

The presence of fibrosis or polymorphonuclear infiltration within the liver in addition to steatosis is also a contraindication to use of a graft. Steatosis is the most common reason for not using liver grafts.

Other criteria that have been put forward to define marginal liver donors include:

- intensive care unit stay >4 days;
- prolonged hypotensive episodes of >1 hour and <60 mmHg with high inotropic drug use – dopamine (DPM) >14 µg/kg/min;
- cold ischaemia time >14 hours;
- peak serum sodium >155 mEq/L.

As a rule, it is recommended not to accumulate risk factors in either the donor or the recipient.

The acceptance policies of European liver transplant centres of these marginal donors are highly variable, both between and within units. However, busy centres tend to be less selective than less busy centres, despite the same donor pool.[60]

Despite the use of marginal grafts, the number of donor organs has only increased slowly. The general impression is that if transplant teams had remained as selective as they were 10 years ago, the number of organs would in fact have decreased.

ANTI-HBC OR ANTI-HCV-POSITIVE DONORS

Donor shortage has also brought into consideration the suitability of using the grafts of anti-HCV-positive donors for anti-HCV-positive recipients provided the grafts do not show features of fibrosis or active hepatitis. The rationale for this approach is that HCV recurs almost systematically even when HCV recipients are transplanted with anti-HCV-negative donors. Initial experience showed no detrimental impact during the first postoperative year.[62] This has been confirmed in several other studies with more prolonged observation periods.[63,64] Although the prevalence of HCV antibodies in the general population is around 1%, it has been estimated that up to 30% of donor livers are declined for liver transplantation because of HCV seropositivity in some areas. The reason for this difference is unclear.

The situation is somewhat different for donors previously exposed to HBV. Hepatitis B core antibody (HBcAb)-positive grafts carry a 25–95% risk for transmitting HBV to recipients. Previous or latent HBV infection in the donor may become reactivated in the recipient, in particular as a result of corticosteroid usage. However, anti-hepatitis B immunoglobulins and lamivudine reduce the risk of contamination so that recipients of these grafts have patient and graft survivals comparable with HBV-positive recipients of HBcAb-negative grafts.[65] HBcAb positivity is probably more frequent than the usual estimate of HBV infection prevalence of 3–5%. Figures as high as 25% have been reported.

Finally, a recent study has even found that donors with both HCV and HBc seropositivity could be used as liver donors without impact on patient or graft survivals.[64]

However, the use of these virally infected grafts in selected recipients has not gained favour in current practice. Large series are emerging from some centres, in particular in the USA and Asia, but the administrative authorities in some countries still prohibit the use of these grafts.

Split-liver transplantation

The concept of split-liver transplantation is derived from the anatomy of the liver, which makes it a paired organ. The left liver (comprising segments 2–4) and the right liver (comprising segments 5–8) represent approximately 40% and 60% of the liver volume respectively. Each hemiliver has its own arterial, portal and biliary system (**Fig. 8.4**).

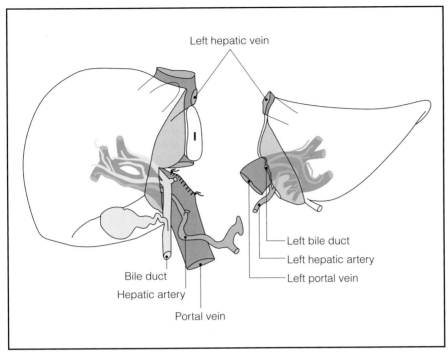

Left hepatic vein

I

Left bile duct
Left hepatic artery
Left portal vein

Bile duct
Hepatic artery
Portal vein

Figure 8.4 • Schematic drawing of two grafts obtained after splitting. Each hemiliver has its own vascular supply and bile duct.

However, there are some differences between the two hemilivers in terms of diameter or length of these branches. The portal branches and bile ducts on the left side are longer than on the right side. Due to anatomical variations, the right portal vein and bile duct is occasionally absent with an immediate bifurcation or confluence from the right anterior and posterior sector. In contrast, the right branch of the hepatic artery has a larger diameter than the left branch. On the drainage side, the left and right hepatic veins clearly belong to the left and right liver respectively. The middle hepatic vein, in contrast, drains both segment 4 (i.e. part of the left liver) and the right anterior sector (i.e. part of the right liver). In any case, a prerequisite to the use of split-liver grafts is the preservation of the recipient's inferior vena cava (see above). Finally, an important consideration is the stability of each hemiliver when they are positioned as orthotopic grafts. The right liver fits perfectly in the right hypochondrium whereas the left liver is occasionally more difficult to position without inducing a twist of the afferent or efferent vessels.

The technique of split-liver transplantation was first described in Europe in 1989.[66,67] In contrast to reduced-size grafts, which are a redistribution of grafts in favour of children, split-liver transplants theoretically double the number of cadaveric grafts and appeared as an ideal technique in the context of donor shortage. In the conventional, ex situ splitting technique, the graft is harvested in a conventional way and its division is performed on the back table under slushed saline. Several potential lines of liver transection have been described (**Fig. 8.5**), either along the falciform ligament or along the main scissura. The portal and arterial structures are divided extraparenchymally. The main portal vein is usually kept with the right-side graft whereas the left graft comprises only the left portal vein as this is usually longer. The coeliac axis usually stays with the left graft as the right hepatic artery is more frequently unique and larger than on the left side. The critical issue is, however, the division of the biliary confluence. We tend to divide it upon completion of the parenchymal transection as this allows a clearer exposure of the hilar plate

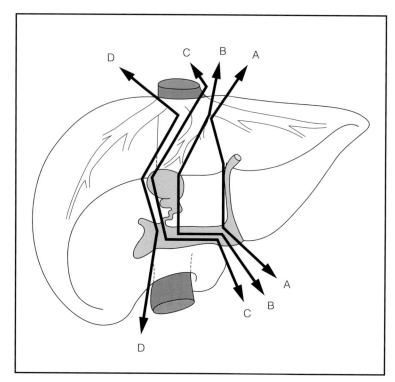

Figure 8.5 • Split-liver graft preparation. Liver surface alternative division lines. A: usual division for transplantation in an infant and an adult. B: variant of A for retaining a larger parenchymal mass for a larger recipient of left graft. C: division line for retaining the middle hepatic vein with the left graft. D: rarely used; this division line would provide a right split graft without vena cava and a rather large left split graft that could be implanted in a large child or a small adult.

and a more precise visualisation of the biliary branches.[68]

 However, the technique of split-liver transplantation has not expanded significantly, although with increased experience the results now match those for whole grafts.[69,70]

Split-liver transplantation accounts for 2% of liver transplants in the USA and 5% in Europe and its evolution over time has been limited. There are several reasons for this limited expansion.

TECHNICAL LIMITATIONS

Splitting requires an additional 2–3 hours to the conventional bench procedure and therefore increases the cold ischaemia time. It also requires additional skills, and there is a clear learning curve to avoid the increased incidence of biliary leaks (as high as 20%) and, most notably, bleeding from the transection surface. Bleeding is usually related to congestion secondary to incomplete drainage of the hemiliver, which will not have the middle hepatic vein. Some of these drawbacks have been reduced

with the use of in situ splitting.[71] Here, the liver is divided in the donor, prior to retrieval. Haemostasis is therefore more effective and a collateral circulation has time to develop as the blood flow persists during the transection as for living-related donors. Also, cold ischaemia times are shortened. The disadvantage of this technique is the prolongation of the donor operation and the potential negative effect on the other organ retrieval teams. It is therefore performed by only very few centres.

RECIPIENTS' LIMITATIONS

Split-liver transplantation was initially designed to avoid discarding the right lobe as was the case with the former size-reduction technique used for paediatric recipients. Hence, experience with split-liver transplantation has mainly been with grafting the right hemiliver and the left lateral sector into an adult and a paediatric recipient respectively. Paediatric recipients, however, account for only 10% (at most) of all transplants. Split-liver transplantation is therefore of limited impact on donor shortage unless it can be expanded for use with two adult recipients. Each graft should account for at least 1% of the recipient's body weight (the liver/body weight ratio in a normal individual is 2%). Hence, splitting grafts for two adult recipients is only possible if the donor is clearly larger than each recipient. Moreover, the donor should have none of the risk factors for a marginal graft so as to ensure optimal postoperative function. It has been estimated that only 10% of donors fulfil these criteria.[72] Hence, split-liver transplantation for two adults is still marginal.

ORGANISATIONAL LIMITATIONS

The final, but not the least, limitation is the difficulty in performing the two transplantations in a single centre. This has been overcome by shipping one of the hemigrafts to another centre. Several studies have shown that shipping the graft does not alter its function but some centres are still reluctant to use grafts that they have not prepared themselves. An interesting protocol is currently adopted in France to stimulate the development of adult splitting. If a donor liver is considered optimal for splitting, this graft is offered as a priority to the centre that agrees to split it.

Management of small-for-size grafts

Experience with resectional surgery of non-cirrhotic livers has shown that up to 75% of the liver mass can be removed without significant prolonged liver dysfunction because the remnant liver undergoes rapid regeneration. This does not appear to be the case in liver transplantation, and recipients of grafts less than 50% of the predicted liver volume of the patient frequently develop primary non-function or dysfunction.[73] This manifests as cholestasis, prolonged coagulopathy, portal hypertension, ascites and, in severe cases, gastrointestinal bleeding, within the first postoperative weeks. It is estimated that 50% of recipients of such small-for-size grafts will die of sepsis 4–6 weeks after liver transplantation. This risk of dysfunction is correlated with the recipient's clinical status. Patients with liver failure and/or hyperdynamic portal flow are at a higher risk of graft failure than patients with stable liver disease and without portal hypertension.[74]

The discrepancy between the minimal volume of a native liver and of a graft is related to the additional injuries that a graft undergoes, such as manipulation, prolonged ischaemia or predonation damage if the donor was septic or haemodynamically unstable. It has been estimated that approximately 50% of the functional mass of a graft is lost during transplantation. Hence, the volume of a liver graft should not be less than 50% of the recipient's theoretical volume, or less than 1% of the recipient's body weight.

One additional problem unique to lobar transplantation relates to hepatic congestion. This congestion is multifactorial and relates to low graft-weight ratio, insufficient venous outflow or excessive portal venous inflow.[75] Increasing disparities of graft-weight ratios exaggerate the importance of the other two factors.

The two most recently advanced methods to avoid failure of small-for-size grafts are based on the reduction of intrahepatic portal flow, although the methods to achieve this differ. One hypothesises that increased portal pressure may directly lead to tissue injury and therefore suggests performing an end-to-side mesenteric-caval shunt at the end of the transplant.[76] Portal flow within the graft is maintained through the splenic, gastric and pancreatic venous drainage. This portal decompression has been shown to be effective in reducing the small-for-size syndrome in both experimental models and the clinical setting.

The second method is derived from the observation that an increased portal blood flow (related to the use of a small-for-size graft) will induce a vasoconstriction of the hepatic artery as part of the buffer response that aims at maintaining a constant hepatic blood flow. Injury to the graft is therefore more the direct consequence of a reduced arterial flow than of an increased portal flow. It is therefore recommended to ligate the splenic artery at the end of the transplant.[77] This will reduce the portal blood flow by interrupting its splenic vein component. In addition, this will direct all the blood from the coeliac trunk into the hepatic artery. Both methods offer considerable hope in the development of split-liver transplantation in adults.

Domino transplantation

Familial amyloidotic polyneuropathy (FAP) is a rare autosomal dominant disease related to a variant of the amyloidogenic transthyretin present in the liver. The deficit of this enzyme results in progressive peripheral and autonomic neuropathy, leading to cardiac, gastrointestinal and urinary dysfunction. Liver transplantation corrects the deficit and allows stabilisation or even remission of neurological symptoms. The livers of these patients have an otherwise normal function. They have therefore been used as grafts for recipients who were either marginal candidates or unlikely to receive a graft in time. These grafts have been shown to function normally and although these recipients are exposed to the risk of developing FAP, the time necessary for symptoms to appear exceeds several decades.[78] The number of patients undergoing liver transplantation for FAP is, however, very low and this technique, although interesting, does not increase the number of grafts significantly. During the past 10 years, there have been less than 250 domino transplantations performed in Europe.

Splitting and domino transplantations have recently been combined during one procedure. A cadaveric donor was transplanted to a patient with FAP, whose liver was split into two grafts, each transplanted to another recipient. Hence, by using one cadaveric graft, three patients were transplanted.[79] This procedure is anecdotal but shows how imaginative surgeons have been in attempting to optimise the use of cadaver grafts.

LIVING-RELATED LIVER TRANSPLANTATION

Living-related liver transplantation (LRLT) was initially described in children for whom graft shortage was the most unacceptable. The first experiences were reported almost simultaneously in 1989 and 1990 from Brazil, Australia, the USA and Japan. The procedure involved resecting the left lateral segment from one parent. With excellent patient and graft survival and donor safety, LRLT for paediatric transplantation has become a routine procedure, not only in Asian countries but also in the Western world.

Besides decreasing waiting-list mortality, LRLT offers specific advantages over cadaveric transplantation. The graft has better viability because the donor is healthy and haemodynamically stable, and the cold ischaemia is much shorter than with cadaveric grafts. Most importantly, the ability to schedule the procedure allows active preparation of the recipients with renutrition and antibiotics. The procedure can always be postponed if the recipient is felt to be in suboptimal condition. In contrast, there does not appear to be any immunological advantage of LRLT over cadaveric transplantation. Several studies have suggested that the outcome following LRLT was superior to that of cadaveric transplantation in paediatric recipients.[80]

However, paediatric liver transplantation accounts for only 10% of all liver transplants and the main shortage is for adults. As the left lateral segment is too small for an adult recipient, the donor procedure has been extended to provide larger grafts. These have included left livers, right livers, without and subsequently with the middle hepatic vein. Even more imaginative has been the use of right lateral sectors[81] or the use of left livers from two donors to be transplanted in a single recipient.[82] As for split grafts, the aim is to provide a graft volume that accounts for approximately 1% of the recipient's body weight. On the donor side, it is estimated that the remnant liver volume should not be less than 30–35% of the initial liver mass. Most LRLTs in adults have been performed using the right liver.

The practice of LRLT is tightly regulated in most countries. Donors are first-degree relatives (occasionally up to third-degree in some countries). There is, however, a growing trend to also consider stable emotionally related individuals such as spouses. Close friends or 'good Samaritans' are even allowed in the USA, and although the latter remain rare, the former account for 19% of donors. In any case, these donors have to give informed consent in full knowledge of the risks.

The prime concern of LRLT is donor safety because the procedure subjects a healthy person to major surgery, potential morbidity and mortality. Donor mortality has indeed been reported in virtually all countries with an active LRLT programme (Germany, France, the USA and Japan) although with different incidences. Overall, this risk is estimated to be 0.4% but the information given to potential donors is that it is around 1%. The incidence of donor morbidity has been very variably reported. A literature review[83] and NIH survey (Dallas, November 2001) quoted figures ranging between 0 and 67% for the morbidity rate and between 0 and 29% for the readmission rate. The ethics surrounding living donation and the considerable media impact of under-reporting some donor deaths have paved the way for a more comprehensive listing of donor complications. The results of three multicentric surveys originating from the USA,[84] Europe[85] and Asia[86] have been disclosed over the past 3 years. The overall incidence of complication was 15% in the North American and Asian surveys and 34% in the European cohort. All three surveys showed comparable figures for the classical complications that were analysed (biliary leak, 6%; biliary stricture, 1–2%). However, the number of items analysed was considerably higher in the Asian report, indicating a greater attention paid to apparently even minor adverse events.

The number of LRLTs performed in adult recipients increased exponentially in the USA and Europe between 1991 and 2001 (1 case per year during 1991–95; 15 and 24 in 1998; 163 and 408 in 2001 in Europe and the USA respectively). This evolution reflected the enthusiasm of both transplantation teams and of the public for this new procedure. One survey even reported that the general public's stated threshold for living donation was a median survival for themselves of only 79%, and that 60% of the surveyed population would prefer to donate and die as a result of the procedure rather than forgo donation and watch a family member die.[87] However, in contrast to initial anticipations, this increase has not persisted and the number of LRLTs is actually slowing down. There are several reasons for this shift. The first is that not all adult transplant candidates have a potential living-related donor. Approximately 50% of the potential recipients have either no family or do not accept that one of their family members donates. In addition, only 50% of identified donors have the requisite blood group and present no medical or anatomical contraindications to donation. Hence one in four transplant candidates at most could be candidates for LRLT.

The second reason is that in contrast to paediatric recipients, the result of LRLT in adults is at best equal to, and probably slightly inferior to, that of cadaveric transplantation. This is related to both an increased incidence of technical complications (biliary leak or stenosis, arterial thrombosis) and insufficient liver volume provided to recipients in poor condition. Finally, LRLT is technically and emotionally demanding. Few centres worldwide can manage to perform more than 50 procedures a year.

Experience also shows that any serious complication or fatality in a donor has a considerable negative impact on the programme.

Nevertheless, with more than 2000 procedures performed worldwide (half in Asia and half in the Western world) living-related liver transplantation has de facto become an established alternative to cadaveric transplantation.

CONCLUSION

Liver transplantation has evolved considerably during the past 10 years, especially on the technical side, to cope with the shortage of cadaveric donors. Another concern is the shortage of trained transplant surgeons, due to the low attractiveness of transplant specialities.[88] It is hoped that this latter problem can be overcome to allow another decade of innovation and evolution.

• Key points

- Liver transplantation is an established treatment for acute and chronic liver disease, with 5-year survival rates greater than 70% for most indications.
- The early post-transplant mortality depends both on the quality of the graft and the general status of the patients. Patients should therefore be referred early for evaluation.
- Transplant surgeons are increasingly using marginal donors and have developed a number of innovative techniques such as split-liver transplantation, domino transplantation or living-related liver transplantation to overcome graft shortage.
- As a rule, these alternatives best suit good-risk recipients. Patients in poor general condition at the time of transplantation should receive optimal grafts
- Allocating grafts to centres rather than to a national waiting list probably allows greater flexibility in the choice of the optimal recipient of a given graft.
- Split-liver transplantation and living-related liver transplants have not achieved, in practice, the anticipated increase in the number of transplantations.

REFERENCES

1. European Liver Transplant Registry. (Chairman Adam R, Hepato-Biliary Center, Hôpital Paul Brousse, 94804 Villejuif, Cedex, France) www.eltr.org

2. Blanch J, Sureda B, Flavia M et al. Psychosocial adjustment to orthotopic liver transplantation in 266 recipients. Liver Transplant. 2004; 10:228–34.

3. Karam VH, Gasquet I, Delvart V et al. Quality of life in adult survivors beyond 10 years after liver, kidney, and heart transplantation. Transplantation 2003; 76:1699–704.

4. Jain AB, Reyes J, Marcos A et al. Pregnancy after liver transplantation with tacrolimus immuno-suppression: a single center's experience update at 13 years. Transplantation 2003; 76:827–32.

5. Ghobrial RM, Gornbein J, Steadman R et al. Pre-transplant model to predict post transplant survival in liver transplant patients. Ann Surg 2002; 236:315–22.

6. Schnitzler MA, Woodwards RS, Brenman DC et al. The economic impact of preservation time in cadaveric liver transplantation. Am J Transplant 2001; 1:360–5.

7. Noun R, Sauvanet A, Belghiti J. Appraisal of the order of revascularization in human liver grafting: a controlled study. J Am Coll Surg 1997; 185:70–3.

8. Sadler KM, Walsh TS, Garden OJ et al. Comparison of hepatic artery and portal vein reperfusion during orthotopic liver transplantation. Transplantation 2001; 72:1680–4.

9. Scatton O, Meunier B, Cherqui D et al. Randomized trial of choledochocholedochostomy with or without a T tube in orthotopic liver transplantation. Ann Surg 2001; 233:432–7.

10. Shaw BW, Martin DJ, Marquez JM et al. Veno-venous bypass in clinical liver transplantation. Ann Surg 1984; 200:649–52.

11. Belghiti J, Noun R, Sauvanet A. Temporary portocaval anastomosis with preservation of caval flow during orthotopic liver transplantation. Am J Surg 1995; 169:277–9.

12. Gonzales FX, Garcia-Valdecassa JC, Grande L et al. Vena cava reconstruction during orthotopic liver transplantation: a comparative study. Liver Transplant Surg 1998; 4:133–40.

13. Lerut JP, Molle G, Donataccio M et al. Cavocaval liver transplantation without venovenous bypass and without temporary portocaval shunting: the ideal technique for adult liver grafting? Transplant Int 1997; 10:171–9.

14. Navarro F, Le Moine MC, Fabre JM et al. Specific vascular complications of orthotopic liver transplantation with preservation of the retrohepatic vena cava: review of 1361 cases. Transplantation 1999; 68:646–50.

A large multicentre survey on the results of caval preservation.

15. Belghiti J, Ettorre GM, Durand F et al. Feasibility and limits of caval-flow preservation during liver transplantation. Liver Transplant 2001; 7:983–7.

16. Figueras J, Llado L, Ramos E et al. Temporary portocaval shunt during liver transplantation with vena cava preservation. Results of a prospective randomized study. Liver Transplant 2001; 7:904–11.

17. Lerut J, Ciccarelli O, Roggen F et al. Cavocaval adult liver transplantation and retransplantation without venovenous bypass and without portocaval shunting: a prospective feasibility study in adult liver transplantation. Transplantation 2003; 75:1740–5.

18. Tzakis A, Todo S, Starzl TE. Orthotopic liver transplantation with preservation of the inferior vena cava. Ann Surg 1989; 210:649–52.

19. Belghiti J, Panis Y, Sauvanet A et al. A new technique of side to side caval anastomosis during orthotopic hepatic transplantation without inferior vena caval occlusion. Surg Gynecol Obstet 1992; 175:271–2.

20. Robles R, Parrilla P, Acosta F et al. Complications related to hepatic venous outflow in piggy-back liver transplantation: two- versus three-suprahepatic-vein anastomosis. Transplant Proc 1999; 31:2390–1.

21. Bismuth H, Houssin D. Reduced-sized orthotopic liver graft in hepatic transplantation in children. Surgery 1984; 95:367–70.

22. Beath SV, Brook GD, Kelly DA et al. Successful liver transplantation in babies under 1 year. BMJ 1993; 307:825–8.

23. Terpstra JL, Schalm SW, Weimar W et al. Auxiliary partial liver transplantation for end-stage chronic liver disease. N Engl J Med 1988; 319:1507–11.

24. Chenard-Neu MP, Boudjema K, Bernuau J et al. Auxiliary liver transplantation: regeneration of the native liver and outcome in 30 patients with fulminant hepatic failure – a multicentre European study. Hepatology 1996; 23:1119–27.

25. van Hoek B, de Boer J, Boudjema K et al. Auxiliary versus orthotopic liver transplantation for acute liver failure. EURALT Study Group. European Auxiliary Liver Transplant Registry. J Hepatol 1999; 30:699–705.

Largest survey on the outcome of auxiliary liver transplantation for fulminant liver failure.

26. Azoulay D, Samuel D, Ichai P et al. Auxiliary partial orthotopic versus standard orthotopic whole liver transplantation for acute liver failure: a reappraisal from a single center by a case-control study. Ann Surg 2001; 234:723–31.

27. Whitington PF, Emond JC, Heffron T et al. Orthotopic auxiliary liver transplantation for Criggler-Najjar syndrome type I. Lancet 1993; 342:779–80.

28. Rela M, Muisan P, Vilca-Melandez H et al. Auxiliary partial orthotopic liver transplantation for Criggler-Najjar syndrome type I. Ann Surg 1999; 229:565–9.

29. Consensus Conference on Indications of Liver Transplantation, Paris, France, June 22–23, 1993. Hepatology 1994; 20:1S–68S.

   Summary of the consensus conference on the indications for liver transplantation.

30. Devlin J, O'Grady J. Indications for referral and assessment in adult liver transplantation: a clinical guideline. Gut 1999; 45(suppl. 6):vi1–vi22.

   Statements on the indication for liver transplantation in the UK.

31. Corpechot C, Carrat F, Bonnand AM et al. The effect of ursodeoxycholic acid therapy on liver fibrosis progression in primary biliary cirrhosis. Hepatology 2000; 32:1196–9.

32. Neuberger J. Liver transplantation for primary biliary cirrhosis: indications and risk of recurrence. J Hepatol 2003; 39:142–8.

33. Vera A, Moledina S, Gunson B et al. Risk factors for recurrence of primary sclerosing cholangitis of liver allograft. Lancet 2002; 360:1943–4.

34. Adam R, McMaster P, O'Grady JG et al. and European Liver Transplant Association. Evolution of liver transplantation in Europe: report of the European Liver Transplant Registry. Liver Transplant 2003; 9:1231–43.

35. Gane EJ, Portmann BC, Naoumov NV et al. Long-term outcome of hepatitis C infection after liver transplantation. N Engl J Med 1996; 334: 815–20.

36. Sanchez-Fueyo A, Restrepo JC, Quinto L et al. Impact of the recurrence of hepatitis C virus infection after liver transplantation on the long-term viability of the graft. Transplantation 2002; 73:56–63.

37. Gane EJ, Naoumov NV, Qian KP et al. A longitudinal analysis of hepatitis C virus replication following liver transplantation. Gastroenterology 1996; 110:167–77.

38. Forman LM, Lewis JD, Berlin JA et al. The association between hepatitis C infection and survival after orthotopic liver transplantation. Gastroenterology 2002; 122:889–96.

   Large study reporting reduced survival in patients transplanted for HCV cirrhosis.

39. Berenguer M, Prieto M, San Juan F et al. Contribution of donor age to the recent decrease in patient survival among HCV-infected liver transplant recipients. Hepatology 2002; 36:202–10.

40. Berenguer M, Ferrel L, Watson J et al. HCV-related fibrosis progression following liver transplantation: increase in recent years. J Hepatol 2000; 32:673–84.

41. Machicao VI, Bonatti H, Krishna M et al. Donor age affects fibrosis progression and graft survival after liver transplantation for hepatitis C. Transplantation 2004; 77:84–92.

42. Berenguer M, Crippin J, Gish R et al. A model to predict severe HCV-related disease following liver transplantation. Hepatology 2003; 38:34–41.

43. Davis GL. Chronic hepatitis C and liver transplantation. Rev Gastroenterol Dis 2004; 4:7–17.

44. Samuel D, Bizollon T, Feray C et al. Interferon-alpha 2b plus ribavirin in patients with chronic hepatitis C after liver transplantation: a randomized study. Gastroenterology 2003; 124:642–50.

45. Dumortier J, Scoazec JY, Chevallier P et al. Treatment of recurrent hepatitis C after liver transplantation: a pilot study of peginterferon alfa-2b and ribavirin combination. J Hepatol 2004; 40:669–74.

46. Mazzaferro V, Regalia E, Doci R et al. Liver transplantation for the treatment of small hepatocellular carcinomas in patients with cirrhosis. N Engl J Med 1996; 334:693–9.

47. Ragni MV, Belle SH, Im K et al. Survival of human immunodeficiency virus-infected liver transplant recipients. J Infect Dis 2003; 188:1412–20.

48. Pruett TL. The allocation of livers for transplantation: a problem of titanic consideration. Hepatology 2002; 35:960–3.

49. Ubel PA, Loewenstein G. Distribution of scarce livers: the moral reasoning of the general public. Soc Sci Med 1996; 42:1049–55.

50. Organ procurement and transplantation network – HRSA. Final rule with comment period. Fed Regist 1998; 63:16296.

51. Lucey MR, Brown KA, Everson GT et al. Minimal criteria for placement of adults on the liver transplant waiting list: a report of a national conference organized by the American Society of Transplant Physicians and the American Association for the Study of Liver Diseases. Liver Transplant Surg 1997; 3:628–37.

52. Sharma P, Balan V, Hernandez JL et al. Liver transplantation for hepatocellular carcinoma: the MELD impact. Liver Transplant 2004; 10:36–41.

53. Cuende N, Grande L, Sanjuan F et al. Liver transplant with organs from elderly donors: Spanish experience with more than 300 liver donors over 70 years of age. Transplantation 2002; 73:1360.

54. Montalti R, Nardo B, Bertelli R et al. Donor pool expansion in liver transplantation. Transplant Proc 2004; 36:520–2.

55. Todo S, Demetris AJ, Makowka L et al. Primary nonfunction of hepatic allografts with preexisting fatty infiltration. Transplantation 1989; 47:903–5.

56. Marsman WA, Wiesner RH, Rodriguez L et al. Use of fatty donor liver is associated with diminished

early patient and graft survival. Transplantation 1996; 62:1246–51.

57. D'alessandro AM, Kalayoglu M, Sollinger HW et al. The predictive value of donor liver biopsies on the development of primary non function after orthotopic liver transplantation. Transplant Proc 1991; 23:1536–7.

58. Adam R, Bismuth H, Diamond T et al. Effect of extended cold ischemia with UW solution on graft function after liver transplantation. Lancet 1992; 340:1373–6.

59. Fishbein TM, Fiel MI, Emre S et al. Use of livers with microvesicular fat safely expands the donor pool. Transplantation 1997; 64:248–51.

60. Mirza D, Gunson B, Da Silva R et al. Policies in Europe on 'marginal quality' donor livers. Lancet 1994; 344:1480–3.

61. Abt PL, Desai NM, Crawford MD et al. Survival following liver transplantation from non-heartbeating donors. Ann Surg 2004; 239:87–92.

62. Vargas HE, Laskus T, Wang LF et al. Outcome of liver transplantation in hepatitis C virus-infected patients who received hepatitis C virus-infected grafts. Gastroenterology 1999; 117:149–53.

63. Velidedeoglu E, Desai NM, Campos L et al. The outcome of liver grafts procured from hepatitis C-positive donors. Transplantation 2002; 73:582–7.

64. Saab S, Chang AJ, Comulada S et al. Outcomes of hepatitis C- and hepatitis B core antibody-positive grafts in orthotopic liver transplantation. Liver Transplant 2003; 9:1053–61.

    Study investigating the impact of using grafts from virologically infected donors.

65. Joya-Vazquez P, Dodson F, Dvorchik I et al. Impact of anti-hepatitis Bc-positive grafts on the outcome of liver transplantation for HBV-related cirrhosis. Transplantation 2002; 73:1598–602.

66. Pichlmayr R, Ringe B, Gubernatis G et al. Transplantation einer Spenderleber auf zwei empfänger (splitting-transplantation) – eine neue methode in der weiterentwicklung der lebersegment-transplantation [Transplantation of a donor liver to two recipients (splitting transplantation) – a new method in the further development of segmental liver transplantation.] Langenbecks Arch Chir 1988; 373:127–30.

67. Bismuth H, Morino M, Castaing D et al. Emergency orthotopic liver transplantation in two patients using one donor liver. Br J Surg 1989; 76:722–4.

68. Balzan S, Farges O, Sommacale D et al. Direct bile duct visualization during the preparation of split livers. Liver Transplant 2004; 10:703–5.

69. Deshpande RR, Bowles MJ, Vilca-Melendez H et al. Results of split liver transplantation in children. Ann Surg 2002; 236:248–53.

70. Broering DC, Topp S, Schaefer U et al. Split liver transplantation and risk to the adult recipient: analysis using matched pairs. J Am Coll Surg 2002; 195:648–57.

    Large study on the results of split-liver transplantation.

71. Rogiers X, Malago M, Gawad K et al. One year experience with extended application and modified techniques of split liver transplantation. Transplantation 1996; 61:1059–61.

72. Toso C, Ris F, Mentha G et al. Potential impact of in situ liver splitting on the number of available grafts. Transplantation 2002; 74:222–6.

73. Emond JC, Renz JF, Ferrell LD et al. Functional analysis of grafts from living donors. Implications for the treatment of older recipients. Ann Surg 1996; 224:544–52.

74. Ben-Haim M, Emre S, Fishbein TM et al. Critical graft size in adult-to-adult living donor liver transplantation: impact of the recipient's disease. Liver Transplant 2001; 7:948–53.

75. Shimamura T, Taniguchi M, Jin MB et al. Excessive portal venous inflow as a cause of allograft dysfunction in small-for-size living donor liver transplantation. Transplant Proc 2001; 33:1331.

76. Boillot O, Delafosse B, Mechet I et al. Small-for-size partial liver graft in an adult recipient; a new transplant technique. Lancet 2002; 359:406–7.

77. Troisi R, Cammu G, Militerno G et al. Modulation of portal graft inflow: a necessity in adult living-donor liver transplantation? Ann Surg 2003; 237:429–36.

    Description of an innovative technique to cope with small-for-size grafts.

78. Ericzon BG, Larsson M, Herlenius G et al. Familial Amyloidotic Polyneuropathy World Transplant Registry. Report from the Familial Amyloidotic Polyneuropathy World Transplant Registry (FAPWTR) and the Domino Liver Transplant Registry (DLTR). Amyloid 2003; 10(suppl1.):67–76.

79. Azoulay D, Castaing D, Adam R et al. Transplantation of three adult patients with one cadaveric graft: wait or innovate. Liver Transplant 2000; 6:239–40.

80. Reding R, de Goyet J de V, Delbeke I et al. Paediatric liver transplantation with cadaveric or living related donors: comparative results in 90 elective recipients of primary grafts. J Pediatr 1999; 134:280–6.

81. Sugawara Y, Makuuchi M, Takayama T et al. Right lateral sector graft in adult living-related liver transplantation. Transplantation 2002; 73:111–14.

82. Lee S, Hwang S, Park K et al. An adult-to-adult living donor liver transplant using dual left lobe grafts. Surgery 2001; 129:647–50.

83. Beavers KL, Sandler RS, Shrestha R. Donor morbidity associated with right lobectomy for living

donor liver transplantation to adult recipients: a systematic review. Liver Transplant 2002; 8:110–17.

84. Brown RS, Russo MW, Lai M et al. A survey of liver transplantation from living adult donors in the United States. N Engl J Med 2003; 348: 818–25.

85. European Liver Transplant Registry (ELTR). Data analysis booklet, June 2002. Available at http://www.eltr.org

86. Lo CM. Complications and long-term outcome of living liver donors: a survey of 1,508 cases in five Asian centers. Transplantation 2003; 75:S12–15.

Results of a large survey of morbidity following living-related liver transplantation.

87. Cotler SJ, McNutt R, Patil R et al. Adult living donor liver transplantation: Preferences about donation outside the medical community. Liver Transplant 2001; 7:335–40.

88. Morris-Stiff GJ, Benson S, Casey J et al. Transplant surgeons in training: is anybody out there? Ann R Coll Surg Engl 1999; 81:191–4.

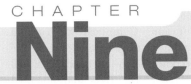

CHAPTER

Nine

Pancreas transplantation

Murat Akyol

Transplantation of the pancreas is the only treatment currently available that reliably offers insulin independence and normal glucose metabolism for patients with type I diabetes mellitus. The first pancreas transplant was performed in the University of Minnesota in 1966.[1] Early experience with pancreatic transplantation was disappointing. This has remained so for many years. Difficulties were related to the management of the exocrine secretions and septic complications and a high incidence of thrombosis, acute rejection and pancreatitis. For the first 22 years of its 37-year history less than 1200 pancreas transplants were performed worldwide. Even after the introduction of ciclosporin, 1-year patient and graft survival rates were only 75% and 37%, respectively, in 1983. In the 1970s and 1980s, therefore, scepticism rather than enthusiasm appeared to be a reasonable standpoint in judging the value of pancreas transplantation.

Throughout the 1990s there was a considerable change. This came about as a consequence of improvements in organ retrieval and preservation methods, refinements in surgical techniques, advances in immunosuppression, advances in the prophylaxis and the treatment of infection, and the experience gained in donor and recipient selection. Success rates following pancreas transplantation are now comparable with other forms of organ transplantation, and more than 20 000 pancreas

transplants have been performed worldwide. Interestingly, as an increasingly common option in the management of diabetes, pancreas transplantation has never been compared with insulin therapy in a prospective controlled trial. It is unlikely that such a trial will ever be performed. However, considerable experience and a substantial body of evidence has accumulated, which now favours the viewpoint of the enthusiasts rather than the sceptics.

INDICATIONS FOR PANCREAS TRANSPLANTATION

Pancreas transplantation for type II diabetes

Pancreas transplantation aims to provide patients with type I diabetes with an alternative source of insulin. In 1998 Sasaki and colleagues reported a small number of patients with insulin-requiring type II diabetes who had received pancreas transplants with short-term success.[2] The long-term outlook for such patients remains unknown. There are a number of theoretical concerns in considering patients with type II diabetes for pancreatic transplantation. The pathogenesis of type II diabetes is fundamentally different from that of type I diabetes.

Patients with type II diabetes have insulin resistance as part of their clinical syndrome and the influence of this on the long-term outlook for pancreas transplantation remains unknown. Furthermore, type II diabetes is much more prevalent than type I diabetes worldwide and carries a different, often much poorer prognosis. The allocation of a scarce resource to such patients at the expense of those with type I diabetes clearly poses ethical difficulty.

Pancreas transplantation from living donors

The pancreas transplant database of all US transplants between 1988 and 2003 records 66 living donor transplants out of approximately 15 000 pancreas transplants.[3,4] The experience regarding perioperative morbidity and the long-term risks for the donor is inadequate to allow comment. The fact that it remains a tiny fringe activity confined to very few centres presumably indicates that living donor pancreas transplantation is not endorsed by the transplantation community in general. This is certainly the view that prevails in the UK and the rest of Europe. The discussion in this chapter is confined to allogeneic pancreas transplantation from cadaveric organ donors.

Patient selection for pancreas transplantation

Pancreas transplantation is performed in three distinct clinical settings, as presented below.

SIMULTANEOUS PANCREAS–KIDNEY TRANSPLANTATION (SPK)

There is little debate that diabetic patients with renal failure should be offered kidney transplantation, and there is good evidence that their prognosis is poor on dialysis.[5] Such patients will already be obligated to immunosuppression on account of kidney transplantation. Combined kidney and pancreas transplantation offers these patients the opportunity to become insulin independent as well as dialysis independent. The risks and potential benefits of SPK transplantation are summarised in **Box 9.1**. The evidence for the risks and benefits alluded to in **Box 9.1** is reviewed in the final part of the chapter.

Experience has taught us the crucial importance of recipient selection to the success of pancreas transplantation. Cardiovascular comorbidity is the most important factor leading to patient death in the early postoperative period after transplantation in diabetic patients. Patient selection needs to include a comprehensive medical evaluation, ideally performed by a multidisciplinary team within each transplant unit. Asymptomatic ischaemic heart disease is not uncommon in diabetics. The cardiac assessment should include as a minimum a 12-lead ECG, echocardiography, exercise tolerance test and a non-invasive test of myocardial perfusion (a radio-isotope scan or dobutamine stress echo). There is insufficient evidence to comment on the value of routine angiography.[6] Any abnormality in non-invasive tests detected should be investigated further including angiography and any correctable coronary artery disease should be dealt with prior to transplantation.[7]

Most pancreas transplant units will have an arbitrary and flexible upper age limit of around 45–50 in determining suitability for SPK transplantation. With increasing experience, criteria for suitability of individuals for SPK transplantation have become more liberal. Previous contraindications have become relative contraindications or risk factors (**Box 9.2**). Strong evidence to differentiate between contraindications and relative contraindications does not exist. Neither blindness nor previous amputation are regarded as contraindications. **Box 9.2** is

Box 9.1 • Potential risks and benefits of simultaneous pancreas–kidney (SPK) transplantation

Risks	Benefits
Perioperative morbidity and mortality	Improved quality of life
Potential for pancreas transplant to adversely affect kidney transplant outcome	Potential benefits on diabetic complications
Consequences of higher immunosuppression	Improved life expectancy

Box 9.2 • Contraindications and risk factors for pancreas transplantation

- Inability to give informed consent
- Active drug abuse
- Major psychiatric illness
- HIV infection
- Recent history of malignancy
- Active infection
- Recent myocardial infarction
- Evidence of significant uncorrectable ischaemic heart disease
- Insufficient cardiac reserve with poor ejection fraction
- Any other illness that significantly restricts life expectancy
- Age greater than 55
- Significant obesity (BMI >30)
- Severe aortoiliac atherosclerosis

intended as a guide only. No attempt has been made to separate absolute and relative contraindications. The use of imprecise definitions such as 'significant', 'severe' or 'recent' is also intentional. Appropriate patient selection requires a balanced assessment by experienced clinicians of the risk factors versus potential benefits.

PANCREAS AFTER KIDNEY TRANSPLANTATION (PAK)

Historically the large majority of pancreas transplants performed have been SPKs. This was largely because of the relatively poor outcomes following solitary pancreas transplantation. Improved success of pancreas transplantation in the last 6 or 7 years has encouraged many transplant units to offer pancreas transplantation for diabetic patients who have previously undergone successful kidney transplantation. Until the end of 2000, PAK transplants constituted 11% of all pancreas transplants performed in the USA and 5% of pancreas transplants performed outside the USA.[8] In the last 2 years nearly a quarter of US pancreas transplants have been solitary pancreas transplants.[9] More detailed analysis of activity and outcome in different forms of pancreas transplantation is given in the next section of the chapter.

Criteria for recipient selection in PAK are not well defined. Contraindications to PAK transplantation are very similar to those for SPK (**Box 9.2**). Within the confines of these contraindications, all diabetics who have previously undergone successful kidney transplantation are potentially suitable candidates for PAK. In practice the procedure is most useful for those diabetics who have a potential living donor for kidney transplantation. With PAK outcomes now approaching those of SPK, an elective and early living donor kidney transplantation has obvious benefits to the potential recipient and has additional benefits to the overall pool of patients awaiting transplantation by releasing another cadaveric kidney. Clearly some time should elapse after kidney transplantation to allow for recovery from surgery and stabilisation of allograft function and immunosuppression. The optimal timing has not been determined. Available data comparing early (within the first few months) with late (more than 4 months after kidney transplantation) PAK do not reveal any significant difference in the incidence of morbidity or outcome.[10]

There are also unique immunological considerations for patients who are being considered for PAK. Previous kidney transplantation may have influenced sensitisation profiles for such patients. In the presence of good renal allograft function and no history of acute rejection following kidney transplantation, shared HLA antigens between the pancreas allograft and the previous renal allograft may have a favourable impact on the outcome, an assertion that remains untested. Whether acute rejection following previous kidney transplantation predisposes PAK recipients to acute rejection of the pancreatic allograft is not known either.

Finally, an important consideration, in particular for patients who are being considered some considerable time after kidney transplantation, is the adequacy of kidney function. Criteria based on strong evidence do not exist but a creatinine clearance of greater than 40 mL/min is commonly quoted as a minimum requirement.[11] For recipients of kidney transplants who are not receiving calcineurin inhibitors, a higher creatinine clearance of not less than 55 mL/min is recommended. A renal allograft biopsy prior to PAK is useful for documentation of the baseline renal reserve and for the monitoring of the progression of allograft nephropathy (diabetic or otherwise).

PANCREAS TRANSPLANTATION ALONE (PTA)

Universally agreed criteria that constitute indications for PTA are more difficult to find compared with those for SPK or PAK. The consideration of risks of surgery for non-uraemic diabetics needs to take account of not only perioperative morbidity but also risks associated with immunosuppression. At present the majority of patients developing type I diabetes will be better served by insulin injections at the onset of disease. Clear indications for PTA are life-threatening complications of diabetes in patients managed with insulin; namely hypoglycaemic unawareness and cardiac autonomic neuropathy. In these two subpopulations of diabetic patients pancreas transplantation is truly life saving. Other indications for PTA are more controversial. The presence of two or more diabetic complications has been advocated as an indication.[12] In the absence of conclusive data on some of the diabetic complications, as reviewed in the final section of this chapter, it is difficult to defend the logic behind the assertion that two or more complications constitute an indication for PTA. Disabling and intractable symptoms of diabetic neuropathy or early nephropathy with preserved renal function may be considered as indications. In diabetics with overt nephropathy and impaired renal function, the nephrotoxicity of the immunosuppressive drugs will need to be considered. Available evidence does not permit precise guidelines but patients with creatinine clearance less than 40 mL/min may be better served by SPK transplantation.

PANCREAS TRANSPLANTATION ACTIVITY WORLDWIDE

At the end of 2003 the total number of pancreas transplants performed worldwide exceeded 20 000.[9] Nearly two-thirds of these have been performed in the USA. The International Pancreas Transplantation Registry (IPTR), based at the University of Minnesota, shares US transplant data with the United Network for Organ Sharing (UNOS). Reporting of data to UNOS is compulsory and IPTR records regarding US pancreas transplantation activity are accurate and complete. Non-US pancreas transplants are reported to the IPTR on a voluntary basis. Some national organisations such as UK Transplant and Eurotransplant, share data with the international registry. The IPTR estimates that >90% of non-US transplants are reported. Despite the probable under-representation of non-US transplants, there seems to be a genuine difference in the utilisation of pancreas transplantation between the USA and the remainder of the world. **Figure 9.1** shows worldwide pancreas transplantation activity as recorded by the IPTR at the beginning of 2003.

SPK transplantation activity reached a peak of 972 transplants in the year 1998 in the USA. Thereafter there has been a small decline, and in the last 4 years the activity has remained stable at a plateau of around 900 SPK transplants per annum. In contrast solitary pancreas transplantation activity (PAK + PTA) continued to increase from 64 in 1992 to 554 in 2002 (**Fig. 9.2**).

The total numbers of pancreas transplants performed in the UK and in the Eurotransplant zone are shown in **Table 9.1** for comparison.[13,14]

The age profile of pancreas transplant recipients has also changed significantly over the last 15 years. In the USA between 1987 and 1992, 9% of pancreas transplant recipients were older than 45; in the period 1999–2002 this proportion had risen to 27%.[9]

Interestingly 5% of patients receiving pancreas transplants in the USA between 1994 and 2002 were classified as having type II diabetes at the time of transplant.[9]

Management of exocrine secretions has also seen significant change. Enteric drainage has always been the predominant method in Europe but in the USA until the mid-1990s less than 10% of pancreas transplants were enterically drained. Enteric drainage has since surged in popularity in the USA also. Between 1996 and 2002 about half of US solitary pancreas transplants and two-thirds of US SPK transplants were enterically drained.

Portal venous drainage gained popularity in the mid-1990s. Utilisation of portal venous drainage has remained relatively constant during the late 1990s and has increased slightly since 1999. In the USA between 1996 and 2002, 1091 of the 4394 (25%) enterically drained primary SPK cases have been performed with the portal venous drainage technique.[9]

Other demographic data for patients transplanted in the USA between 1996 and 2002 are summarised in **Table 9.2**.

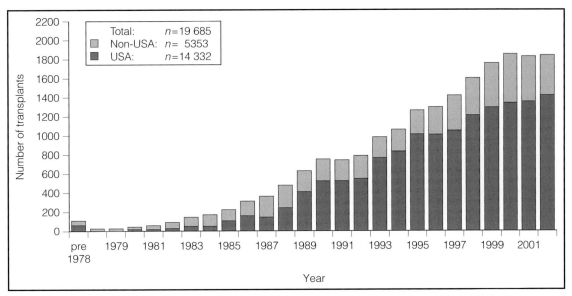

Figure 9.1 • Pancreas transplants reported to the International Pancreas Transplant Registry (June 2003).

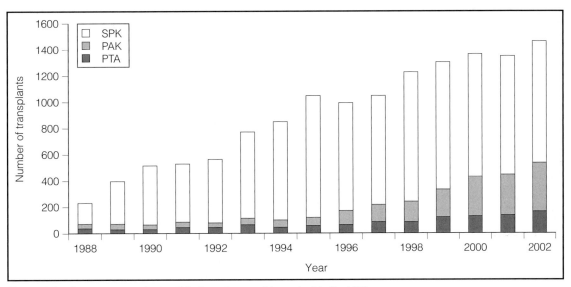

Figure 9.2 • Pancreas transplant activity by category of transplant in the USA.

Table 9.1 • Pancreas transplantation activity in Eurotransplant and the UK

Year	Eurotransplant*	UK[†]
1998	236	22
1999	288	31
2000	309	32
2001	267	41
2002	212	52

*Eurotransplant zone includes Austria, Belgium, Germany, Luxembourg, The Netherlands and Slovenia.
[†]UK transplants referred to are SPK transplants only.

THE PANCREAS DONOR AND THE ORGAN RETRIEVAL PROCEDURE

Criteria for eligibility for pancreas donors

Absolute contraindications to organ donation are human immunodeficiency virus (HIV) infection, diagnosis of Creutzfeldt–Jakob disease (CJD), history of malignancy (except non-melanoma skin cancer and certain primary central nervous system tumours) and active systemic sepsis. Additional specific contraindications for pancreas donors are diabetes mellitus and gross pancreatic disease in the donor (including trauma, acute or chronic pancreatitis, excessive fatty infiltration). Neither hyperglycaemia nor hyperamylasaemia should preclude pancreas donation providing the pancreas appears normal on inspection. Increasing donor age, cerebrovascular/cardiovascular cause of death and donor obesity are associated with poorer pancreas transplant outcomes.[9] A precise upper age limit for pancreas donors is difficult to define because of many confounding variables, the retrospective nature of the studies and small sample sizes of individual reports. IPTR analyses use 45 as the age cut-off distinguishing 'young' and 'old' donors. Only 3% of the US pancreas donors were older than 50.[9] In practice an upper age limit of 45–55 is used by most transplant units and the general consensus is that the ideal pancreas donor will be younger than 45.

It is similarly difficult to quote an acceptable weight limit for donors. BMI >30 should be regarded as a contraindication. Pancreas grafts from paediatric donors (age >4 years) and selected non-heart-beating donors can be used with excellent results.[15]

Table 9.2 • Demographics of pancreas transplant recipients for US cadaveric primary pancreas transplants 1/96–7/02

	SPK	PAK	PTA
No. of transplants	6032	1081	471
Recipient age (years)	39.3 ± 7.9	41.1 ± 7.5	38.8 ± 9.0
Male recipients (%)	59	58	39
% Minorities	12	7	3
Diabetes duration (years)	26 ± 8	28 ± 7	24 ± 10
% Enterically drained	65	50	46
Preservation time (h)	13 ± 6	15 ± 6	16 ± 6
Donor age (years)	27 ± 12	27 ± 11	27 ± 12
No. of HLA A, B donor mismatches	4.5 ± 1.3	3.9 ± 1.3	3.7 ± 1.5
Waiting list time (median days)	302	140	105
Interquartile range	98–455	55–330	47–255

SPK, simultaneous pancreas–kidney transplants; PAK, pancreas after kidney transplants; PTA, pancreas transplantation alone.

Pancreas retrieval operation

The pancreas is a close neighbour of the liver and shares important vascular structures. During multi-organ retrieval procedures priority clearly needs to be given to the liver. The key to successful retrieval of both the liver and the pancreas is good cooperation between the two retrieval teams. The optimum scenario is for both organs to be retrieved and transplanted by the same team. Specific anomalies in the arterial blood supply to the liver that preclude successful liver and successful pancreas transplantation are very rare.

It is not intended to give a detailed description of the surgical procedure for pancreas retrieval in this section, but several pertinent points about pancreatic retrieval from multiorgan donors are highlighted below.

University of Wisconsin solution was first developed as a pancreatic preservation solution[16] and remains the benchmark for pancreas preservation. Other preservation solutions have been used but experience with these is limited.[17]

The cold ischaemia tolerance of the pancreas is somewhere between that of the liver and the kidney. In pancreas allografts perfused with UW solution, 20–24 hours appears to be the limit for successful preservation, beyond which a time-dependent deterioration in outcome is demonstrable.[18]

The pressure gradient between mean arterial pressure and portal venous pressure that maintains blood flow through the pancreas can be significantly diminished during the perfusion of the abdominal organs in retrieval operations. Particular attention is required to maintain an adequate gradient if a cannula for perfusion is placed in the portal venous system as well as the aorta. Many transplant units perfuse abdominal organs with an aortic cannula only. Some evidence supports the view that additional portal perfusion is unnecessary.[19] For the interests of the pancreatic allograft, aortic perfusion alone is the most 'physiological' state that allows satisfactory perfusion and adequate drainage of the effluent.

It is common practice to flush the donor duodenum through a nasogastric tube with an antiseptic or antibiotic solution during the retrieval operation. No evidence exists to demonstrate the superiority of any solution used for duodenal decontamination.

Povidone–iodine during cold storage may be toxic to duodenal mucosa.[20] If povidone–iodine is used for flushing the allograft duodenal segment during organ retrieval, further flushing of the duodenal segment with preservation solution on the back table should be considered.

Donor duodenal contents should be submitted for bacterial and fungal culture. The results may be important in guiding the management of infection in pancreas transplant recipients.[21]

- Careful and minimal handling of the pancreas during retrieval is important. Removal of the spleen and the pancreatico-duodenal graft en bloc with the liver is the quickest and the safest method for both organs. The organs are then easily and quickly separated on the back table at the retrieval centre.
- Further back-table preparation of the pancreas, which takes place in the recipient centre, is a crucial part of the procedure and takes a minimum of 2 hours. The short stumps of the proximal superior mesenteric artery (SMA) and splenic artery should be marked with fine polypropylene sutures at the time of retrieval. Demonstration of good collateral circulation between these two arteries by flushing them individually at the back table is reassuring. An iliac artery Y graft of donor origin anastomosed to the SMA and the splenic artery is the most common method of reconstruction for the graft arterial inflow (**Fig. 9.3**). Meticulous dissection and ligation of the lymphatic tissue and small vessels around the pancreas is important to prevent haemorrhage upon reperfusion of the graft in the recipient. Particular attention should be paid to secure the duodenal segment staple lines by inversion with further sutures.

THE PANCREAS TRANSPLANT OPERATION

General considerations

In simultaneous pancreas–kidney transplantation, pancreatic implantation is usually performed first because of the lower ischaemia tolerance of the pancreas. It is easier to implant the pancreatic graft on the right side. The renal allograft can also be

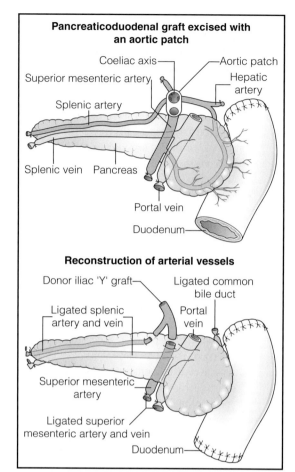

Pancreaticoduodenal graft excised with an aortic patch

Coeliac axis

Superior mesenteric artery

Splenic artery

Aortic patch

Hepatic artery

Splenic vein   Pancreas

Portal vein

Duodenum

Reconstruction of arterial vessels

Donor iliac 'Y' graft

Ligated splenic artery and vein

Ligated common bile duct

Portal vein

Superior mesenteric artery

Ligated superior mesenteric artery and vein

Duodenum

Figure 9.3 • In the absence of an aortic patch containing hepatic artery and the gastroduodenal artery, the pancreatic graft reconstruction requires a donor iliac 'Y' graft.

placed intra-abdominally with anastomoses to the left iliac vessels. Alternatively, and perhaps more easily, an extraperitoneal renal transplant on the left side can be performed using the same incision or through a separate left iliac fossa incision.

In PAK transplantation, even in the presence of a right-sided renal allograft, the preferred site for the pancreas would be on the righthand side cranial to the renal allograft. The arterial inflow to the pancreatic allograft usually comes from the right common iliac artery. Unless the lower aorta is clamped or unless the allograft renal artery has previously been anastomosed end to end to the internal iliac artery the renal graft does not suffer any ischaemia during pancreatic implantation.

Severely atherosclerotic and calcified vessels in some diabetic recipients can be a challenge during pancreatic implantation. Iliac Y grafts for back-table reconstruction offer greater flexibility in choosing a suitable arterial anastomotic site in the recipient vessels.

In the last 10 years the most common technique used for pancreas transplantation has been intra-abdominal implantation of the whole pancreas together with a donor duodenal segment. A list of previously employed techniques is given below. These are all associated with poorer outcomes and are rarely performed nowadays.

- segmental pancreas transplantation using only the tail and the body of the pancreas;
- pancreatic duct occlusion or ligation;
- free drainage of exocrine secretions into the peritoneal cavity;
- direct anastomosis of the transected pancreatic head into the bladder;
- utilisation of a small duodenal button.

Currently the choices available to the surgeon are related to the management of the exocrine secretions and the management of the venous drainage, as discussed below.

Management of exocrine secretions

Drainage of the exocrine secretions of pancreatic grafts into the recipient's bladder was the most common technique, accounting for 90% of US pancreas transplants during the 1980s and early 1990s.[22] The popularity of this technique was due to its perceived safety, primarily less serious consequences of anastomotic leaks (compared with enteric drainage) in the days of higher corticosteroids and unrefined immunosuppression. The ability to monitor amylase levels in the urine has been considered an additional advantage of bladder drainage. The latter point is contentious. The evidence with respect to the usefulness of urinary amylase monitoring is reviewed later in this chapter (see p. 198). The unphysiological diversion of pancreatic exocrine secretions into the urinary bladder causes frequent complications often leading to chronic and disabling symptoms. As a consequence conversion of the urinary diversion to enteric drainage is required in many patients. Complications of pancreatic transplantation, including specific problems associated with bladder drainage, are discussed in detail later in the chapter (see p. 198).

Enteric drainage has been gaining in popularity during the last 10 years. In the USA two-thirds of primary SPK transplants and half of solitary pancreas transplants performed between 1996 and 2002 were enterically drained.[4,9] Data regarding the prevalence of enteric versus bladder drainage for pancreas transplantation in Europe are not easy to find. Historically enteric drainage has been the preferred method in Europe and it is likely that the large majority of European pancreas transplant units employ this technique.

Any part of the recipient's small bowel can be used for the anastomosis to the allograft duodenum. No data exist to demonstrate the superiority of one particular site over others. Roux-en-Y loops, which were commonly used, are becoming rare and a simple side-to-side entero-enterostomy is preferred.[12] The correct alignment of the vascular anastomoses is also easier with enteric drainage.

Delayed endocrine function from the transplanted graft is rare and insulin infusion should be discontinued at the time of reperfusion. Achieving insulin independence for the first time in many years in the recipient is a gratifying part of the operation for the surgeon. Patients can become hypoglycaemic at this stage. Blood sugar levels should be checked frequently and a low rate of dextrose infusion is often required.

Management of the venous drainage

Drainage of the venous outflow from pancreas grafts into the portal circulation was first described by Calne in 1984.[23] This complex surgical technique using a segmental graft and gastric exocrine diversion in a paratopic position has never gained popularity. Drainage of the venous outflow into the systemic circulation at the level of the lower inferior vena cava (IVC) has been the norm in pancreatic transplantation. Since the mid-1990s there has been a resurgence of interest in portal venous drainage (PV). The technique described by Shokouh-Amiri et al.[24] involves placement of the graft slightly more cranially in the abdominal cavity with the utilisation of the superior mesenteric vein for the venous drainage. Several studies, including prospective randomised comparisons,[25–27] have shown that this offers at least equivalent outcome to that of systemic venous drainage (SV) with no compromise in safety. The impetus for PV drainage was to achieve a more physiological insulin delivery. A theoretical benefit was considered to be avoidance of hyperinsulinaemia, which has been linked with atherogenesis.[28] Systemic drainage does not always cause hyperinsulinaemia. Nor may it be the only factor since hyperinsulinaemia occurs in non-diabetic recipients of kidney transplants receiving steroids.[29,30] None of the studies of metabolic function after PV drainage have shown a clear benefit in terms of glucose metabolism, lipid profiles or atherogenesis. There is, however, evidence suggestive of an immunological advantage to PV drainage in the form of a reduction in the incidence of acute rejection. The mode of antigen delivery is known to modulate the immune response, which has been proposed as the mechanism responsible for the observed reduction in acute rejection rates in portal venous drained grafts.[12,25–27]

Technically PV drainage may be attractive for re-transplants or for patients who have had previous lower abdominal surgery. It requires a long donor iliac Y graft but offers greater flexibility in choosing a suitable arterial anastomotic site on the recipient vessels. In obese patients and in those with thickened or foreshortened bowel mesentery the SMV may not be easily accessible and PV drainage may be difficult to perform.

IMMUNOSUPPRESSION IN PANCREAS TRANSPLANTATION

Historically there is ample evidence that the incidence of acute rejection is higher after pancreas transplantation compared with kidney transplantation.[12,18,22] The reasons for this difference are not clear. Nevertheless there has been general acknowledgement of the higher immunological risk of pancreas transplantation. This has resulted in the evolution of strategies that employ more intense immunosuppressive protocols for pancreas transplantation compared with kidney transplantation.

In Europe immunosuppressive protocols in organ transplantation in general have been less aggressive compared with the USA. In the evolution of immuno-suppression for pancreas transplantation tacrolimus has largely replaced ciclosporin starting from the mid-1990s (**Fig. 9.4**). Similarly mycophenolate mofetil (MMF) has replaced azathioprine in most immunosuppressive protocols. Steroids remain part of the initial immunosuppression in the large majority of cases. Interleukin 2 (IL-2) receptor anti-bodies have gradually replaced ATG or OKT3 in induction therapy in the last 5 years. In general there has been a small decline in the use of antibody induction, from 90% in 1987–93 to 83% in 1994–97 and 76% in 2001 in the USA.[4] There is a sound evidence base for this evolution. This evidence, reviewed below, has been provided not only by single-centre reports or registry analyses but also by prospective randomised trials.

Studies of induction therapy with ATG or OKT3 were conducted in the early 1990s, in the ciclosporin era. Two prospective multicentre randomised trials[31,32] show that these agents delay the onset and lessen the severity of rejection episodes at the expense of increased cytomegalovirus (CMV) disease but with no demonstrable influence on patient survival. Pancreas graft survival at the medium term in this Sandimmun era was also improved with ATG or OKT3 induction.

Two prospective randomised multicentre studies were published in 2003 investigating the role of induction therapy combined with tacrolimus- and MMF-based immunosuppression. Stratta and colleagues reported a significant reduction in the

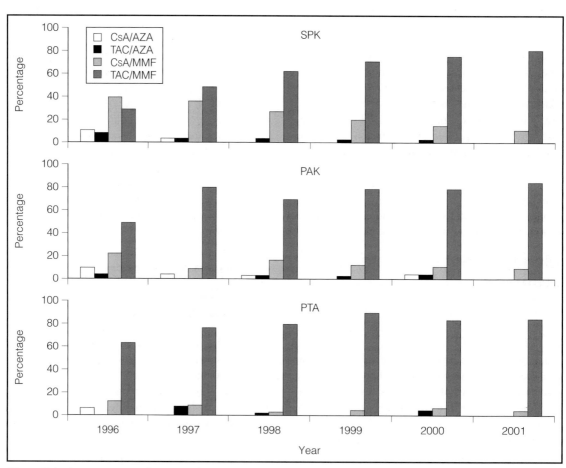

Figure 9.4 • Immunosuppressive protocols used in pancreas transplant recipients in the USA – International Pancreas Transplant Registry database.

incidence of kidney and pancreas rejection with daclizumab induction.[33] Adverse events, including infectious complications, were not different with or without induction therapy. A modified two-dose daclizumab regime gave overall better results than the standard five-dose regime. Another prospective randomised trial at 18 US centres compared induction using any one of the biological agents (OKT3, ATG, basiliximab or daclizumab) with no induction.[34] A trend towards reduction in the incidence of acute rejection by induction therapy was seen. The 1-year incidence of acute rejection (kidney or pancreas) was 24.6% and 31.2% in induction therapy and control groups respectively ($P = 0.28$). The incidence of biopsy-confirmed acute kidney allograft rejection was 13.1% and 23% ($P = 0.08$).

MMF has been shown to reduce the incidence of acute rejection compared with azathioprine in two large prospective randomised trials in the USA and Europe in kidney transplant recipients[35,36] and one prospective randomised trial in pancreas transplant recipients.[37]

Two other prospective controlled studies and many single-centre reports and registry analyses demonstrate improved outcomes with tacrolimus in pancreas transplant recipients compared with ciclosporin.[38–40] Experience with islet transplantation[41] and solid organ pancreatic transplantation[42] suggests that sirolimus in combination with induction therapy and calcineurin antagonists may be as effective as other current regimens in preventing acute rejection. It remains to be seen whether the effect of sirolimus on wound healing will be an impediment for its routine use as primary immunosuppression in whole-organ pancreas transplant recipients.

ACUTE REJECTION FOLLOWING PANCREAS TRANSPLANTATION

Diagnosis of acute rejection

One of the notable features about pancreas transplantation over the last decade has been the considerable reduction in the incidence of acute rejection. In 1992 74% of SPK transplant recipients

and 50% of solitary pancreas transplant recipients (this probably underestimates the true incidence) were reported to have received antirejection therapy.[8,12,18] This had reduced to 19% and 17% respectively by 2000.[3,9]

An important feature of pancreatic graft rejection for the purposes of patient management is the lack of a reliable early marker. In SPK transplants diagnosis of acute rejection almost completely relies on monitoring of the renal allograft by serum creatinine levels and further assessment when indicated by renal biopsy. Discordant rejection of allografts is thought to occur rarely following SPK transplantation. Isolated rejection of the pancreas is said to represent no more than 5–10% of acute rejection episodes.[12,43] Direct evidence from series with simultaneous kidney and pancreas biopsies is very limited. Experimental work in dogs by the Westmead Team in Sydney showed isolated pancreas rejection to occur with an incidence of no more than 2% following combined kidney and pancreas transplantation.[44] The most convincing evidence for the security of the implied diagnosis of rejection in the pancreas by diagnosing kidney rejection comes from consistent clinical observations of higher pancreatic graft survival rates following SPK transplantation compared with solitary pancreas transplantation. Monitoring for acute rejection and patient management in the early postoperative period is therefore a particular challenge in solitary pancreas transplants.

Acute rejection of the pancreas affects the exocrine pancreas first. The inflammation may cause pain and a low-grade fever associated with a rise in serum amylase. These symptoms and signs are non-specific, can be subtle and do not distinguish between acute rejection and other causes of graft inflammation (such as ischaemia–reperfusion injury or allograft pancreatitis). Islets of Langerhans are scattered sparsely throughout the exocrine pancreas and beta cells have considerable functional reserve. Therefore dysfunction of the majority of islets manifesting as hyperglycaemia as a consequence of rejection occurs only very late in the course of acute rejection. Imaging modalities such as computed tomography (CT) or magnetic resonance imaging (MRI) visualise the pancreas and may be helpful to exclude other pathology (such as lack of perfusion, which may be segmental or intra-abdominal collections). However, there are no specific signs of acute rejection on any radiological investigation. Unlike the kidney, the pancreas lacks a firm capsule. Therefore vascular resistance is not reliably altered as a consequence of inflammation and duplex scan monitoring is not useful. Detection of urinary amylase in bladder-drained grafts is a sensitive indicator of function. However, detection of hypoamylasuria lacks specificity. Factors other than acute rejection such as diuresis or fasting also cause hypoamylasuria.[45] Greater than 25% reduction in urinary amylase correlates with acute rejection in no more than half of the cases when assessed by biopsy.[46] A stable urinary amylase may therefore be helpful in excluding acute rejection but detection of hypoamylasuria is unhelpful. Other tests have been shown to be better correlated with early endocrine dysfunction of pancreas grafts such as glucose disappearance rate or insulin secretion dynamics following an intravenous glucose load.[47,48] Owing to their complexity and lack of availability, such tests are not practical for use as routine daily monitoring tools in patient management.

Pancreas allograft biopsy has recently become established as a reliable and safe technique and is the gold standard in the diagnosis of acute rejection in solitary pancreas transplants. Percutaneous biopsy under ultrasound or CT guidance is the most common method. Histological criteria for the diagnosis and grading of rejection have been standardised.[49]

Management of acute rejection

Recipients of pancreas transplants have more to lose than recipients of other organ transplants from unnecessary treatment for acute rejection. Diagnosis of acute rejection of the pancreas should always be confirmed histologically prior to the institution of treatment.

The first-line management of acute rejection of pancreas allografts is high-dose corticosteroids. Pancreatic rejection episodes concurrent with the rejection of the kidney usually resolve with steroids. In many transplant centres anti-T-cell agents are used for the management of acute rejection in solitary pancreas transplants, for recurrent acute rejection or for moderate to severe rejection. IPTR

data show that steroids were used in 85% of SPK and 80% of solitary pancreas transplant recipients diagnosed as having acute rejection.[3] However, 48% of SPK recipients and 80% of solitary pancreas recipients with acute rejection are recorded as having had anti-T-cell agents also, suggesting that many patients are given both.

Acute rejection in pancreas allografts is not life threatening and caution is advised against over-immunosuppression. If diagnosed before the onset of hyperglycaemia most rejection episodes are reversible.

Impact of acute rejection on outcome

The UNOS data for 4251 patients who received SPK transplants between 1988 and 1997 were analysed by Reddy and colleagues in order to determine the influence of acute rejection on long-term outcome.[50] Acute rejection of either graft increased the relative risk of pancreas and kidney graft failure at 5 years. The relative risks, adjusted for other risk factors, were 1.32 and 1.53 for pancreas and for kidney, respectively, if acute rejection occurred. In this analysis 45% of the cohort had no acute rejection. The worst outcome was in patients who had both kidney and pancreas rejection.

COMPLICATIONS OF PANCREAS TRANSPLANTATION

Introduction

Pancreas transplantation is associated with a higher incidence and a greater range of complications than kidney transplantation, and the postoperative patient management constitutes a greater challenge (Box 9.3). Between a fifth and a quarter of patients require relaparotomy following pancreas transplantation to deal with complications. Part of the reason for the increased incidence of complications is the higher level of immunosuppression in a high-risk diabetic population who already exhibit impaired infection resistance, poor healing and a high prevalence of comorbidity. Other factors relate to the allograft, which unlike kidney or liver allografts is

Box 9.3 • Complications of pancreas transplantation

Infective complications

- Systemic infection (opportunistic infections associated with immunosuppression)
- Local infections (peritonitis, localised collections, enteric or pancreatic fistulas)

Vascular complications

- Haemorrhage: early haemorrhage from allograft vessels and late haemorrhage (rupture of pseudoaneurysms)
- Thrombosis: allograft arterial or venous thrombosis

Allograft pancreatitis

- Ischaemia/reperfusion injury or reflux pancreatitis (especially after bladder drainage)

Complications specific to bladder drainage

- Chronic dehydration, acidosis, recurrent urinary tract infections, haematuria, chemical cystitis, urethral strictures or urethral disruption

not sterile and uniquely possesses rich proteolytic enzymes, making it susceptible to specific complications such as pancreatitis, leaks and fistula formation. The blood flow to the pancreas is much lower compared with the kidney, and this is a further risk factor specifically for thrombotic complications. Finally, bladder drainage of the exocrine secretions is associated with a high incidence of complications unique to this unphysiological diversion.

Infective complications

CMV disease is more common after pancreas transplantation compared with kidney or liver transplantation. Antiviral prophylaxis in CMV-mismatched donor/recipient pairs is mandatory. Unique to pancreatic transplantation are intra-abdominal septic complications that occur as a consequence of bacteria or fungi transmitted from the donor via the allograft or those that occur as a consequence of anastomotic leaks. Patients on peritoneal dialysis at the time of transplantation may have a higher rate of intra-abdominal infection compared with those on haemodialysis.[18]

It is not known whether duodenal decontamination during organ retrieval has any influence

on recipient intra-abdominal or wound infections. A bacteriology specimen of the donor duodenal contents should be used to guide antimicrobial therapy in the event of intra-abdominal sepsis. Abdominal lavage with warm saline or antibiotic/antifungal solutions is also common practice after implantation of pancreatic allografts. There are no controlled trials demonstrating their efficacy.

Vascular complications

THROMBOSIS

Allograft venous or arterial thrombosis occurs more commonly following pancreatic transplantation compared with kidney transplantation. Retrospective analysis of data reported to registries regarding the causes of graft loss is understandably prone to error and difficult to interpret. Nevertheless graft thrombosis appears to be one of the two most common causes of early graft loss following pancreas transplantation.[9,18] A predisposing factor could be the use of venous extension grafts for the portal vein anastomosis, which should be only very rarely required. Concern about a potentially higher incidence of thrombosis following portal venous drainage has not been borne out by clinical experience. There is no difference in the incidence of technical failure rate with portal venous drainage compared with systemic venous drainage. Routine use of heparin for prophylaxis against allograft vascular thrombosis is associated with increased haemorrhage. Most transplant centres do not use heparin; however, authors from the largest pancreas transplant unit in the world have reported a small reduction in the incidence of graft thrombosis with heparin.[18]

Table 9.3 illustrates the relative prevalence of some of the complications leading to graft loss in the IPTR database. Graft thrombosis stands out as a much more common cause of graft loss than any other complication. None of the complications occurs more commonly in bladder-drained grafts compared with enterically drained grafts.

HAEMORRHAGE

Release of the vascular clamps and reperfusion of the pancreatic allograft during the recipient operation can be a tricky moment, with potential for bleeding from multiple points on the allograft. The

Table 9.3 • Technical failures as causes of graft loss in US cadaveric primary pancreas transplants 1/1/96–10/7/02

	SPK			PAK			PTA		
	BD	ED	*P*	BD	ED	*P*	BD	ED	*P*
Graft thrombosis	5.1%	6.3%	0.073	6.3%	9.6%	0.059	7.1%	10.8%	0.166
Infection/pancreatitis	0.8%	1.4%	0.090	0.8%	2.9%	0.178	1.2%	1.5%	0.83
Anastomotic leak	0.4%	0.9%	0.036	0.6%	1.0%	0.471	0.8%	1.47%	0.665
Bleeding	0.3%	0.3%	0.935	0.4%	0.2%	0.569	0.0%	0.0%	–

SPK, simultaneous pancreas–kidney transplants; PAK, pancreas after kidney transplants; PTA, pancreas transplantation alone; BD, bladder drained; ED, enterically drained.

key to avoiding this is meticulous preparation of the allograft on the back table prior to implantation.

Late haemorrhage following pancreas transplantation is an uncommon but catastrophic complication, often due to the rupture of a pseudoaneurysm or direct erosion of one of the anastomoses secondary to a leak. Any unexplained fever, tachycardia, leucocytosis or abdominal pain in recipients of pancreas transplants should lead to investigations in order to detect or exclude a leak or an intra-abdominal collection.

Allograft pancreatitis

Cold storage and ischaemia reperfusion injury inevitably result in a degree of oedema of the pancreatic allograft. This is a commonly encountered finding if a relaparotomy becomes necessary in the first few postoperative days and it is not always associated with an elevation in serum amylase. There is no universally agreed definition of allograft pancreatitis. The condition has a different clinical course to native pancreatitis. It is rarely severe or life threatening. Ischaemia–reperfusion injury may be the cause or a predisposing factor. It is not known (although likely) whether drugs associated with native pancreatitis can also cause allograft pancreatitis. Bladder drainage (especially with autonomic neuropathy and high intravesical pressures) can be associated with recurrent episodes of allograft pancreatitis due to reflux. Catheter drainage of the bladder for at least 7–10 days is usually adequate for the management of the acute episode but ultimately enteric conversion may be required.

During the pancreas transplant operation the allograft exocrine function starts very promptly upon revascularisation and the duodenal segment fills with the pancreatic juice quickly. Excessive distension of the duodenal segment and the consequent reflux could cause postoperative pancreatitis. Even if the exocrine diversion is not going to be performed straight away, the duodenal segment should be decompressed and excessive distension of the graft duodenum should be avoided during the recipient operation.

The distinction between allograft pancreatitis and acute rejection in the presence of an oedematous pancreas, abdominal pain and a slightly raised serum amylase is a difficult clinical diagnosis, which was discussed earlier (see p. 197).

Complications specific to bladder drainage

The most common consequence of the diversion of the exocrine pancreatic secretions into the bladder is a chemical cystitis, which predisposes patients to infection, persistent haematuria and troublesome dysuria. Dysuria is more troublesome in men, with urethritis that can progress to urethral disruption. Failure of reabsorption of the exocrine secretions results in chronic dehydration and acidosis. Urinary tract infections are much more common compared with intestinal drainage. Persistent haematuria can require repeated blood transfusions. In the presence of autonomic neuropathy, repeated episodes of reflux allograft pancreatitis are another potential complication. As a consequence of one or more of these complications enteric conversion of the exocrine drainage may become necessary. The enteric conversion rate in bladder-drained pancreas transplants increases with increasing follow-up and could be as high as 40% at 5 years.[12]

OUTCOME FOLLOWING PANCREAS TRANSPLANTATION

Introduction

There is little doubt that patient and graft survival rates following pancreas transplantation continued to improve throughout the 1990s. Detailed analyses of outcomes reported to the IPTR have been published by Gruessner and Sutherland annually in *Clinical Transplants* for many years.[8] They remain as valuable sources of data. The IPTR reports, however, refer to short- or medium-term outcome and should be interpreted within the context of their limitations. The analysis of 1996–2000 US pancreas transplants refers to 5276 transplants performed in this period. The outcome figures were based on data from 4073 of these patients for whom complete information was available. It is not mentioned what information was missing in the remaining 1203 patients.

Table 9.4 summarises the improvements observed in the success rate of pancreatic transplantation in the USA between 1987 and 2000.

Continuing improvement in short-term and medium-term pancreas transplant outcomes is also illustrated in **Figs 9.5, 9.6 and 9.7.**

Another comprehensive database that is readily accessible on the internet and regularly publishes and updates pancreas transplantation activity and outcome from the USA is the OPTN/SRTR (Organ Procurement and Transplantation Network/Scientific Registry of Transplant Recipients) database.[3,4]

Table 9.5 summarises patient survival and graft survival data from the database as of August 2002.

Short-term patient survival and graft survival rates remain as the standard primary outcome measure in organ transplantation. In common with other solid organ transplants, these rates have improved considerably in pancreas transplantation to the extent that demonstration of any further significant improvement as a consequence of any intervention requires prospective studies with very large patient groups. In order to circumvent this difficulty in kidney transplantation, surrogate endpoints (or secondary outcome measures) such as the incidence of acute rejection or the quality of graft function have been used. Similar surrogate outcome measures applicable to pancreas transplantation are more difficult to define. As an example of difficulties with the interpretation of data, one may recall the evidence previously discussed from several single-centre reports demonstrating immunological benefits of portal venous drainage. The fact that this is not reflected in improved graft survival rates may indeed be a genuine finding. However, it could also be attributed to already excellent graft survival rates with systemic venous drainage and the relatively infrequent application of portal venous drainage in possibly selected patients. Distorted reporting with less incomplete data in the registry from the portal-drained subgroup of patients may also be a confounding factor.

Any enquiry into the outcome of pancreas transplantation worldwide also suffers from the lack of a truly representative international database. The IPTR and the OPTN/SRTR databases have given us a

Table 9.4 • Improvements observed in 1-year survival rates of pancreatic transplantation in the USA between 1987 and 2000

	SPK		PAK		PTA	
	1987–1990	1998–2000	1987–1990	1998–2000	1987–1990	1989–2000
Patient survival	89%	95%	91%	94%	93%	100%
Pancreas graft survival	72%	82%	52%	74%	47%	76%
Kidney graft survival	84%	92%	–	–	–	–

SPK, simultaneous pancreas–kidney transplants; PAK, pancreas after kidney transplants; PTA, pancreas transplantation alone.

remarkably useful insight into the picture in the USA. Information with respect to the outcome of pancreas transplantation outside the USA is more sketchy. The responsible attitude for the pancreas transplantation community worldwide should be to regard complete and accurate reporting of pancreas transplantation activity and outcome as an indispensable priority.

Factors influencing pancreas transplantation outcome

Knowledge regarding the recipient- and donor-related factors that influence the outcome of pancreas transplantation relies largely on the IPTR and the OPTN/SRTR databases.

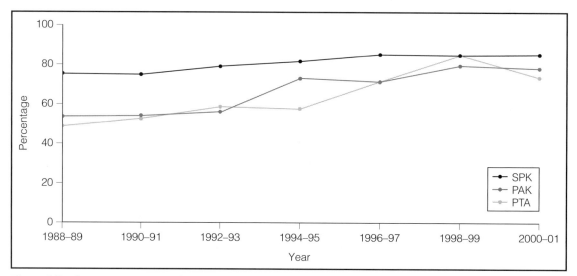

Figure 9.5 • One-year pancreas graft function.

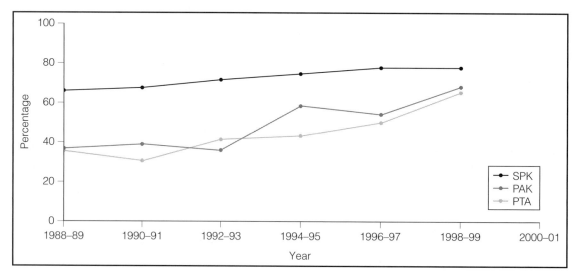

Figure 9.6 • Three-year pancreas graft function.

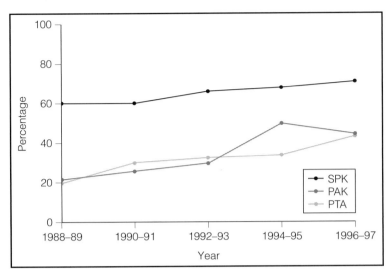

Figure 9.7 • Five-year pancreas graft function.

Table 9.5 • Patient and graft survival based on data from the OPTN/SRTR database at August 2002

	Patient survival (%)			Graft survival (%)		
	1-year	3-year	5-year	1-year	3-year	5-year
SPK	95.1 N = 1823	89.2 N = 1803	82.6 N = 1749	83.8 N = 1840	76.9 N = 1817	69.2 N = 1763
PAK	95.5 N = 374	89.3 N = 205	77.3 N = 132	78.3 N = 519	60.2 N = 287	45.5 N = 178
PTA	98.6 N = 222	86.0 N = 121	77.8 N = 72	81.2 N = 242	57.1 N = 135	32.4 N = 81

SPK, simultaneous pancreas–kidney transplants; PAK, pancreas after kidney transplants; PTA, pancreas transplantation alone.
One-year data in this analysis refer to the outcome (actual survival rates) for the cohort transplanted in 1999–2000. Three-year data give the outcome for transplants performed in 1997–1998. Five-year data refer to the outcome of transplants performed in 1995–1996. The number of patients included in each of the analyses is shown.

RECIPIENT AGE

Increasing recipient age is a small but significant risk factor in the outcome of pancreas transplantation. Historically patient and graft survival rates have been higher in younger recipients. In the last few years more careful patient selection has influenced the outcome in older recipients favourably to the extent that the short-term outcome following pancreas transplantation is no different for patients older than 45 at the time of transplant compared with those who are younger than 45.[9] The number of patients in solitary pancreas transplant categories is smaller and most patients receiving solitary trans-

plants tend to be in the younger age group. As a consequence the influence of recipient age is more readily demonstrable in simultaneous pancreas–kidney transplantation and becomes more pronounced with longer follow-up. Five years after simultaneous pancreas–kidney transplantation patient survival is 82% for recipients aged 35–49 at the time of transplantation compared with 75% for those aged 50 or older.[3]

RE-TRANSPLANTATION

Re-transplantation appears as a consistent and significant risk factor for graft survival in all

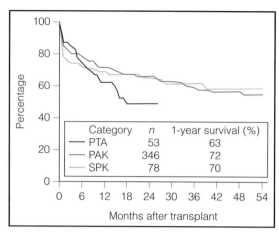

Figure 9.8 • Pancreas *re-transplant* graft function. These are US cadaveric re-transplants from January 1996 to July 2003.

categories. One-year pancreas graft survival rates after re-transplants in SPK, PAK and PTA categories are 70%, 72% and 63% respectively[9] (**Fig. 9.8**).

HLA MATCHING

HLA (human leucocyte antigen) matching has a small influence on the outcome of pancreas transplants depending on the category. In SPK transplantation the outcome appears to be independent of HLA. Similarly in PAK transplantation no influence of HLA matching on outcome is demonstrable. However, in pancreas transplants alone the 2-year graft survival rates in the IPTR database are quoted as 89%, 75%, 71%, 65% and 57% for 0, 1, 2, 3 and 4 HLA mismatches respectively.[9]

MANAGEMENT OF EXOCRINE SECRETIONS: MANAGEMENT OF VENOUS DRAINAGE

The surgical technique employed for the exocrine diversion has no influence on outcome in SPK transplantation and pancreas transplantation alone. There may be a small survival advantage (graft survival) in favour of bladder-drained grafts in PAK transplantation.[9]

Portal venous drainage versus systemic venous drainage made no difference to the outcome in SPK transplantation and PAK transplantation.[9] In pancreas transplantation alone 1-year graft survival was superior after portal venous drainage (81% PV versus 70% SV).

IMMUNOSUPPRESSION

Immunosuppressive therapy has a major influence on the outcome of pancreas transplantation. As illustrated in **Fig. 9.4**, a combination of prednisolone, tacrolimus and MMF is the most successful protocol for maintenance immunosuppression. It has virtually replaced all others for pancreas transplantation in the USA over the last few years. The use of rapamycin has been reported in over 400 transplants, but this drug has not yet been included in the IPTR outcome analyses.[9]

OTHER FACTORS

Other factors that are variably associated with increased risk of graft failure or patient death are donor age (>45 years), donor cause of death (cardiovascular), donor obesity (BMI >25) and recipient obesity (BMI >25).

LONG-TERM OUTLOOK FOLLOWING PANCREAS TRANSPLANTATION

Pancreas transplantation and life expectancy

Clearly one of the most important factors for patients considering pancreas transplantation is whether their life expectancy will be influenced by the transplant. Numerous studies and analyses of databases have consistently shown that successful pancreas transplantation is associated with improved survival prospects in diabetic patients. No prospective controlled study has ever been carried out that compares pancreas transplantation with insulin therapy. Hence all available evidence is subject to selection bias. It would be reasonable to expect that in clinical practice younger fitter patients with lower risk would have been chosen for pancreas transplantation, creating bias in favour of this group. Nevertheless a strong body of indirect evidence suggests that successful pancreas transplantation may truly increase life expectancy as well as improving quality of life.

Several studies have addressed the question of the impact of pancreas transplantation on long-term mortality in a number of different ways. The University of Wisconsin experience in 500 SPK transplant recipients published in 1998[51] simply quotes a 10-year patient survival rate of 70%. This is matched in their experience only by recipients of living-donor kidney transplants. Unsurpassed as they are, these results were obtained in a highly selected group of young patients with a relatively short duration of diabetes and kidney failure and strict eligibility criteria excluding those with ischaemic heart disease.

A large registry analysis from the USA published in 2001 by Ojo et al. looked at the outcome in 13 467 adults with type I diabetes registered in kidney and SPK transplant waiting lists between 1988 and 1997.[52] Adjusted 10-year patient survival was 67% for SPK transplant recipients, 65% for living-donor kidney (LKD) transplant recipients and 46% for cadaveric kidney (CAD) transplant recipients. Taking the mortality of patients who remained on dialysis as reference, the adjusted relative risk of 5-year mortality was 0.40, 0.45 and 0.74 for SPK, LKD and CAD recipients. Another large review of the UNOS database published by Reddy et al.[53] in 2003 analysed long-term survival in 18 549 type I diabetic patients transplanted between 1987 and 1996. There was a long-term survival advantage in favour of pancreas transplant recipients (8-year crude survival rates: 72% for SPK, 72% for LKD and 55% for CAD). This diminished but persisted after adjusting for donor and recipient variables and kidney graft function. Tyden and colleagues from Sweden demonstrated a striking difference in long-term survival in a small group of diabetic patients transplanted between 1982 and 1986 and followed up for at least 10 years.[54] Fourteen patients received successful SPK transplants. The control group consisted of 15 patients who had undergone the same assessment, had been accepted for SPK transplants but either declined pancreas transplantation or received SPK but lost the pancreas graft within the first year because of a technical complication. Ten years later three of the SPK transplant recipients had died (20%) compared with 12 of the 15 kidney transplant recipients (80%). Another interesting study addressing the long-term survival after transplantation in type I diabetics came from The Netherlands. Smets et al. studied all 415 adults with type I diabetes who started renal replacement therapy in The Netherlands between 1985 and

1996. Patients were divided into two groups depending on where they lived. The basis for this was the fact that in the Leiden area the treatment of choice for such patients was SPK transplantation (73% of transplants), whereas in the remainder of Holland kidney transplantation alone was the predominant type of therapy and SPK was performed uncommonly (37%). They demonstrated that the relative risk of death for patients who lived outside the Leiden area was 1.9. When the transplanted patients only were analysed the mortality ratio was 2.5 for those outside the Leiden area.[55]

Influence of pancreas transplantation on diabetic complications

NEPHROPATHY

There is convincing evidence that successful pancreas transplantation can stop the progression of diabetic nephropathy and reverse associated histological changes. This evidence largely comes from studies that have assessed the course of diabetic nephropathy in kidney allografts in SPK or PAK transplant recipients.[56,57] Fioretto et al. have shown that established lesions of diabetic nephropathy in native kidneys can be reversed with successful pancreas transplantation (PTA).[58] In the setting of clinical transplantation the beneficial effect of the pancreas graft is counterbalanced by the nephrotoxicity of the immunosuppressive drugs.

RETINOPATHY

Patients with type I diabetes often quote preservation of their eyesight as one of the main reasons for considering pancreas transplantation. There is insufficient evidence to reassure patients that diabetic retinopathy will improve following successful pancreas transplantation. Chow et al. have published the Westmead experience with diabetic retinopathy after SPK transplantation, and a balanced review of the available data is discussed by these authors.[59] Pancreas transplantation for the preservation of poor eyesight with current evidence is not justified. Importantly, preoperative stabilisation of any proliferative retinopathy is necessary in order to prevent the risk of further deterioration following pancreas transplantation. It is unlikely that pancreas transplantation will have a significant beneficial or adverse influence within the first 2 years. Like nephropathy and neuropathy, any benefit to retinopathy as a consequence of better blood glucose control takes more than 2 years to become evident.[60] Most patients are likely to achieve stabilisation of retinopathy in the medium term. Comparisons with the alternative of remaining on insulin therapy in the long term are scarce but patients with successful pancreas transplants may fare better beyond 5 years.[61]

NEUROPATHY

Patients with end-stage renal failure and type I diabetes almost universally exhibit an autonomic and peripheral (somatic) diabetic polyneuropathy as well as uraemic neuropathy. Improvement in neuropathy following SPK transplantation using objective measures of nerve function has been demonstrated by several transplant centres.[62,63] For individuals with intractable and distressing symptoms of neuropathy the clinical benefit may be considerable. Obesity, presence of advanced neuropathy and poor renal allograft function may be predictors of poor recovery in nerve function after SPK transplantation.[64]

CARDIOVASCULAR DISEASE

Pancreas transplantation has demonstrable benefit on microangiopathy in diabetics.[65] Some of its effects on retinopathy, nephropathy and neuropathy may be mediated through this mechanism. It has been more difficult to demonstrate any improvement in macroangiopathy. The enhanced survival prospects after pancreas transplantation ought to be at least in part due to the improvement in the cardiovascular risk profile. Evidence to support this is accumulating. Fiorina and colleagues in Milan demonstrated favourable influences of pancreas[66] and islet[67] transplantation on atherosclerotic risk factors including plasma lipid profile, blood pressure, left ventricular function and endothelial function.

This translates into reduced cardiovascular death rate.[68,69] Similar improvement occurs in early non-uraemic diabetics after PTA.[70]

Key points

- By the end of 2003, over 20 000 pancreas transplants had been reported to the International Registry.
- The outcome following pancreas transplantation has improved considerably in the last 10 years. It is now comparable to the outcome for other solid organ transplants.
- The number of SPK transplants has remained stable for the last 5 years whilst solitary pancreas transplantation activity continues to increase.
- Prednisolone/tacrolimus/MMF is by far the most common maintenance immunosuppression protocol used for pancreas transplantation. There has been a small reduction in the utilisation of antibody induction in recent years.
- Over the last decade preference for the management of exocrine secretions in pancreas transplantation has gradually changed in favour of enteric drainage. Bladder drainage now accounts for a small minority.
- Portal venous drainage introduced in the mid-1990s is gaining popularity and currently accounts for about a quarter of the pancreas transplants.
- Evidence regarding the influence of pancreas transplantation on diabetic complications and life expectancy is not available from prospective controlled trials. Nevertheless accumulating evidence from many studies strongly suggests that successful pancreas transplantation has a favourable influence on diabetic complications and survival prospects for patients.

REFERENCES

1. Kelly KD, Lillehei KC, Merkle FK et al. Allo-transplantation of pancreas and duodenum along with kidney in diabetic nephropathy. Surgery 1967; 61:827–37.

2. Sasaki TM, Gray RS, Ratner RE et al. Successful long term kidney-pancreas transplants in diabetic patients with high C-peptide levels. Transplantation 1998; 65:1510–12.

3. HHS/HRSA/OSP/DOT and UNOS. 2000 Annual Report of the US Scientific Registry of Transplant Recipients and the Organ Procurement and Transplantation Network. Rockville, MD and Richmond, VA, 16 February 2001.

4. URREA, UNOS. 2003 Annual Report of the US Organ Procurement and Transplantation Network and the Scientific Registry of Transplant Recipients. http://www.OPTN.org

   Comprehensive report of US transplant activity and outcomes, including detailed explanation of methodology and authorship of individual sections. Note large file size.

5. McMillan MA, Briggs JD, Junor BJ. Outcome of renal replacement treatment in patients with diabetes mellitus. BMJ 1990; 301:540–4.

6. Rabbat CG, Treleaven DR, Russell DJ et al. Prognostic value of myocardial perfusion studies in patients with end-stage renal disease assessed for kidney or kidney-pancreas transplantation: a meta-analysis. J Am Soc Nephrol 2003; 14:431–9.

7. Lin K, Stewart D, Cooper S et al. Pre-transplant cardiac testing for kidney-pancreas transplant candidates and association with cardiac outcomes. Clin Transplant 2001; 15:269–75.

8. Gruessner AC, Sutherland DER. Pancreas transplant outcomes for United States (US) cases reported to the United Network for Organ Sharing(UNOS) and non-US cases reported to the International Pancreas Transplant Registry (IPTR) as of October 2000. Clinical Transplants 2000:45–72.

9. International Pancreas Transplant Registry. 2002 Annual Report, vol. 15, no. 1, August 2003. http://www.iptr.umn.edu

   The latest annual report from the International Pancreas Transplant Registry. Contains links to previous reports, interim report for the current year and printed copies of the information contained within the website.

10. Humar A, Sutherland DE, Ramcharan T et al. Optimal timing for a pancreas transplant after successful kidney transplant. Transplantation 2000; 70:1247–50.

11. Hariharan S, Pirsch JD, Lu CY et al. Pancreas after kidney transplantation. J Am Soc Nephrol 2002; 13:1109–18.

   Detailed review article about PAK transplantation with authoritative and representative contributions from the large US centres.

12. Odorico JS, Sollinger HW. Technical and immuno-logical advances in transplantation for insulin dependent diabetes mellitus. World J Surg 2002; 26:194–211.

   Review article with an extensive list of references, from one of the leading North American pancreas transplant units.

13. http://www.uktransplant.org.uk/statistics/statistics. htm

14. http://www.eurotransplant.org/index.php?id= statistics

15. Krieger NR, Odorico JS, Heisey DM et al. Underutilization of pancreas donors. Transplantation 2003; 75:1271–6.

16. D'Allessandro AM, Stratta JR, Sollinger HW et al. Use of UW solution in pancreas transplantation. Diabetes 1989; 38(suppl. 1): 7–9.

17. Potdor S, Eghtesad B, Jain A et al. Comparison of early graft function and complications of pancreas transplant recipients in Histidine-Tryptophan-Ketoglutarate (HTK) solution and University of Wisconsin (UW) solutions. Transplantation 2003; 76:S28.

18. Sutherland DER, Gruessner RW, Dunn DL et al. Lessons learned from more than 1000 pancreas transplants at a single institution. Ann Surg 2001; 233:463–501.

   The largest single-centre pancreas transplantation experience in the world from the pioneers of pancreas transplantation.

19. DeVilleDeGoyet J, Hausleithner V, Malaise J et al. Liver procurement without in-situ portal perfusion. Transplantation 1994; 57:1328–32.

20. Olson DW, Kadota S, Cornish A et al. Intestinal decontamination using povidone iodine compromises small bowel storage quality. Transplantation 2003; 75:1460–2.

21. Woeste G, Wallstein C, Vogt J et al. Value of donor swabs for intra-abdominal infection in simultaneous pancreas kidney transplantation. Transplantation 2003; 76:1073–8.

22. Pancreas transplants for United States (US) and non-US cases as reported to the International Pancreas Transplant Registry (IPTR) and to the United Network for Organ Sharing (UNOS). Clinical Transplants 1997:45–59.

23. Calne RY. Para-topic segmental pancreas grafting: a technique with portal venous drainage. Lancet 1984; 1:595–7.

24. Shokouh-Amiri MH, Gaber AO, Gaber LW et al. Pancreas transplantation with portal venous

drainage and enteric exocrine diversion: a new technique. Transplant Proc 1992; 24:776–7.

25. Petruzzo PA, Palmina A, DaSilva MA et al. Simultaneous pancreas-kidney transplantation: portal versus systemic venous drainage of the pancreas allografts. Clin Transplant 2000; 14:287–91.

26. Stratta RJ, Shokouh-Amiri MH, Egidi MF et al. A prospective comparison of simultaneous kidney-pancreas transplantation with systemic-enteric versus portal-enteric drainage. Ann Surg 2001; 233:740–51.

27. Stratta RJ, LoA, Shokouh-Amiri MH et al. Improving results in solitary pancreas transplantation with portal enteric drainage, thymoglobulin induction and tacrolimus/mycophenolate mofetil based immunosuppression. Transplant Int 2003; 16;154–60.

28. Despres JP, Lamarche B, Mauriege P et al. Hyper-insulinemia as an independent risk factor for ischaemic heart disease. N Engl J Med 1996; 334:952–7.

29. Ost LD, Tyden G, Fehrman I. Impaired glucose tolerance in Ciclosporine-prednisolone treated renal allograft recipients. Transplantation 1988; 46:370–2.

30. Christiansen E, Vestergaard H, Tibell A et al. Impaired insulin-stimulated non-oxidative glucose metabolism in pancreas-kidney transplant recipients: dose-response effects of insulin on glucose turnover. Diabetes 1996: 45:1267–75.

31. Wadstrom J, Brekke B, Wrammer L et al. Triple versus quadruple induction immunosuppression in pancreas transplantation. Transplant Proc 1995; 27:1317–18.

32. Cantarovich D, Karam G, Giral-Classe M et al. Randomized comparison of triple therapy and anti-thymocyte globulin induction treatment after simultaneous pancreas kidney transplantation. Kidney Int 1998; 54:1351–6.

33. Stratta RJ, Alloway RR, Lo A et al. Two dose daclizumab regimen in simultaneous kidney pancreas transplant recipients: primary endpoint analysis of a multi-center randomised study. Transplantation 2003; 75:1260–6.

34. Kaufman DB, Burke GW, Bruce DS et al. Prospective randomised multi-center trial of antibody induction therapy in simultaneous kidney-pancreas transplantation. Am J Transplant 2003; 3:855–64.

35. European Mycophenolate Mofetil Co-operative Study Group. Placebo controlled study of mycophenolate mofetil combined with Ciclosporine and corticosteroids for prevention of acute rejection. Lancet 1995; 345: 1321–5.

36. Sollinger HW for the US Renal Transplant Mycophenolate Mofetil Study Group. Mycophenolate mofetil for the prevention of acute rejection in primary cadaveric renal allograft recipients. Transplantation 1995; 60:225–32.

37. Merion RM, Henry ML, Melzer JS et al. Randomized prospective trial of mycophenolate mofetil versus azathioprine for prevention of acute renal allograft rejection after simultaneous kidney-pancreas transplantation. Transplantation 2000; 70:105–11.

38. Stratta RJ. Review of immunosuppressive usage in pancreas transplantation. Clin Transplant 1999; 13:1–12.

39. Gruessner RWG. Tacrolimus in pancreas transplantation: A multi-center analysis. Clin Transplant 1997; 11:299–312.

40. Bartlett ST, Schweitzer EJ, Johnson LB et al. Equivalent success of simultaneous pancreas-kidney and solitary pancreas transplantation. A prospective trial of tacrolimus immunosuppression with percutaneous biopsy. Ann Surg 1996; 224:440–9.

41. Shapiro AMJ, Lakey JRT, Ryan EA et al. Islet transplantation in seven patients with Type 1 diabetes mellitus using a glucocorticoid free immunosuppressive regimen. N Engl J Med 2000, 343:230–8.

42. Knight RJ, Kerman RH, Zela S et al. Thymoglobulin, Sirolimus and reduced dose Ciclosporine provides excellent rejection prophylaxis for pancreas transplantation. Transplantation 2003; 75:1301–6.

43. Allen RDM. Pancreas transplantation. In: Forsythe JLR (ed.) Transplantation surgery, 1st edn. London: WB Saunders, 1997; pp. 167–201.

44. Hawthorne WJ, Allen RDM, Greenberg ML et al. Simultaneous pancreas and kidney transplant rejection: separate or synchronous events. Transplantation 1997; 63:352–8.

45. Munn SR, Engen DE, Barr D et al. Differential diagnosis of hypoamylasuria in pancreas allograft recipients with urinary exocrine drainage. Transplantation 1990; 49:359–62.

46. Benedetti E, Najarian JS, Gruessner A et al. Correlation between cystoscopic biopsy results and hypoamylasuria in bladder drained pancreas transplants. Surgery 1995; 118:864–72.

47. Elmer DS, Hathaway DK, Bashar AA et al. Use of glucose disappearance rates (kG) to monitor endocrine function of pancreas allografts. Clin Transplant 1998; 12:56–64.

48. Osei K, Henry ML, O'Dorioso TM et al. Physiological and pharmacological stimulation of pancreatic islet hormone secretion in Type 1 diabetic pancreas allograft recipients. Diabetes 1990; 39:1235–42.

49. Drachenberg G, Klassen D, Bartlett S et al. Histologic grading of pancreas acute allograft rejection

in percutaneous needle biopsies. Transplant Proc 1996; 28:512–13.

50. Reddy KS, Davies D, Ormond D et al. Impact of acute rejection episodes on long term graft survival following simultaneous kidney pancreas transplantation. Am J Transplant 2003; 3:439–44.

51. Sollinger HW, Odorico JS, Knechtle SJ et al. Experience with 500 simultaneous pancreas-kidney transplants. Ann Surg 1998; 228:284–96.

    At the time of reporting this was the largest series of SPK transplants published. Detailed analysis of this selected series of patients with excellent outcome.

52. Ojo AO, Meier-Kriesche H, Hanson J et al. The impact of simultaneous pancreas kidney transplantation on long-term patient survival. Transplantation 2001; 71:82–9.

53. Reddy KS, Stablein D, Taranto S et al. Long-term survival following simultaneous kidney-pancreas transplantation versus kidney transplantation alone in patients with type 1 diabetes mellitus and renal failure. Am J Kidney Dis 2003; 41:464–70.

54. Tyden G, Bolinder J, Solders G et al. Improved survival in patients with insulin-dependent diabetes mellitus and end-stage diabetic nephropathy 10 years after combined pancreas and kidney transplantation. Transplantation 1999; 67:645–8.

55. Smets YFC, Westendorp RGJ, Van der Pijl JW et al. Effect of simultaneous pancreas-kidney transplantation on mortality of patients with Type 1 diabetes and end stage renal failure. Lancet 1999; 353: 1915–20.

56. Wilczek HE, Jaremko G, Tyden G et al. Evolution of diabetic nephropathy in kidney grafts. Transplantation 1995; 59:51–7.

57. El-Gebely S, Hathaway DK, Elmer DS et al. An analysis of renal function in pancreas kidney and diabetic kidney alone recipients at two years following transplantation. Transplantation 1995; 59:1410–15.

58. Fioretto P, Steffes MW, Sutherland DER et al. Reversal of lesions of diabetic nephropathy after pancreas transplantation. N Engl J Med 1998; 339:69–75.

59. Chow VCC, Pai RP, Chapman JR et al. Diabetic retinopathy after combined kidney-pancreas transplantation. Clin Transplant 1999; 13:356–62.

60. Frank RN. Medical progress: diabetic retinopathy. N Engl J Med 2004; 350:48–58.

61. Pearce IA, Ilango B, Sells RA et al. Stabilisation of diabetic retinopathy following simultaneous pancreas and kidney transplant. Br J Ophthalmol 2000; 84:736–40.

62. Cashion AK, Hathaway DK, Milstead EJ et al. Changes in patterns of 24 hour heart rate variability after kidney and kidney-pancreas transplant. Transplantation 1999; 68:1426–30.

63. Hathaway DK, Abell T, Cardoso S et al. Improvement in autonomic and gastric function following pancreas-kidney versus kidney alone transplantation and the correlation with quality of life. Transplantation 1994; 57:816–22.

64. Allen RDM, Al-Harbi IS, Morris JG et al. Diabetic neuropathy after pancreas transplantation: Determinants of recovery. Transplantation 1997; 63:830–8.

65. Abendroth D, Schmand J, Landgraf R et al. Diabetic microangiopathy in Type 1 (insulin-dependent) diabetic patients after successful pancreatic and kidney or solitary kidney transplantation. Diabetology 1991; 34:131–4.

66. Fiorina P, LaRocca E, Venturini M et al. Effects of kidney-pancreas transplantation on atherosclerotic risk factors and endothelial function in patients with uraemia and Type 1 diabetes. Diabetes 2001; 50:496–501.

67. Fiorina P, Folli F, Maffi P et al. Islet transplantation improves vascular diabetic complications in patients with diabetes who underwent kidney transplantation: a comparison between kidney-pancreas and kidney alone transplantation. Transplantation 2003; 75:1296–301.

68. LaRocca E, Fiorina P, DiCarlo V et al. Cardiovascular outcomes after kidney-pancreas and kidney alone transplantation. Kidney Int 2001; 60:1964–71.

69. Jukema JW, Smets YF, van der Pijl JW et al. Impact of simultaneous pancreas and kidney transplantation on progression of coronary atherosclerosis in patients with end-stage renal failure due to type 1 diabetes. Diabetes Care 2002; 25:906–11.

70. Copelli A, Giannarelli R, Mariotti R et al. Pancreas transplant alone determines early improvement of cardiovascular risk factors and cardiac function in type 1 diabetic patients. Transplantation 2003; 76:974–6.

Ten

Islet transplantation

John J. Casey and
A.M. James Shapiro

The World Health Organisation defines diabetes as a metabolic disorder of multiple aetiology characterised by chronic hyperglycaemia with disturbances of carbohydrate, protein and fat metabolism resulting from defects in insulin secretion, insulin action or both. Classically, diabetes presents insidiously with polydipsia, polyuria and weight loss and is confirmed by measuring plasma glucose. It is estimated that by 2010 three million patients in the UK will be diagnosed as diabetic, and the incidence of diabetes is increasing in children at a rate of 3–4% per year.[1] Five percent of the total National Health Service (NHS) budget is spent treating diabetes and its complications and although much of this is used in the community, 10% of inpatient hospital resources is taken up in the treatment of diabetes.[2]

Insulin is secreted by beta (β) cells found in the islets of Langerhans in the pancreas. Type I diabetes is thought to occur as a result of autoimmune destruction of the islets, and it is estimated that after 80% of beta cells have been destroyed, the classical features of diabetes present. The treatment of type I diabetes with insulin injections is life saving; however, secondary complications of diabetes such as nephropathy, retinopathy, neuropathy and vasculopathy still occur in up to 40% of type I diabetic patients. The Diabetes Control and Complications Study Group Trial demonstrated that the incidence of these complications can be reduced by tight glycaemic control but the risk of severe hypoglycaemic reactions is then increased.[3]

Transplantation of the whole pancreas (normally simultaneously with a kidney transplant) is now an established treatment option for some type I diabetics. But this is only an option for a small group of diabetic patients with advanced disease, and even in the most experienced hands it has a high morbidity and modest mortality (40% and 3–5% respectively).[4] The pancreatic islets only account for around 1% of the volume of the pancreas and so transplantation of the exocrine pancreatic tissue is unnecessary and carries added risk. Transplantation of islets alone offers an attractive alternative to whole pancreas transplantation and may be associated with a lower incidence of serious complications.

The first islet transplant was attempted in 1893 in Bristol – 28 years before the discovery of insulin – whereby fragments of a sheep's pancreas were implanted in the subcutaneous tissues of a 15-year-old boy dying from uncontrolled ketoacidosis.[5] This xenograft was destined to fail without immunosuppression. The era of experimental islet research began in 1911 when Bensley stained islets within the guinea pig pancreas using a number of dyes, and was able to pick free the occasional islet for morphological study.[6] Mass isolation of large numbers of viable islets from the human pancreas has proven to be a challenge ever since. The average adult human pancreas weighs 70 g and contains an average of 1 to 2 million islets of average diameter 157 μm, constituting 0.8–3.8% of the total mass of the gland.[7] The techniques used today for the mass isolation of human islets evolved from earlier techniques used to prepare islets in rodent models.

Islet transplantation for type I diabetes mellitus has been attempted in many units over the last 10–15 years with poor long-term success. Of over 400 islet transplants reported to the International Transplant Registry between 1990 and 2000, less than 10% resulted in long-term insulin independence.[8] These transplants were carried out on a heterogeneous group of diabetic patients and, in the majority of cases, included glucocorticoids in the immunosuppression protocol.

THE EDMONTON PROTOCOL

A report published by the Edmonton group of seven consecutive type I diabetic patients who attained long-term insulin independence after islet transplantation renewed interest in islet transplantation as a feasible option for a select group of diabetic patients.[9] These patients were all transplanted using a glucocorticoid-free immunosuppressive regimen. The islets were infused into the portal vein after cannulation of the vein under fluoroscopic control by a radiologist. The Edmonton protocol included several changes to previous islet transplant protocols:

1. 'Islet alone' transplants were carried out in patients with severe hypoglycaemic unawareness, labile diabetes or progressive secondary complications without another organ graft. Patients with concurrent renal failure were not transplanted. The patients included in this series were judged to be at greater immediate risk due to severe diabetic complications than the risk presented by transplantation and subsequent immunosuppression.

2. The immunosuppression protocol consisted of daclizumab – anti-interleukin 2 receptor monoclonal antibody (anti-IL-2R mAb) – induction followed by sirolimus and low-dose tacrolimus, without the use of steroids. This potent immunosuppressive regimen reduces the metabolic demands on the newly transplanted

islets normally incurred by the use of steroids and reduces the likelihood of calcineurin inhibitor-induced nephropathy and diabetes.

3. The islet isolation procedure was carried out using further refinements of the Ricordi method[23] and controlled perfusion of the pancreatic duct. These developments in the islet isolation procedure have allowed the isolation of large numbers of highly purified islets to be transplanted in a small tissue volume. In the current Edmonton series, around 350 000 islet equivalents were isolated on average from each pancreas with an average purity of 60% in an average tissue volume of 4 mL. Although these data are encouraging, this still represents less than a third of the potential islet mass of the pancreas.

 4. Two pancreases, transplanted sequentially, were required for insulin independence in the majority of patients.

Three patients required three infusions and one patient has required four pancreases. This variation results from differing patient weights and the variability in the number of islets isolated per pancreas. It appears that insulin independence is only obtained when at least 9000 islet equivalents (IE)/kg are transplanted. The islet infusions were carried out sequentially when donor pancreases became available (on average 29 days apart). It should be noted, however, that complete correction of hypoglycaemia was seen in all patients after the first islet transplant despite the continuing need for insulin at a reduced dose (one-fifth to three-quarters of the pretransplant dose).

 5. Immunogenic xenoproteins were eliminated from islet preparations.

It has been suggested that coating of islets with xenogenic proteins commonly used in cell preparation such as bovine serum albumin and fetal calf serum may enhance the immunogenicity of the islets. These proteins have been eliminated from the cell preparation media used by the Edmonton group and replaced by human products such as human serum albumin.

PATIENT SELECTION FOR ISLET TRANSPLANTATION

Patients can be considered for either islet transplantation alone or for islet transplantation while immunosuppressed for another organ transplant, usually kidney. The results of combined islet and kidney transplantation now match those of islet alone,[10,11] and recent data suggest that islets transplanted with a kidney may prolong the patient and kidney graft survival and protect against diabetic vascular complications.[12,13] Inclusion criteria for islet transplantation are outlined in **Box 10.1**. The major indications for islet transplantation are hypoglycaemic unawareness and metabolic lability. Assessment of these complications is subjective and a number of scoring systems have been devised to allow quantification of these problems. The mean amplitude of glycaemic excursion (MAGE) using 14 blood glucose values over a 2-day period has previously been used in the assessment of potential recipients;[14,15] however, it has been superseded recently by the combination of a lability index (LI) and composite HYPO score based on 4 weeks of glucose values.[16] (The HYPO scoring system takes into account the frequency, severity and degree of unawareness of hypoglycaemia, and has not been shown to be significantly higher in islet transplant patients pre-transplant. It becomes normal post islet transplant.) Ryan and colleagues suggest that this provides a more objective assessment of the metabolic instability of an individual patient and allows pre- and post-transplant comparison. Patients must be assessed by an endocrinologist and have continuing problems despite an optimum insulin regimen. Ultimately, the decision whether to offer islet transplantation depends on the individual patient and should be arrived at by balancing the risks of the islet transplant procedure itself and potentially lifelong immunosuppression against the daily risks taken by a patient with type I diabetes. It should not be forgotten that diabetes mellitus (DM) is the commonest cause of renal failure in the UK and the commonest cause of blindness in those over 60 years old. In addition, patients with diabetes are three times more likely to suffer a stroke and five times more likely to have a myocardial infarct, reducing their life expectancy by 20%.[1]

THE DONOR

Successful islet isolation depends on the selection of suitable donors and meticulous surgical technique during the retrieval process. Donor criteria for islet isolation are similar to those for solid pancreas transplantation but a number of variables appear to be unique to islets (**Table 10.1**).[17] Pancreases from older donors with a high BMI appear to have a higher rate of successful isolation. These data have resource implications since pancreases that may not be suitable for solid pancreas transplantation may still be used for islet isolation. The surgical technique for removal of the pancreas for islets should be the same as that for solid pancreas

Box 10.1 • Indications for islet-alone transplantation

- Age 18–65 years
- Type I diabetes mellitus for more than 5 years
- C-peptide negative
- Evidence of good compliance
- Type I diabetes mellitus complicated by:
  - hypoglycaemic unawareness (absence of adequate autonomic symptoms at blood glucose levels <3.0 mmol/L)
  - metabolic lability (lability index, HYPO score)
  - progressive secondary complications

Despite intensive insulin management defined by monitoring of blood glucose values no less than four times each day and by the administration of three or more insulin injections each day.

Table 10.1 • Donor-related variables predicting isolation success (Lakey et al.[17])

Variable	*P*-value	*R*-value	Odds ratio
Donor age (years)	<0.05	0.18	1.10
Body mass index	<0.01	0.19	1.30
Local vs. distant procurement team	<0.01	0.21	7.04
Min. blood glucose	<0.01	−0.24	0.68
Duration of cardiac arrest	<0.01	−0.17	0.81
Duration of cold storage	<0.05	−0.13	0.86

transplantation taking care to avoid direct handling of the pancreas and keeping the capsule intact.[17] The pancreas can be removed before or after the liver, or en bloc with the liver and separated on the back table. Care should be taken to keep the pancreas cold after cross-clamping and during back-table preparation and packaging of the organ as this has been shown to double the yield of viable islets.[18] Ryan et al. have shown that the ischaemia index, which is the cold ischaemic time for a given transplanted islet mass, correlates with insulin secretion.[19] Ideally, the cold ischaemia time should not exceed 8–12 hours; however, it has been demonstrated that suspending the explanted pancreas in a bilayer of oxygenated perfluorochemical (PFC) and University of Wisconsin (UW) solution during or after transport allows satisfactory islet preparations to be obtained from suboptimal pancreases and may even increase yields from pancreases with long ischaemia times (**Fig. 10.1**).[20,21] PFC-based preservation may also help to expand the donor pool by allowing islet isolation from non-heart-beating pancreases and older donors.[22]

ISLET ISOLATION

A modern human islet isolation facility must comply with current Good Manufacturing Practice (cGMP) requirements for tissue preparation and as such is expensive to construct from scratch. In the UK, the Medicines Control Agency regulates the processing of tissues and cells for human use and will certify and monitor facilities for islet processing.

The currently used semiautomated process for human islet isolation was described by Camillo Ricordi (**Fig. 10.2**) and is based on combined collagenase digestion and mechanical dissociation of the donor pancreas.[23–25] First, the pancreas is distended with cold collagenase via the pancreatic duct and then transferred to the Ricordi digestion chamber and circuit. Here the temperature of the collagenase is raised to 37°C to allow activation of the enzyme and digestion of the pancreas. The digest is regularly sampled so that digestion can be stopped when the intact islets are free from the surrounding exocrine tissue. This part of the isolation process requires some skill and experience and is critical to the whole process. The production of consistently good islet preps has been hampered

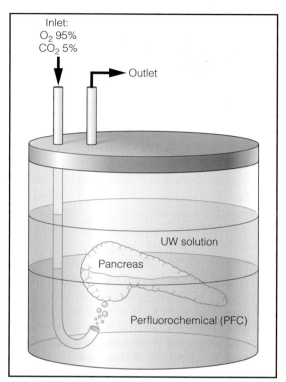

Figure 10.1 • The perfluorochemical (PFC) 'two-layer' method for pancreas preservation.

over the years by the inherent batch-to-batch variation in collagenase activity. The introduction of Liberase HI (Roche), which has more consistent collagenase activity combined with neutral protease activity and low endotoxin levels, has reduced this variability but is costly.[26] Newer enzyme blends such as Collagenase NB1 (Serva) are now coming onto the market with the promise of consistent enzyme activity coupled with product quality to cGMP requirements, but collagenase consistency is still the biggest obstacle to successful islet isolation.

The crude pancreatic digest must be purified to separate the islets from other products of digestion such as ductal tissue, lymphoid tissue and necrotic cells. Transplantation of unpurified digests can result in insulin independence; however, this approach increases the risk of portal vein thrombosis, portal hypertension and disseminated intravascular coagulation (DIC).[27–29] There is also some evidence to suggest that low-purity preps result in impaired islet engraftment and function.[30–32] Modern islet purification techniques rely on the fact

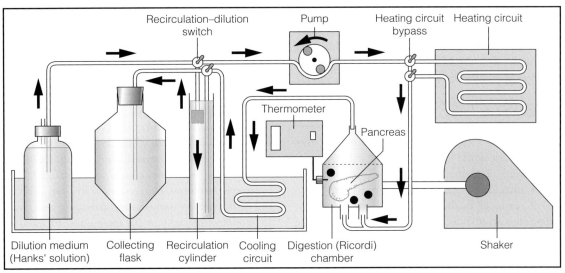

Figure 10.2 • The 'Ricordi' digestion circuit. Copyright © 1988 American Diabetes Association. From Diabetes 1988; 37:413–20.[23] Reprinted with permission from *The American Diabetes Association*.

that islets are less dense than exocrine tissue and can be separated using a density gradient.[33] The crude islet preparation is therefore passed along a continuous Ficoll density gradient created on a Cobe 2991 cell separator and centrifuged at 2400 rpm for 5 minutes. The temperature of the preparation is maintained at 4–10°C during this process either by core cooling of the Cobe 2991 or by carrying out the purification in a specially designed cold room.[34]

The resulting purified islet prep is then washed, counted and assayed to make sure that it meets the product release criteria of the isolation facility. These criteria are essential to ensure that a safe, pure and effective islet preparation is consistently produced by the isolation facility (**Box 10.2**). Safety is measured by negative Gram stain and endotoxin assay and islet purity (ideally >50%) determined by eye although computerised counting software is currently under evaluation. The likely potency of an islet preparation is difficult to determine prior to transplantation and several investigations are under-way to develop reliable assays of islet function. Current practice is to use a combination of islet counts and cell viability stains such as fluorescein diacetate/propidium iodide and SytoGreen/ethidium bromide to determine the viable beta cell mass. Islet function is quantified by glucose-stimulated insulin

Box 10.2 • Islet product release criteria

- Sufficient islet mass: 5000 IE/kg
- ABO blood group matched
- Gram stain negative
- Endotoxin load <5 endotoxin units (EU/kg)
- Islet packed cell volume <5 cc (normally 2–3 cc)
- Purity >30% (usually >50%)

release assays.[35–37] Newer techniques, such as islet oxygen consumption rate and beta cell ATP content, show good correlation between product testing and in vivo islet function in animal studies and may be useful in the future, but they are time consuming and expensive. The Minnesota group has recently demonstrated good correlation between marginal mass islet transplants in diabetic nude mice and outcome of human islet transplants from the same donor.[38]

Patients transplanted under the initial Edmonton protocol received islet infusions immediately after purification. Recent evidence, however, suggests that a period of culture may enhance the purity of the islet prep without loss of potency. Data from the Miami programme suggest that a period of culture of 24–48 hours increases islet purity and reduces the infused volume but can result in insulin independence in the majority of recipients.[39] This ability to culture islets has implications for both immunomodulation of the islet prep and the graft recipient and for effective product release testing.

THE ISLET TRANSPLANT

In contrast to solid pancreas transplantation, islet recipients can expect to spend no more than 24 hours in hospital. The main portal vein is cannulated under ultrasound and fluoroscopic control using a 4 Fr catheter in the radiology department. The Edmonton group have reported 100% success using this route and have found that avoiding aspirin and completely occluding the catheter track with fibrin glue markedly reduces the risk of bleeding following percutaneous implantation.[40] Alternatively, the portal vein can be cannulated at laparotomy via a mesenteric or omental vein. The intraportal site for islet embolisation was recognised to be the most efficient location for islet implantation in the rodent, with the benefit of high vascularity, proximity to islet-specific nutrient factors and physiological first-pass insulin delivery to the liver.[41] While many different sites have been tried for islet implantation, the optimal site appears to be through portal venous embolisation. Attempts to embolise the spleen have led to significant life-threatening complications of splenic infarction, rupture and even gastric perforation.[42]

Once implanted in the liver, the islets undergo a process of angiogenesis, which, in animal models, is complete within 14 days.[43] Most groups are now using a closed bag system for islet infusion with gravity drainage rather than a syringe to infuse the cells. This minimises trauma to the islets during implantation, and allows continuous monitoring of portal pressure. The closed bag system also ensures that the islet preparation remains in a sterile environment and complies with cGMP guidelines.[44] Prior to infusion unfractionated heparin is added to the islet prep (35 U/kg if the packed cell volume is less than 5 cc and 70 U/kg if greater than 5 cc) to minimise the risk of portal vein thrombosis.[45]

Portal vein pressures increase during the islet infusion and this is particularly marked in patients receiving their second and third islet transplants. Portal venous pressure should therefore be monitored throughout the islet infusion and if excessive changes in portal pressure are detected the infusion can be slowed down or stopped.[45]

IMMUNOSUPPRESSION

Anti-IL-2R mAb (daclizumab in the Edmonton series) is administered at 1 mg/kg pretransplant, then repeated at 2-weekly intervals post-transplant for a total of five doses.[9] In cases where a second islet graft was given beyond the 10-week induction window, the induction course of daclizumab was repeated. Sirolimus is given as a loading dose of 0.2 mg/kg orally immediately pretransplant, with maintenance initially at 0.1 mg/kg/day adjusted to 24-hour target serum trough levels of 12–15 ng/mL for 3 months, then reduced to 7–10 µg/L thereafter. Low-dose tacrolimus is initiated at 2 mg orally given twice daily, but adjusted to target 12-hour trough levels of 3–6 µg/L – representing between a quarter and half of the usual standard dose for other transplants.[9] This regimen appears to provide adequate immunosuppression while avoiding the diabetogenic side effects of glucocorticoids and tacrolimus. Newer biological agents such as infliximab (anti-TNF-α mAb) and Campath 1H are also being evaluated in islet transplantation in an attempt to aid islet engraftment and induce tolerance respectively. An exciting new agent in islet transplantation is the hOKT3γI (Ala-Ala) antibody. This antibody appears to regulate autoimmunity in type I diabetes and is associated with promotion of CD25+ regulatory T cells.[38]

OUTCOMES OF ISLET TRANSPLANTATION POST-EDMONTON PROTOCOL

In the initial Edmonton series all seven patients remained insulin independent at 1 year with complete correction of hypoglycaemic unawareness.[9] The experience at Edmonton has now been expanded to over 60 patients, with 1-year insulin independence reported at 80% and two of the initial patients remaining insulin free for longer than 4 years (unpublished data). Cumulative data of over 75 patients treated since 1999 at Edmonton, Miami and Minnesota have now been reported, with primary islet function in 99% of patients, and 96% of patients remaining C peptide-positive at

1 year. Insulin independence is reported at 85% at 1 year and 70% at 2 years in this combined series. Preliminary results of the ITN nine-site trial of the Edmonton protocol demonstrates that the success of the initial Edmonton report can be reproduced in centres with adequate experience of islet isolation and of the immunosuppressive protocol.[46]

It appears that a minimum of 9000 IE/kg is required to produce insulin independence and the majority of patients still require two or occasionally three pancreases to attain this.[9] Recent data from the ITN study, however, suggest that by matching larger donors with low-weight, insulin-sensitive recipients, 38% of patients can be rendered insulin independent with single-pancreas infusions.[46] Indeed, a recent series from the Minnesota group has reported long-term insulin independence in four out of six single-pancreas islet recipients using a combination of strategies to optimise islet single-donor success.[38]

The results of metabolic studies on successful islet recipients have been reported by Ryan et al. and demonstrate that in patients who have labile diabetes or hypoglycaemic problems the results are excellent. Even in those patients using insulin again, the glucose profiles are more stable than pretransplant.[47,48] In addition, health-related quality of life data indicate that fear of hypoglycaemic reactions is significantly reduced in islet recipients.[49] Despite this, however, the majority of patients continue to demonstrate impaired glucose tolerance, and this may reflect the fact that the mass of islets transplanted represents about 75% of the number of islets present in the non-diabetic pancreas.[9,48]

The overall procedural complication rate is low for percutaneous islet transplantation (**Table 10.2**). The more serious procedure-related complications of segmental portal vein thrombosis and bleeding have been reported at 4% and 10% respectively.[45,47] The risk of portal vein thrombosis can be minimised by heparinisation of the recipient and by using only low-volume high-purity preps. Bleeding from the liver puncture can be avoided by using a fine-bore (4 Fr) cannula and by ablating the track in the liver using coils, thrombostatic agents or a coagulative laser.[40] The short-term risks of the immuno-suppression protocol appear low, with no reports of malignancy or post-transplant lymphoproliferative disease (PTLD) and no reported cases of cyto-

Table 10.2 • Significant complications of islet transplantation in the first 50 Edmonton recipients

Complication	Procedures (102)	Patients (50)
Mouth ulceration	–	38 (76%)
Dyslipidaemia	–	23 (46%)
Liver function test rise	–	24 (48%)
Liver bleeds	7 (7%)	7 (14%)
Severe neutropenia	–	3 (6%)
Pneumonia	–	2 (4%)
Elevated creatinine	–	2 (4%)
Segmental portal vein thrombosis	2 (2%)	2 (4%)
Ileal ulceration	–	2 (4%)
Haemobilia	1 (1%)	1 (2%)
Sensitisation	–	1 (2%)

megalovirus (CMV) disease although one would anticipate that the long-term risk of malignancy is at least similar to those transplant patients on conventional immunosuppression. No mortality has been reported to date. Significant elevation of liver enzymes is seen in over 50% of patients receiving intraportal islet grafts. This is more pronounced after the first graft and resolves spontaneously in the majority of patients by 4 weeks. The long-term effect of islets transplanted into the liver remains to be seen but periportal hepatosis is seen in animal models of islet transplantation and as such may have implications for long-surviving grafts in humans.[50]

FUTURE DEVELOPMENTS

Optimal use of the donor pool

The worldwide shortage of cadaveric donors and the expansion in potential islet recipients means that the current need for two or even three donors to achieve insulin independence is not sustainable. Substantial steps have been taken towards single-donor islet transplantation by the Minnesota group using a combination of careful donor and recipient selection and meticulous islet preparation.[38] Improved laboratory preparation of islets coupled with more reliable and effective collagenases are also required to ensure that the maximum number of functioning islets are retrieved from all available pancreases.

New sources of islets

The shortage of organ donors coupled with the increased demand for islets has led to much research into alternative sources of insulin-producing cells, which would be renewable and not depend solely on the availability of human cadaveric donors. The use of fetal or adult porcine islets for human xeno-transplants has been explored. However, the high levels of immunosuppression required and the risk of transmission of porcine viral infections means that xenotransplantation is still some way in the future. Stem cells are capable of both self-renewal and multilineage differentiation. They have the potential to proliferate and differentiate into any type of cell and to be genetically modified in vitro, thus providing a renewable source of cells for trans-plantation. Pancreatic islets have been produced in animal models by in vitro manipulation of both embryonic stem cells and adult pancreatic ductal stem cells. Islets produced in these experiments have been shown to produce endocrine hormones and islet differentiation markers and release insulin in response to glucose stimulation in vitro. In vivo, they can reverse experimentally induced diabetes in mice and maintain vascularised islet-like clusters.[51,52] The production of functional beta cells for trans-plantation is the goal of many research laboratories; however, it is unclear whether transplanted beta cells will function adequately or maintain hypo-glycaemic counter-regulation outside the islet cluster.

Better immunosuppression

Sirolimus-based steroid-free immunosuppression has been central to the success of the Edmonton protocol. However, chemical immunosuppression and the associated long-term risks of infection and malignancy are major barriers to the wider application of islet transplantation. Calcineurin inhibitor-free regimens including agents such as hOKT3γ1 (Ala-Ala) and Campath 1H are showing some promise and may be effective in reducing recurrence of autoimmunity as well as suppressing the rejection response. Manipulation of islets in culture to alter antigen presentation or co-stimulation is an attractive strategy for inducing tolerance, and the development of effective culture media for islets containing insulin–transferrin–selenium makes this a more achievable goal.

• Key points

- Islet transplantation is now a viable option in the treatment of selected patients with type I diabetes.
- The Edmonton protocol has been successfully reproduced in several centres worldwide: outcomes are now comparable with solid pancreas transplantation.
- Protocols are emerging that allow single-donor islet transplants. However, better immuno-suppression and alternative sources of islets are required to allow the application of islet transplantation to a wider population of diabetic patients.

REFERENCES

1. Amos AF, McCarty DJ, Zimmel P. The rising global burden of diabetes and its complications: estimates and projections to the year 2010. Diabet Med 1997; 14(suppl. 5):51–85.

2. Department of Health. National Service framework for diabetes: standards. London: DOH, 2001.

3. The Diabetes Control and Complications Trial Research Group. The effect of intensive treatment of diabetes on the development and progression of long-term complications in insulin dependent diabetes mellitus. N Engl J Med 1993; 329:977–86.

4. Sutherland DER, Gruessener RWG, Gruessener AC. Pancreas transplantation for the treatment of diabetes mellitus. World J Surg 2001; 25:487–96.

5. Williams P. Notes on diabetes treated with extract and by grafts of sheep's pancreas. Br Med J 1894; 2:1303–4.

6. Bensley RR. Studies on the pancreas of the guinea pig. Am J Anat 1911; 12:297–388.

7. Robertson GS, Dennison AR, Johnson PR et al. A review of pancreatic islet autotransplantation. Hepatogastroenterology 1998; 45(19):226–35.

8. Brendel M, Hering B, Schulz A et al. International Islet Transplant Registry Report. Giessen, Germany: University of Giessen, 2001.

9. Shapiro AM, Lakey JR, Ryan EA et al. Islet transplantation in seven patients with type 1 diabetes mellitus using a glucocorticoid-free immunosuppressive regimen. N Engl J Med 2000; 343(4):230–8.

Seven consecutive patients rendered insulin independent for >1 year post-islet transplantation. This paper demonstrated that islet transplantation is a viable treatment option for type I diabetes and served as the catalyst for the increase in islet transplant activity over the past 4 years.

10. Kaufman DB, Baker MS, Chen X et al. Sequential kidney/islet transplantation using prednisolone free immunosuppression. Am J Transplant 2002; 2:674–7.

11. Toso C, Morel P, Bucher P et al. Insulin independence after conversion to tacrolimus and sirolimus based immunosuppression in islet-kidney recipients. Transplantation 2003; 76:1133–4.

12. Fiorina P, Folli F, Zerbini G et al. Islet transplantation is associated with improvement of renal function among uraemic patients with type I diabetes mellitus and kidney transplants. J Am Soc Nephrol 2003; 14:2150–2158.

13. Fiorina P, Folli F, Maffi P et al. Islet transplantation improves vascular diabetic complications in patients with diabetes who underwent kidney transplantation: a comparison between kidney-pancreas and kidney-alone transplantation. Transplantation 2003; 14:1296–301.

14. Service FJ, O'Brien PC, Rizza RA. Measurements of glucose control. Diabetes Care 1987;10(2):225–37.

15. Service FJ, Molnar GD, Rosevear JW et al. Mean amplitude of glycaemic excursions, a measure of diabetic instability. Diabetes 1970; 19(9):644–55.

16. Ryan EA, Shandro T, Green K et al. Assessment of the severity of hypoglycaemia and glycaemic lability in type I diabetic subjects undergoing islet transplantation. Diabetes 2004; 53:955–62.

17. Lakey JR, Warnock GL, Rajotte RV et al. Variables in organ donors that affect the recovery of human islets of Langerhans. Transplantation 1996; 61(7): 1047–53.

This univariate and multivariate analysis of factors affecting the number and functional quality of islets from locally retrieved and imported pancreases has been used to define the optimal donor characteristics for islet isolation. Some of the factors such as long cold ischaemic time can now be compensated for by the use of PFC storage.

18. Lakey JR, Kneteman NM, Rajotte RV et al. Effect of core pancreas temperature during cadaveric procurement on human islet isolation and functional viability 1. Transplantation 2002; 73(7):1106–10.

19. Ryan EA, Lakey JR, Rajotte RV et al. Clinical outcomes and insulin secretion after islet transplantation with the Edmonton protocol. Diabetes 2001; 50(4):710–19.

20. Deai T, Tanioka Y, Suzuki Y et al. The effect of the two-layer cold storage method on islet isolation from ischemically damaged pancreas. Kobe J Med Sci 1999; 45(3-4):191–9.

21. Tsujimura T, Kuroda Y, Kin T et al. Human islet transplantation from pancreases with prolonged cold ischaemia using additional preservation by the two layer (UW solution/perfluorochemical) cold storage method. Transplantation 2002; 74:1687–91.

22. Ricordi C, Fraker C, Szust J et al. Improved human islet isolation from marginal donors following addition of oxygenated perfluorocarbon to the cold storage solution. Transplantation 2003; 75:1524–7.

23. Ricordi C, Lacy PE, Scharp DW. Automated islet isolation from human pancreas. Diabetes 1988; 37:413–20.

The method described here for the first time by Camillo Ricordi for human islet isolation is now adopted in every major islet isolation facility worldwide and is the 'gold standard' for comparison of newer isolation techniques.

24. Toomey P, Chadwick DR, Contractor H et al. Porcine islet isolation: prospective comparison of automated and manual methods of pancreatic collagenase digestion. Br J Surg 1993; 80(2):240–3.

25. Lakey JR, Warnock GL, Shapiro AM et al. Intra-ductal collagenase delivery into the human pancreas using syringe loading or controlled perfusion. Cell Transplant 1999; 8(3):285–92.

26. Linetsky E, Bottino R, Lehmann R et al. Improved human islet isolation using a new enzyme blend, liberase. Diabetes 1997; 46(7):1120–3.

27. Shapiro AM, Lakey JR, Rajotte RV et al. Portal vein thrombosis after transplantation of partially purified pancreatic islets in a combined human liver/islet allograft. Transplantation 1995; 59(7):1060–3.

28. Walsh TJ, Eggleston JC, Cameron JL. Portal hypertension, hepatic infarction, and liver failure complicating pancreatic islet autotransplantation. Surgery 1982; 91(4):485–7.

29. Froberg MK, Leone JP, Jessurun J et al. Fatal disseminated intravascular coagulation after autologous islet transplantation. Hum Pathol 1997; 28(11):1295–8.

30. Gray DW, Sutton R, McShane P et al. Exocrine contamination impairs implantation of pancreatic islets transplanted beneath the kidney capsule. J Surg Res 1988; 45:432.

31. Gotoh M, Maki T, Satomi S et al. Immunological characteristics of purified pancreatic islet grafts. Transplantation 1986; 42:387.

32. Downing R, Morrissey S, Kiske D et al. Does the purity of intraportal islet isografts affect their endocrine function? J Surg Res 1986; 41:41.

33. Lacy P, Kostianovsky M. Method for the isolation of intact islets of Langerhans from adult rat pancreases. Diabetes 1967; 16:35.

34. Lake SP, Bassett PD, Larkins A et al. Large-scale purification of human islets utilizing discontinuous albumin gradient on IBM 2991 cell separator. Diabetes 1989; 38(suppl. 1):143–5.

35. Ricordi C, Gray DWR, Hering BJ et al. Islet isolation in man and large animals. Acta Diabetol Lat 1990; 27:185–95.

36. Gray DWR, Morris PJ. The use of fluorescein diacetate and ethidium bromide as a viability stain for isolated islets of Langerhans. Stain Technol 1987; 62:379–81.

37. Bank HL. Assessment of islet cell viability using fluorescent dyes. Diabetologica 1987; 30:812–17.

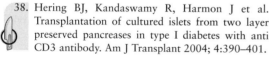

38. Hering BJ, Kandaswamy R, Harmon J et al. Transplantation of cultured islets from two layer preserved pancreases in type I diabetes with anti CD3 antibody. Am J Transplant 2004; 4:390–401.

   This paper describes the Minnesota experience of a combination of strategies to optimise success with single-donor islet transplantation. The group used two-layer PFC organ preservation and culture post-isolation in insulin-transferrin-selenium-supplemented media. Immunosuppression included hOKT3γ1 (Ala-Ala) antibody and four of six patients achieved long-term insulin independence.

39. Alejandro JV, Ferreira A, Caulfield T et al. Insulin independence in 7 patients following transplantation of cultured human islets. Am J Transplant 2002; 2:227.

40. Owen RJ, Ryan EA, O'Kelly K et al. Percutaneous transhepatic pancreatic islet cell transplantation in type 1 diabetes mellitus: radiologic aspects. Radiology 2003; 229:165–70.

41. Kemp C, Knight M, Scharp D et al. Effect of transplantation site on the result of pancreatic islet isografts in diabetic rats. Diabetologia 1973; 9:486–91.

42. White SA, London NJ, Johnson PR et al. The risks of total pancreatectomy and splenic islet autotransplantation. Cell Transplant 2000; 9(1):19–24.

43. Menger MD, Vajkoczy P, Beger C et al. Orientation of microvascular blood flow in pancreatic islet isografts. J Clin Invest 1994; 93(5):2280–5.

44. Biadal DA, Froud TA, Ferreira JV et al. The bag method for islet cell infusion. Cell Transplant 2003; 12:809–13.

45. Casey JJ, Lakey JRT, Ryan EA et al. Portal venous pressure changes following sequential clinical islet transplantation. Transplantation 2002; 74:913–15.

46. Shapiro AM, Ricordi C, Hering BJ et al. International multicentre trial of islet transplantation using the Edmonton protocol in patients with type I diabetes. Am J Transplant 2003; 3:152

47. Ryan EA, Lakey JR, Paty BW. Successful islet transplantation: continued insulin reserve provides long-term glycaemic control. Diabetes 2002; 51:2148–57.

   This paper describes the technical and metabolic outcomes of 54 islet transplant procedures in 30 consecutive patients followed up for at least 1 year and up to 34 months. The paper describes the metabolic function of the islet grafts and the procedure-related risks of islet transplantation in the Edmonton programme.

48. Ryan EA, Lakey JR, Rajotte RV et al. Clinical outcomes and insulin secretion after islet transplantation with the Edmonton protocol. Diabetes 2001; 50:710–19.

49. Johnson JA, Kotovych M, Ryan EA et al. Reduced fear of hypoglycaemia in successful islet transplantation. Diabetes Care 2004; 27(2):624–5.

50. Rafael E, Ryan EA, Paty BW et al. Changes in liver enzymes after clinical islet transplantation. Transplantation 2003; 76:1280–4.

51. Ramiya VK, Maraist M, Arfors KE et al. Reversal of insulin dependent diabetes using islets generated in vitro from pancreatic stem cells. Nature Med 2000; 6:278–82.

52. Lumelsky N, Blondel O, Laeng P et al. Differentiation of embryonic stem cells to insulin secreting structures similar to pancreatic islets. Science 2001; 292:1389–94.

Eleven
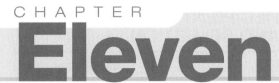

Cardiothoracic transplantation

Stephen C. Clark and
Asif Hasan

It is more than three decades since the first cardiac transplant was undertaken. During this period it has evolved from a headline-grabbing experimental procedure to an effective therapy for end-stage heart disease. In the current era heart transplant programmes around the world are showing medium-term survival in excess of 80%.[1] Nevertheless, the success of heart transplantation has raised expectations that under present circumstances it cannot fulfil. On one hand, due to improved management of ischaemic heart disease and increased longevity, the number of patients with heart failure is growing.[2] On the other hand, there is a decrease in the number of cardiac transplantations due to donor organ constraints. This disparity between the number of donors and potential recipients has stimulated research to find new alternatives to transplantation. However, these have yet to make an impact on the current practice of heart transplantation. The contemporary practice of heart transplantation with respect to indications, surgical techniques and donor and recipient management will now be reviewed.

INDICATIONS FOR HEART TRANSPLANTATION

The reason for undertaking heart transplantation is to prolong life and to improve its quality. The indications for adult heart transplantation have remained essentially unchanged over the last 20 years and at present are equally distributed between coronary heart failure and non-coronary cardiomyopathy (45% each). Valvular (4%), adult congenital (2%) and re-transplantation (2%) constitute the rest.

The indications for paediatric heart transplantation (<16 years) are different to adults. In our series of 107 paediatric heart transplants (1987–2003) 60% were undertaken for cardiomyopathy and 40% for congenital heart disease.

AETIOLOGY OF HEART DISEASE

Ischaemic heart disease

This constitutes the largest group requiring heart transplantation. These patients can present in a variety of ways from being acutely ill after myocardial infarction on mechanical support to being chronically ill with heart failure with or without previous surgical or catheter-based intervention. Unfortunately there are no prospective studies comparing conventional treatment methods with heart transplantation to provide guidance in risk–benefit assessment. A digest of current thinking would indicate that heart transplantation would definitely be indicated in a patient with severe heart failure with poor ventricular function (ejection fraction <15%), symptoms of heart failure with little or no angina, diffuse coronary artery disease, absence of reversible ischaemia and/or poor right ventricular function (ejection fraction <35%). What is clear is that patients with ischaemic cardiomyopathy who develop heart failure are likely to have a worse prognosis than non-ischaemic patients.[3]

Non-ischaemic cardiomyopathy

This group includes a variety of aetiologies with marked left and/or right ventricular dysfunction. The disease processes that result in changes in heart muscle are classified as: (a) dilated cardiomyopathy; (b) hypertrophic cardiomyopathy; (c) restrictive cardiomyopathy; and (d) arrhythmogenic right ventricular dysplasia. In patients with non-ischaemic cardiomyopathy, transplantation is indicated if there is failure of aggressive medical treatment.

Certain types of cardiomyopathies can show reversibility, and a period of observation with medical treatment should be tried before listing. These include lymphocytic myocarditis, peripartum cardiomyopathy, hypertensive cardiomyopathy and alcoholic cardiomyopathy.[4]

Indications for paediatric patients are similar; however, the risk of death is highest during the first 3 months after presentation, therefore failure of aggressive medical treatment early in the course of the disease should lead to early listing for transplantation. Acute myocarditis needs a special mention as the finding of acute inflammation on biopsy is a favourable prognostic sign for subsequent recovery.[5]

Congenital heart disease

In the present era the diagnosis of congenital heart disease is as common as cardiomyopathy as an indication for heart transplantation in children. This group is likely to grow as paediatric cardiac surgery becomes more successful in its outcome. The indications for transplantation in this group can be for either life-saving reasons or for improvement in quality of life.

RECIPIENT EVALUATION AND SELECTION

Patients are evaluated for transplantation once a referral has been made. We admit the patient for a few days for assessment. During this period there is a systematic evaluation of both the physical and psychological state of the patient; it also gives an opportunity to develop a rapport between the patient, relatives and the multidisciplinary team. The protocol used in our own centre for assessment is summarised in **Box 11.1**. The assessment process is designed to answer the following questions:

1. Does the patient fulfil the selection criteria for heart transplantation?
2. Are there any contraindications to transplantation?
3. Is there any possibility of any other treatment option?

Selection criteria

The process of selection of patients for transplantation remains an inexact science. In the majority of cases the referral for transplantation is of a patient with chronic heart failure. In these cases there is remarkable divergence of opinions when a patient should be listed for heart transplantation, further compounded by a lack of evidence to guide day-to-day clinical practice.

 Mancini et al. showed that patients with a peak exercise oxygen consumption of <14 mL/kg/min had a significantly higher mortality than patients with a peak exercise oxygen consumption of >14 mL/kg/min.[6]

The limitation of this technique is that it can be influenced by body composition, motivation or deconditioning. Some centres have incorporated the heart failure survival score (HFSS) to their preoperative assessment. The score consists of using seven variables – resting heart rate, left ventricular ejection fraction, mean arterial blood pressure, interventricular conduction delay, peak exercise oxygen consumption (VO_2), serum sodium and ischaemic cardiomyopathy. Using these variables Aaronson et al. developed a mathematical model to predict outcome with medical management.[7] This score

Box 11.1 • Recipient assessment protocol for heart transplantation

1. Full medical assessment

Full history and physical examination. Investigations include:

- Full blood count, platelets and coagulation screen
- Blood group
- Urea and electrolytes, liver function and thyroid function
- Microbiology – sputum, midstream specimen of urine (MSU), nose/throat/axilla/perineum swabs for culture
- Full viral screen (with patient consent)
- Fasting glucose and lipids
- 12-lead ECG
- Chest X-ray (PA and LAT)
- Spirometry
- Echocardiogram
- Chromium EDTA glomerular filtration rate (GFR) (renal opinion and abdominal ultrasound would be required if GFR <32.5 mL/min)
- Estimation of peak oxygen consumption (VO_{2max})
- Right heart catheter to assess filling pressures and calculate pulmonary vascular resistance, after discussion with the transplant cardiologist (as per protocol)
- Bone density (if >50 years or symptoms)
- Urine flow rate/residual (if male >50 years or symptoms)
- Carotid/peripheral artery Doppler (if symptoms)

2. A structured educational package – provided by the transplant coordinator

Discussion points include:

- Patient's understanding of his or her illness
- Donor compatibility
- Introduction to the concept of transplantation
- Preparation for admission
- Reason for assessment
- Travelling arrangements
- Explain investigations and visits
- Accommodation
- Survival figures
- Outpatient routine
- Waiting lists and waiting period
- Adjusting to family life
- Bleeper
- Driving
- Returning to work

3. Social assessment

This looks at both practical and emotional aspects of the transplant process with the patient and carer. Areas covered include:

- Feelings about what is happening to them
- Social security benefits
- Support networks
- Coping strategies

The aim is to evaluate whether the patient understands and whether he or she will cope with having a transplant and to prepare the ground for future involvement throughout the patient's contact with the transplant team

4. Physiotherapy assessment

An assessment and education package from the transplant physiotherapist with regard to exercise pre- and post-transplant, and postoperative chest care

---

along with maximal oxygen consumption (VO_{2max}) and clinical assessment can bring some rigour to the selection process for transplantation.

Recently Deng et al. have raised questions regarding the selection criteria for transplantation by showing that cardiac transplantation did not benefit patients with medium and low risk as assessed by calculation of heart failure survival score.[8] This landmark paper is the publication of the COCPIT study (Comparative

Outcome and Clinical Profiles in Transplantation) from German transplant centres and shows survival benefit only in patients with high risk of dying on the waiting list.

Contraindications

Contraindications to heart transplantation are summarised in **Box 11.2**. These can be classed in three groups:

Box 11.2 • Contraindications for heart transplant

Factors increasing perioperative mortality

- Irreversible pulmonary hypertension:
  - PVR >6 Wood units despite standardised reversibility testing protocol
  - TPG >14 mmHg
- Active infection
- Recent peptic ulcer disease
- Severe obesity (>140% ideal body weight)
- Cachexia (<80% ideal body weight)
- Pulmonary infarction within 6–8 weeks

Factors affecting long-term prognosis

- Age >65 years
- Severe renal impairment measured by EDTA GFR and kidney biopsy
- Brittle diabetes
- Active or recent malignancy
- Significant chronic lung disease, FEV_1 <40% predicted, FVC <50% of normal and DL_{CO} <40% of predicted
- Severe peripheral vascular disease
- Significant hepatic impairment

Factors that impair compliance

- Active mental illness
- Drug abuse within last 6 months refractory to treatment
- Chronic illness affecting function

DL_{CO}, carbon monoxide diffusing capacity; FEV_1, forced expiratory volume in 1 second; FVC, forced vital capacity; GFR, glomerular filtration rate; PVR, pulmonary vascular resistance (see Box 11.3); TPG, transpulmonary gradient (see Box 11.3).

1. Factors that increase perioperative mortality, e.g. elevated pulmonary vascular resistance.
2. Factors affecting long-term prognosis.
3. Factors related to life-threatening non-compliance.

These exclusion criteria have continued to change with improvement in medical treatment and increasing experience with heart transplantation, and now successful outcome can be obtained in cases previously excluded. Some of the contra-indications deserve special mention.

Box 11.3 • Definitions

Pulmonary vascular resistance
(PVR; Wood units) = [PA mean − pulmonary capillary wedge pressure (PCW)]/CO

Pulmonary vascular resistance index
(PVRI; Wood units/m^2) = (PA mean − PCW)/CI = PVR BSA

Transpulmonary gradient
(TPG; mmHg) = PA mean − PCW

Pulmonary vascular resistance (**PVR**) of more than 6 Wood units has been considered an absolute contraindication to heart transplantation but with the introduction of nitric oxide, use of a bicaval anastomotic technique, early implantation of ventricular assist devices and increasing use of peri-operative phosphodiesterase inhibitors, good results can be obtained in patients who formerly would not have been offered the opportunity of transplantation. Nevertheless, the presence of an elevated PVR should not be taken lightly as the donor right ventricle generally tolerates a systolic pressure of more than 50 mmHg poorly and would acutely fail. In our own practice a PVR >3 Wood units would be considered a relative contraindication to transplantation. The **transpulmonary gradient** (**TPG**) (see **Box 11.3**) represents the pressure gradient across the pulmonary vascular bed and is independent of the pulmonary blood flow. Some consider the elevation of this above 14 mmHg as a more useful indication of raised PVR as this is independent of the cardiac output, which may be poor in these patients. We rely more on this criterion and would consider a fixed TPG of 12 mmHg and above as an absolute contraindication. In paediatric patients a higher TPG can be considered as it could be overcome with a larger sized donor. Heterotopic transplantation can also be undertaken in these circumstances to overcome elevated pulmonary vascular resistance.[9]

Renal dysfunction is one of the most common problems encountered in the assessment of these patients. Multiple studies have shown that it is a major risk factor for mortality after heart transplantation. A common dilemma is to distinguish between renal dysfunction due to intrinsic renal disease or severe heart failure and aggressive diuretic therapy. We undertake measurement of glomerular filtration rate (GFR) using ethylenediamine tetraacetate (EDTA). A low GFR may indicate renal biopsy to further elucidate the problem. Others have used measurement of effective renal plasma flow (ERPF) as an investigative modality, and less than 200 mL/min is considered indicative of major intrinsic renal dysfunction and an indication for combined heart and kidney transplantation.

Compliance is the neurobehavioural capacity to adhere to a complex lifelong medical regimen. Non-compliance following heart transplantation can lead to major morbidity or death. Unfortunately there are no proven psychological or sociological factors to predict poor compliance or adverse outcome after transplantation. Adherence to medical treat-ment and ability to keep appointments can provide some pointers towards compliance. Psychiatric disorders that impair compliance, such as severe depression or untreated schizophrenia, are contra-indications to heart transplantation.[10]

Other options

It is not unusual to find patients who have been referred for transplantation to be suitable for alter-native treatments. In addition there are newer methods of treatment of heart failure in both medical and surgical disciplines being developed, and some of these patients could derive benefit from them. Two developments are worth mentioning.

BIVENTRICULAR PACING

In 20–30% of patients with symptomatic heart failure there is a prolonged PR interval, wide QRS complexes and intraventricular conduction disorders leading to a discoordinate contraction pattern. The result is earlier atrial contraction causing mitral regurgitation. This is further compromised by paradoxical septal motion due to wide QRS and conduction abnormalities. Biventricular pacing has been shown to synchronise contractility and improve the functional class of patients.[11] We have used biventricular pacing in several of our patients with improvement in functional class and subsequent delisting from transplantation.

PARTIAL LEFT VENTRICULECTOMY

Batista et al. first reported the use of resection of a segment of the left ventricular wall between the papillary muscles in patients with dilated cardio-myopathy to treat heart failure.[12] This was based on LaPlace's law, which relates wall tension to chamber radius. There was initial enthusiasm for the procedure, with several centres embarking on this operation. The results have been mixed and show early failure rates with a high requirement for ventricular assist devices.[13] There were, however, some spectacular successes. It is possible that the indication for this form of surgery needs defining more precisely and there may be a selected group who could benefit from this.

DONOR SELECTION AND MATCHING

Donor allocation for hearts in the UK is run by UK Transplant (UKT). The hearts are allocated on a pro rata basis; however, a category of 'urgent' was created in the year 1999 to deal with acutely ill patients. Once a donor is identified certain criteria apply before acceptance.

Donor age

An upper limit of 60 years is used by our own unit but there is variation in other centres. It is important that donor age should not be viewed in absolute terms but should be considered along with other factors such as cardiac function, recipient urgency and projected ischaemic times. However, older donors are more likely to have coronary artery disease and there is increased mortality for the recipient if the heart has come from a donor over 40 years of age.[1] The presence of coronary artery disease should not be considered as an exclusion criterion as satisfactory outcomes can be achieved with concomitant coronary revascularisation.[14] United Network for Organ Sharing (UNOS) data from the USA show that in 1982 2.1% of donors were aged 50 years or greater but by 1994 this percentage had increased to 8.9%.[15]

Cardiac function

Brain death leads to myocardial changes with abnor-malities seen on ECG of ST segment elevation, T wave inversion and Q waves. Events following brain death, namely prolonged hypotension, cardio-pulmonary resuscitation and high-dose inotropic support also contribute to cardiac dysfunction. The assessment of cardiac function is undertaken by echocardiogram, Swan–Ganz catheter and finally by the surgeon procuring the organ. Troponin I may be useful in detecting donor myocardial injury and elevated levels are associated with impaired cardiac function.[16]

There is no consensus on what degree of inotropic support correlates with structural and functional damage sufficient to compromise graft function. It has been recommended that hearts should not be used if the inotropic requirements exceed 20 µg/kg/min of dopamine. Often, inotropes are used in conjunction with fluid infusions to fill a vasodilated circulation and bolster perfusion pressure. We utilise arginine vasopressin under these conditions and wean the inotropes. Failure to wean the inotropes under these conditions is a bad prognostic sign and suggests cardiac dysfunction. Donor hearts developing arrhythmias are not considered suitable.

Donor disease

Donors with an active infective focus are usually turned down. However, donors with a history of meningitis that has been adequately treated are considered for donation. Hepatitis C patients are not considered unless the recipient is positive for hepatitis C or is acutely ill on the urgent list. Hepatitis B donors with positive surface antigen are avoided, but core antibody-positive donors (surface antigen-negative) can be considered.

Donor hearts from donors with primary brain tumours are considered for transplantation. Astrocytomas with recurrence and shunts are not considered.

A history of intravenous drug abuse would disqualify the donor but an exception can be made in the very ill recipient and a normal echocardiogram of the donor heart in the presence of negative serological viral testing. Chronic cocaine use causes cardiomyopathic changes and caution should be used in accepting these hearts from such donors.

Size matching

As a general rule for routine adult heart transplantation with a normal PVR 30% undersizing is acceptable, although much smaller donors have been reported with satisfactory outcome.[17] In patients with a raised PVR deliberate oversizing is routinely undertaken to overcome pulmonary vascular resistance. In the paediatric group oversizing is often done to utilise all available hearts. In our last 30 consecutive paediatric transplants the average size discrepancy between donor and recipient was 150%, and in a cohort of patients who had a failing Fontan circulation as an indication for transplantation, the oversizing was 250%. The adverse consequences of oversizing are delayed sternal closure, collapse of the left lower lobe and systemic hypertension. However, all these factors can resolve with time and appropriate treatment.

ABO compatibility

ABO compatibility is required to avoid hyperacute or accelerated acute rejection. Rhesus incompatibility is acceptable. The only ABO exception would be the A_2 subgroup as donors with this subgroup may be less prone to producing hyperacute rejection, because A_2 antigen is not readily displayed on the endothelial surface of the heart. However, in the paediatric group successful heart transplantation has been undertaken in the presence of ABO incompatibility.[18] This is possible as the immune system in infants is immature and their anti-A and anti-B titres remain low until 12–14 months of age. We have successfully undertaken three transplants in children with ABO incompatibility. The oldest was 18 months old when heart transplantation was undertaken.

Immunological matching

The rationale for undertaking immunological testing is to identify potential recipients with circulating anti-HLA antibodies to avoid mismatch between donor and recipient that could lead to hyperacute or accelerated acute rejection. Sensitisation is determined by the panel reacting antibody test (PRA).

Common causes of sensitisation are pregnancy, prior blood transfusion or insertion of a ventricular assist device. Rarely a patient may be sensitised for unknown reasons. The test is considered positive if a 10% threshold is reached on testing the donor serum with the control group. When the recipient has a positive PRA, a prospective crossmatch is undertaken, which has implications regarding the timing of transplantation and in our experience does disadvantage the recipient. The long-term results of recipients having more than 25% PRA show that they are more prone to rejection.[19]

DONOR HEART PROCUREMENT

It is important to optimise the haemodynamic, metabolic and respiratory condition of the donor to maximise the yield of donor organs. This may entail using a multidisciplinary team to manage and optimise the donor before retrieval. Some poorly functioning hearts could be resuscitated by careful manipulation of inotropes and loading conditions of the heart. Using this strategy up to 30% of such hearts can be successfully 'resuscitated' and used for transplantation.[20]

The thoracic organs are accessed by midline sternotomy; this might have already been undertaken by the liver retrieval team. It is important to secure haemostasis carefully due to coagulopathy and volume replacement should continue actively. Whilst the abdominal dissection is being undertaken the pericardium is opened and the heart is inspected for its functional state as well as the presence of any congenital abnormality. The heart is palpated to feel any thrill for valvular heart disease or any coronary plaques. When the mobilisation of abdominal organs is completed, heparin at a dose of 300 units/kg is administered. If a central line is in place, it is withdrawn. The superior vena cava is ligated and inferior vena cava is completely divided. This allows the heart to exsanguinate into the right pleural cavity. The aorta is now clamped and cardioplegic solution is infused via the aortic root. We use one litre of St Thomas' cold crystalloid cardioplegic solution; this is augmented with cold topical saline. The dose for paediatric donors is 30 mL/kg. During the administration of cardioplegia the right superior pulmonary vein is incised to decompress the left side of the heart. Once the cardioplegia has been given the cardiectomy can proceed further. The superior vena cava is incised above the previous ligature. The aorta is now divided below the innominate artery; this exposes the pulmonary artery, which is divided on the left side where the left pulmonary artery is attached to the pericardial reflection and the right pulmonary artery is divided behind the aorta. The left atrium is now incised at the level of the pericardial reflection. The heart is now inspected for the presence of a patent foramen ovale and if found is oversewn. The heart is now packed inside three bags with cold saline in the intervening bags. The heart is then placed in a transport cooler packed in ice to be transported.

HEART TRANSPLANTATION
(Figs 11.1 and 11.2)

The classical technique of orthotopic heart transplantation as described by Lower et al. has remained the standard operation for 30 years.[21]

However, a recent modification has been the use of a bicaval technique. This results in less tricuspid regurgitation and better haemodynamic performance of the implanted heart.[22]

The operation is undertaken with a midline sternotomy. Cardiopulmonary bypass (CPB) is established with right atrial venous cannulation to allow decompression of the heart; this allows for easier cannulation of superior and inferior venae cavae. The patient is then cooled to 32°C. The

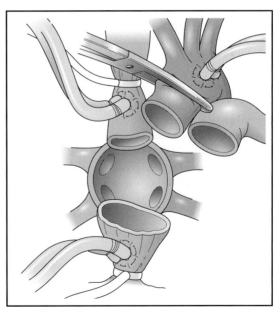

Figure 11.1 • Division of the right atrium to create superior and inferior vena caval cuffs for bicaval technique. The great vessels are divided as in the standard orthotopic method.

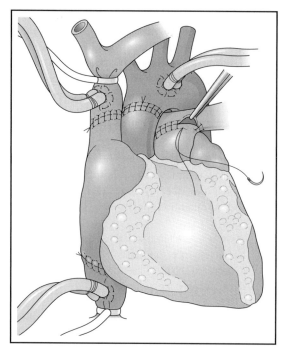

Figure 11.2 • Completion of bicaval transplant technique, showing the inferior vena caval, aortic and pulmonary artery anastomoses. From Kirklin JK, Young JB, McGriffin DC. Heart transplantation. Edinburgh: Churchill Livingstone, 2002, Ch. 10.8, p. 343, with permission.

The donor heart is now prepared for implantation. The pulmonary veins are joined together by incisions removing any excess tissue, the pulmonary artery is cut back to its bifurcation, and a dose of blood cardioplegia is given in the aortic root. The donor and recipient atria are anastomosed with 3/0 polypropylene, care is taken not to leave excess tissue behind as it could be thrombogenic or can obstruct the pulmonary venous orifices. The suture line is not completed as a vent is left in the left atrium to take away the warm blood. The aortic anastomosis is now undertaken with a 4/0 polypropylene suture. At this stage the aortic cross-clamp can be removed to reduce the donor ischaemic time. De-airing is undertaken through the aortic root and a dose of steroids is given before the clamp is removed. This is a critical period as the heart has been reperfused after a prolonged period of ischaemia. The heart usually starts to beat, but if ventricular fibrillation occurs the heart is promptly defibrillated. Careful attention is paid to the perfusion pressures and the ventricle is kept decompressed; the atrial vent is left in until satisfactory contractility is resumed. The pulmonary artery anastomosis is next undertaken, care being taken in trimming of the pulmonary arterial cuff to avoid redundancy. The IVC and then the superior vena caval anastomoses are completed.

Once the implantation is complete the body temperature is brought back to normothermia. We would reperfuse the heart for at least 10 minutes of every hour of ischaemic time before making an attempt at weaning CPB. Weaning from CPB is undertaken carefully avoiding distension of the right ventricle. Before closure of the chest, ventricular and atrial temporary pacing wires are attached, and a left atrial monitoring line is left in situ.

SPECIAL SITUATIONS

Heart transplantation for congenital heart disease

This group of patients presents special technical challenges due to unusual anatomy, previous operations and raised pulmonary vascular resistance. Heart transplantation can be undertaken to overcome most structural abnormalities.[23]

cavae are now snared and the aorta is clamped. To facilitate bicaval anastomosis it is recommended that at this stage the interatrial groove is dissected to develop a cuff of left atrium. The cardiectomy proceeds with a right atrial incision, which runs parallel to the atrioventricular groove; care is taken at the inferior caval end of this incision to preserve as much tissue as possible to facilitate inferior caval anastomosis. An incision is then made in the roof of the left atrium to further decompress the heart before dividing the aorta just above the aortic valve. Retracting the heart downwards now exposes the pulmonary artery, which is again divided above the pulmonary valve. The superior vena cava is now divided just at its right atrial junction. The heart is now only attached to the pulmonary veins and via a small bridge of tissue to the inferior vena cava. The inferior caval attachment is divided, again being mindful of the inferior vena cava (IVC) cuff; the incision in the left atrium is now extended to encircle the pulmonary veins, leaving behind two pulmonary veins on each side attached with a bridge of tissue.

Heterotopic heart transplantation

This describes the placement of the donor heart in parallel with the native heart. In the current era there are two possible indications for this procedure:

1. if the pulmonary vascular resistance is high (pulmonary artery pressure >60 mmHg) and cannot be manipulated by the use of nitric oxide;
2. if the donor is considerably smaller than the recipient.

The results of heterotopic transplantation have been generally inferior to orthotopic heart transplantation. However, this technique is still worth consideration whilst there remains a considerable differential between availability and requirement for donor hearts.[24]

PERIOPERATIVE MANAGEMENT

The principles of early management of the heart transplant patient are: (a) to maintain graft function; (b) to establish adequate immunosuppression; (c) to prevent and treat early infections; and (d) to allow recovery of other system functions, such as renal function.

Graft function

Most patients will have reduced myocardial function after heart transplantation and would require inotropic support, which is usually weaned over 24–48 hours. However, some patients develop either right or left ventricular dysfunction. Development of right ventricular dysfunction is related to the level of PVR after transplantation, inadequate myocardial preservation and discrepancy in size of the donor (smaller donor). The management of this would consist of adjusting preload and inotropic support. If the PVR is elevated nitric oxide is added and in extreme cases a right ventricular assist device is used. It is important that an anastomotic complication is excluded by measuring the pressure gradient across the pulmonary artery suture line; surgical revision is indicated if the systolic gradient is >10 mmHg.

Left ventricular dysfunction is again managed with adjustment in inotropic support; under rare circumstances the dysfunction can be life threatening and left ventricular assist may be required.

Immunosuppression

Triple therapy consisting of ciclosporin, azathioprine and steroids is the standard regimen used by most centres. We employ induction therapy using equine antithymocyte globulin (ATG) in the paediatric group and in patients with severe renal impairment who are intolerant of ciclosporin. Tacrolimus has been used as a substitute for ciclosporin in patients with persistent rejection and in children with side effects of ciclosporin, that is, gingival hypertrophy and hirsutism. Newer immunosuppressive agents, such as mycophenolate mofetil, rapamycin and interleukin 2 (IL-2) receptor antibodies (basiliximab and daclizumab) are being used in heart transplant rejection prophylaxis and treatment but have not yet found their place in routine immunosuppression protocols, despite a number of promising studies (see Chapter 5).

Monitoring of rejection following heart transplantation is crucial to short- and long-term survival of patients. The gold standard of rejection monitoring is endomyocardial biopsy. However, the histological findings of rejection are not uniformly present throughout the myocardium, and a high degree of clinical vigilance is needed in post-transplant follow-up of these patients.

Infection prophylaxis and treatment

Nearly 30% of patients have one or more infective episodes after heart transplantation. The most common type of infection is bacterial (50%) followed by viral (40%), fungal (5%) and protozoal (5%). The commonest single organism causing infection after heart transplantation is cytomegalovirus (CMV).[25]

SURVIVAL

The Registry of the International Society for Heart and Lung Transplantation (ISHLT) collects data on heart transplantation performed worldwide. The data have been collected since 1980; the latest report published in 2003 has 63 000 patients.[1] The survival data show 5-year survival of approximately 65%, at 10 years approximately 45% and at 15 years 23%. The median survival time is 9.3 years. For patients who are alive at 1 year, the median survival time is 12 years.

In our own centre, we have undertaken 554 adult heart transplantations between 1985 and 2003. Amongst these patients 147 have survived more than 10 years and 24 more than 15 years. During a similar period we have also undertaken 107 heart transplants in the paediatric group (<16 years). In this group 24 patients are alive at 10 years and 3 at 15 years.

CAUSE OF DEATH AFTER HEART TRANSPLANTATION

This information is available from the ISHLT registry but needs to be considered in the context of inherent difficulties associated with registry information, namely non-uniformity of definitions, validity of information, etc. The distribution of causes, modes and mechanisms of mortality after heart transplantation are time related. During the first 30 days after heart transplantation, graft failure accounts for 41% of the deaths, followed by non-CMV infection (14.2%) and multiorgan failure (13.9%). After 30 days and up to 1 year, non-CMV infection accounts for almost 35% of deaths, followed by graft failure (19%) and acute rejection (12%). Beyond 5 years, cardiac allograft vasculopathy (CAV) and late graft failure (possibly due to CAV) result in 31% of deaths. Cancers account for 24% and non-CMV infections 10% of deaths.[1]

Cardiac allograft vasculopathy

This is an unusually accelerated and diffuse form of obliterative coronary artery arteriosclerosis and is the commonest cause of graft failure in the long term after heart transplantation. Coronary arterial disease begins to develop relatively early after heart transplantation and nearly all patients after 1 year would show some histopathological evidence of this

disease.[26] Two different types of lesions develop. Type A are discrete stenoses of proximal and middle thirds of epicardial arteries. Type B are present in the distal coronary arteries and consist of tubular constrictions. Small vessels of less than 100 μm in diameter are not involved. CAV is probably due to a complex interplay between immunological and non-immunological factors. Viral infections, immunosuppressive drugs, dyslipidaemias and oxidant stress may all play a part.[27] Risk factors within 5 years of heart transplantation include pretransplant coronary artery disease, PRA positivity of >20% and donor hypertension. Female donors yield a weakly protective effect.[1] Beyond 5 years, hospitalisation for rejection within 5 years of transplantation and donor mass index also become additional risk factors.

Early identification of CAV is necessary as patients generally remain asymptomatic due to cardiac denervation; moreover, early recognition can improve long-term prognosis. Surveillance for CAV can be undertaken by several techniques, including intravascular ultrasound (IVUS), determination of coronary flow reserve and dobutamine stress echocardiography. However, coronary angiography remains the commonest form of investigation. IVUS is a much more sensitive tool in the detection of early intimal thickening.[28] However, it suffers from theoretical shortcomings of a lack of universal grading system and absence of an initial estimate of intimal thickening of donor arteries. In addition the size of available catheters means that they can only be used in vessels exceeding 1.5 mm in diameter. Dobutamine stress echocardiography has the advantage of non-invasive monitoring of CAV but its reported sensitivity of 72%[29] does not make it a suitable tool for replacement of angiography. Angiography is generally undertaken on an annual basis but if new lesions are identified it can be repeated more frequently. We would also undertake a baseline study if the presence of atherosclerosis is suspected in the donor heart at the time of transplant operation.

There is no conventional treatment for CAV and the emphasis has been on prevention of progression. The usual preventative measures of coronary artery disease have limited value. Calcium channel blockers, especially diltiazem and statins, have been shown to be effective.[30,31]

Newer immunosuppressive agents like everolimus, due to its proliferation inhibitor properties, also offer hope for the future.[32] In a prospective randomised study comparing everolimus with azathioprine the incidence of CAV was significantly lower in the group receiving everolimus.

Malignancy

The incidence of malignancy after heart transplantation is three to four times higher than the general population. The three common cancers after heart transplantation in order of frequency are cutaneous malignancies, post-transplant lymphoproliferative disorder (PTLD) and lung cancers. The risk factors for development of malignancies are presence of pretransplant malignancy, pretransplant coronary artery disease and increasing age. Female gender, use of mycophenolate mofetil and tacrolimus seem to have protective effects.[1] The probability of dying from malignancy after heart transplantation at 7 years is 8%.

The incidence of PTLD with ciclosporin-based immunosuppression is 2–4%.[33] Epstein–Barr virus (EBV)-negative PTLD has been described after heart transplantation but is considerably less common. There is a wide spectrum of presentation of PTLD from pulmonary, gastrointestinal, tonsillar to central nervous system involvement. Disseminated PTLD is associated with a poor prognosis. PTLD may respond to reduction of immunosuppression, and lymphomas showing CD20 expression can be successfully treated with CD20 antibody (rituximab)[34] (see Chapter 12).

Hypertension

Most patients will develop arterial hypertension after heart transplantation. It is of interest to note that in the pre-ciclosporin era the incidence of hypertension was 20%; now all patients are expected to have it at 2 years following transplantation.[32] Hypertension needs to be aggressively treated in these patients to prevent CAV and renal dysfunction. The treatment consists of sodium restriction with addition of calcium channel blockers and ACE (angiotensin-converting enzyme) inhibitors.

Chronic renal dysfunction

Chronic renal failure is a well-recognised complication after heart transplantation. The incidence of this is 10.9% at 60 months after transplantation.[35] Our incidence of dialysis is 10% at 10 years. The causation is multifactorial with preoperative renal dysfunction, perioperative haemodynamic insult, hypertension and diabetes mellitus all contributing in some measure, but the principal cause is calcineurin inhibitor treatment. The major decline in renal function occurs during the first 12 months after transplantation; thereafter there is gradual working of dysfunction. Unless there is pre-existing intrinsic renal disease, early renal dysfunction following transplantation is not a predictor of chronic renal failure.

The management of chronic renal impairment consists of preventative measures with close monitoring of calcineurin inhibitors levels, treatment of hypertension and avoidance of other nephrotoxic agents. Calcium channel blockers and ACE inhibitors have been proposed as agents to reduce renal toxicity of ciclosporin, possibly by reduction of afferent arteriolar tone, but clinical trials have failed to substantiate this claim.[36] It is hoped that the use of newer immunosuppressive agents such as sirolimus may lead to less renal toxicity.

HEART AND LUNG TRANSPLANTATION (HLT)

This form of pulmonary transplantation has had a transformation in its indications and the frequency with which it is done since it was first undertaken in 1982. At its inception it was the commonest form of pulmonary transplantation but with the success of isolated lung transplantation the indications are now mainly confined to pulmonary hypertension without congenital heart disease and pulmonary hypertension associated with Eisenmenger's syndrome and congenital heart disease. The annual activity in heart–lung transplantation has been halved since 1995.[37] A minority of centres have continued to use heart–lung transplantation in patients with cystic fibrosis (CF), utilising the healthy recipient heart as a domino procedure (healthy recipient heart is donated to a cardiac recipient).

Recipient selection criteria

The selection criteria for patients requiring HLT are similar to isolated lung transplantation. We have an upper limit of 50 years for acceptance to the transplant list. Specific guidelines for selection of patients in this group are as follows.

PULMONARY HYPERTENSION WITHOUT CONGENITAL HEART DISEASE

These patients have either pulmonary hypertension as a result of thromboembolic disease, veno-occlusive disease or collagen vascular disease. Patients are considered for transplantation when they become symptomatic and in spite of medical or surgical treatment remain in New york Heart Association (NYHA) grade III or IV. They should be resistant to vasodilator treatment with either prostacyclin or calcium channel blockers. Useful parameters for acceptance include cardiac index <2 L/min/m^2, right atrial pressure of >15 mmHg and a mean pulmonary artery pressure of >55 mmHg.[38]

EISENMENGER'S SYNDROME

These patients behave differently from the above group in several ways. With a similar degree of pulmonary hypertension these patients have better cardiac function and better prognosis. The predictors of survival are also less reliable. The selection criteria are unclear but severe progressive symptoms with NYHA grade III or IV symptoms despite optimum medical treatment would constitute an indication for transplantation.

Heart–lung operation

The operation is undertaken via sternotomy. Cardiopulmonary bypass is similar to heart implantation. The heart is excised first as it improves visualisation for pneumonectomy. Both the phrenic and vagus nerves are carefully preserved while pneumonectomy is undertaken. The recurrent laryngeal nerve is particularly at risk while the left pulmonary artery is being divided as the pulmonary artery is markedly enlarged due to pulmonary hypertension. A cuff of pulmonary artery can be left around the ligamentum arteriosum region to add to protection. The trachea is divided two rings above the carina.

The implantation proceeds with tracheal anastomosis, which is similar to bronchial anastomosis

as described with lung transplantation (see below). The left and right lungs are carefully placed in their respective cavities behind the phrenic nerves, taking care to avoid hilar torsion. The aortic and caval anastomoses are undertaken to complete the operation. Often the donor atrial appendage has been divided at the time of procurement of organs to decompress the heart and requires securing.

The postoperative care is similar to patients who have had heart transplantation.

Survival

The results of HLT are not dissimilar to pulmonary transplantation. Survival at 1 and 5 years is 61% and 40% respectively.[37] Recipients with Eisenmenger's syndrome have a better prognosis than patients with primary pulmonary hypertension (PPH).

FUTURE DIRECTION IN HEART TRANSPLANTATION

It is gradually being recognised that the number of heart transplant procedures is unlikely to exceed the present numbers of <3000 in the USA and <300 in the UK. Unfortunately the demand for donor hearts continues to escalate.

Alternatives to heart transplantation are being explored worldwide with research programmes exploring novel strategies including cell transplantation and regrowth of heart muscle, mechanical circulatory support and use of neurohumoral blockers to treat end-stage heart failure.

Xenotransplantation has continued to raise hopes for an unlimited supply of donor hearts. However, the feasibility of translating this technology into good long-term outcome in the foreseeable future looks rather remote. Presently the median time of survival of transgenic pig hearts in baboon is only 76 days.[39] According to a committee of the International Society for Heart and Lung Transplantation (ISHLT), the current experimental results do not justify initiating a clinical trial.[40] The future of xenotransplantation for hearts is still indeterminate.[41]

LUNG TRANSPLANTATION

The lung has historically been the most challenging of the human organs to be successfully transplanted in clinical practice. It took almost two decades since the first successful renal transplant before it was accepted that this procedure may bring significant improvements in quality of life to some recipients.[41] Since Hardy undertook the first single lung transplant in 1966[42] the operation has continued to be challenged by the frequent occurrence of bronchiolitis obliterans leading to the progressive onset of respiratory failure in the longer term.

Demographically, the International Society for Heart and Lung Transplantation registry indicates that 78% of recipients in Europe were between 35 and 65 years of age with the majority receiving their transplant for chronic obstructive pulmonary disease (COPD), cystic fibrosis or pulmonary fibrotic disease (**Fig. 11.3**). Only 4.1% were re-transplant procedures.

It is possible to transplant lungs singly (SLT) or sequentially as a bilateral lung transplant (BSLT) depending on patient characteristics and the nature of the pathological lung condition present. In some situations combined transplantation of the heart and lungs en bloc is necessary, as previously described.

CHOICE OF LUNG TRANSPLANT PROCEDURE

Bilateral sequential lung transplantation is performed where it is clinically necessary to remove all native lung tissue. In the context of chronic lung sepsis in cystic fibrosis or bronchiectasis, single lung transplantation would fail as infection may cross-contaminate from the native remaining lung into the graft. Similarly, extensive destruction of both lungs in emphysema may suggest the need for bilateral replacement to avoid air trapping in a remaining overly compliant native lung, resulting in mediastinal shift and compromise of the contra-lateral graft.

Single lung transplantation (SLT) is an attractive approach to the treatment of lung failure. The operation can often be performed without the acute lung injury and other attendant risks associated with cardiopulmonary bypass. There is an economy in the use of scarce donor organs, with two lung recipients benefiting from each donor and, in the event of acute or chronic injury to the graft, some viable native lung tissue will remain. Fibrotic lung conditions with normal pulmonary vasculature, a relatively immobile mediastinum and no native overinflation are most suited to this type of pulmonary transplant procedure. However, SLT is used with varying enthusiasm between centres for selected patients with emphysema (with or without α_1-antitrypsin deficiency) and sarcoidosis.

A controversial area is lung transplantation for primary pulmonary hypertension. Here, in the absence of structural problems in the heart, bilateral lung transplantation may suffice although many centres still advocate combined heart and lung transplantation. Some centres are performing SLT alone in these circumstances.[43] Survival for all three modalities of treatment for primary pulmonary hypertension is similar.

Transplantation of both lungs en bloc with the heart for pulmonary pathology is becoming less popular although this was the early means of lung replacement. Some centres still use this approach in circumstances where total lung replacement is required (the same indications as for bilateral lung transplantation). Although at first sight this may seem wasteful of scarce donor hearts where sequential lung transplantation will suffice, the structurally normal recipient heart is harvested and

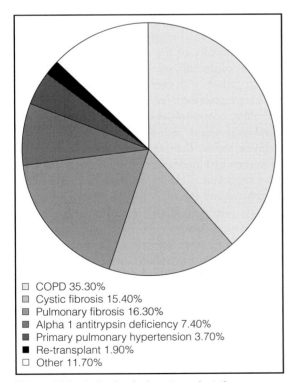

□ COPD 35.30%
▨ Cystic fibrosis 15.40%
▨ Pulmonary fibrosis 16.30%
▨ Alpha 1 antitrypsin deficiency 7.40%
▨ Primary pulmonary hypertension 3.70%
■ Re-transplant 1.90%
□ Other 11.70%

Figure 11.3 • Indication for lung transplantation.

used for a heart transplant candidate (the 'domino' operation).[44]

LUNG RECIPIENT ASSESSMENT AND SELECTION

The general aspects of assessment for lung transplantation are identical to those for heart assessment including a chromium EDTA glomerular filtration rate (GFR) to determine renal function. Again, after inpatient assessment, a recommendation is made to the patient by the surgeon after ensuring that all conventional treatments have been exhausted, and in terms of patient prognosis, that the timing for listing for transplantation is appropriate. Lung transplant assessment tests will typically also include sputum tests for *Aspergillus* and *Aspergillus* precipitins.

A six-minute walk test is performed, which measures the distance a patient is able to walk in a given time and the degree of arterial desaturation that results during this exertion. Not only does this give a measure of symptomatic restriction but it also has prognostic value. Values of less than 300 m are seen in patients in end-stage pulmonary failure.[45]

Computed tomography (CT) is used to study the texture of lung parenchyma and identify areas of maximal lung destruction or bullous disease accurately. This, along with the results of ventilation–perfusion scanning, assists with the decision of whether to perform BSLT or SLT in those conditions where either might be considered and, if SLT is selected, which side should be transplanted. For SLT it is usual to replace the lung that has the poorer perfusion. It is always preferable to explant a lung if there is evidence of chronic sepsis within it or if there is a bulla that is likely to rupture. These investigations also help to identify those emphysematous patients who might be suitable for lung volume reduction surgery as an alternative to transplantation with the aim of improving their ventilatory mechanics with symptomatic relief.

Detailed microbiological screening is an essential part of the assessment with attention also paid to cultures performed over the preceding months and years at the referring centre. This information identifies patients likely to be colonised with multiply resistant organisms (especially pseudomonads in the cystic population) and helps direct antibiotic prophylaxis in the perioperative period.

Of late, the particular importance of colonisation with *Burkholderia cepacia* has been recognised as an important predictor of post-transplant mortality,[46] which may influence acceptance or postoperative management.

In the cystic patient population with chronic sepsis and malabsorption, a nutritional assessment is vital since wound healing is impaired and the loss of muscle bulk may result in insufficient respiratory effort to permit weaning from the ventilator in the postoperative period.

Cardiopulmonary bypass is used routinely for BSLT and in about 20% of cases undergoing SLT. Therefore, identifying coincidental cardiac disease is important. Older patients and those with relevant risk profiles should undergo cardiac catheterisation with coronary angiography. Right heart catheterisation is undertaken in patients considered for lung transplantation for pulmonary hypertension. This can be supplemented by pulmonary angiography if pulmonary thromboendarterectomy might be considered as an alternative to transplantation.

The remainder of the assessment is designed to identify contraindications to organ replacement. Unlike patients with cardiac failure most candidates for lung replacement have preserved renal function. Absolute contraindications to pulmonary transplantation might include multiorgan failure and ongoing sepsis. Current malignancy, active peptic ulceration and inadequate conventional therapy are also important. Relative contraindications include peripheral and cerebral vascular disease, diabetes, obesity, osteoporosis and ischaemic heart disease. On occasion patients who have acute pulmonary failure – e.g. acute respiratory distress syndrome (ARDS) – and are ventilator-dependent are referred to be considered for transplantation.[47] Pulmonary transplantation is seldom successful under these circumstances as sepsis and multiorgan failure are common. However, if attempted, it is worth considering single lung replacement since the potential for recovery in the native lung is present in many cases of acute respiratory disease.

LUNG DONOR CRITERIA AND SELECTION

Specific considerations for lung donation must include a demonstration of good gas exchange with no evidence of aspiration, embolism or pneumonia. Smokers and patients with a history of mild asthma may still be considered as potential lung donors. In practice, only a minority of multiorgan donors are suitable for lung donation as potential lung injury may arise in a number of ways. After chest trauma, a haemothorax and fractured ribs may indicate parenchymal damage, but this is not always so and the contralateral lung may be uninjured and available for use. Aspiration of gastric contents at the time of injury or cardiac arrest is not uncommon. Injudicious fluid replacement during the patient's care may lead to pulmonary oedema, and the transfusion of blood and blood products in large volumes also predisposes to lung injury (sometimes becoming apparent only after implantation). Fat embolus from long-bone fractures with catastrophic results has also been reported. In all these circumstances, infection in the donor is more likely and will compound the injury to the lung.

Examination of the chest radiograph is essential. Aspirates taken from the endotracheal tube should be examined microscopically and Gram stained at the donor hospital. Mixed Gram-negative and Gram-positive organisms and numerous polymorphs in the aspirate may indicate potentially unacceptable infection. Previous culture results should be requested and considered. Use of broad-spectrum antibiotics in the absence of specific organism sensitivities should also be treated with caution. Flexible bronchoscopy can be useful to facilitate full expansion of the lungs and obtain good specimens of pulmonary secretions.

Lung function is assessed by gas exchange. A useful standardised measure is the P_aO_2 with the donor ventilated on 100% oxygen and with 5 mmHg of positive end-expiratory pressure to optimise ventilation. A value of <35 kPa is an indicator of significant lung injury, and many centres will not use lungs where a value of <50 kPa is recorded. The aspiration of blood from individual upper and lower lobe pulmonary veins is often useful when evaluating single lungs, where 45 kPa is a reasonable level of acceptability.[48]

Final assessment of the lungs is performed by the donor surgeon, who can see bullae and traumatised lung and feel areas of consolidation. Oedematous lungs feel heavy and spongy and may lead the donor team to reject the organs for use.

LUNG RECIPIENT–DONOR MATCHING

As with heart donors, matching of donor and recipient for lung transplantation is largely a crude process focusing on blood group and dimensions with no prospective match for tissue type.

Size can be assessed in a number of ways including comparison of measurements taken from donor and recipient chest radiographs. Donor and recipient heights are a useful guide to matching, with a 10–15% mismatch permissible. However, it is now generally recognised that donors should be matched to the predicted lung size of the recipient rather than the pathological size since thoracic capacity and chest wall mechanics will normalise after transplantation.

CMV status is an important consideration. CMV mismatch here has greater implications for a lung recipient in the event of seroconversion or reactivation in the grafted tissue.

LUNG RETRIEVAL AND PRESERVATION

As with heart retrieval, the median sternotomy is completed after initial mobilisation of the liver. Both pleurae are now opened widely and the lungs inspected. Any adhesions between visceral and parietal pleura are divided with electrocautery. The inferior pulmonary ligament on each side is divided up to the inferior pulmonary vein. The innominate vein is now ligated between ligatures and the pericardium is opened with the incision being continued up along the innominate artery, which is similarly divided. For this reason central venous access must be via the right internal jugular vein and arterial monitoring from the left radial artery. The pericardium is now opened and the aorta, superior vena cava (SVC) and inferior vena cava (IVC) are mobilised as before. Once the superior vena cava has been mobilised the azygos vein can be identified, ligated and divided behind the SVC to facilitate the future removal of the bloc. It is now possible to mobilise the trachea above the aortic arch. It is important not to denude the trachea of its blood supply and a tape is simply passed around it. Perfusion cannulas are now inserted into the ascending aorta and into the main pulmonary artery.

When perfusion apparatus has been set up for perfusion of the abdominal organs, removal of the heart and lung bloc can proceed. The SVC is divided between ligatures and the IVC is clamped above the diaphragm. The aorta is now cross-clamped and the heart is cardiopleged as described above for solitary heart transplant organ retrieval. However, under these circumstances the cardioplegia is vented from the heart by incision of the tip of the left atrial appendage leaving the pulmonary veins intact. Once electromechanical arrest has been achieved, infusion of preservative into the lungs can proceed through the pulmonary artery catheter. Simultaneous topical cooling of heart and lungs with cold saline solution proceeds throughout this time.

Pulmonary preservative solutions exist in many forms. Traditionally Euro-Collins solution has been used, which essentially has an intracellular fluid electrolyte composition. Recently, other preservatives based on extracellular fluids have been used, such as low-potassium dextran, with more encouraging results and the potential to extend organ ischaemic times.[49]

Prostaglandins may help prevent leucocyte sequestration and also optimise perfusion of the pulmonary capillary bed, and are given before infusion of the pulmoplegic solution. Preservation is achieved by cooling with extracorporeal circulation in some centres but most units use a hypothermic cold flush perfusion technique. Ischaemic times of 6–8 hours can be safely achieved.

The anaesthetist is now asked to ventilate the lungs by hand with air to prevent alveolar collapse. Occasional cessation of ventilation will facilitate excision of the bloc, which is undertaken when cardioplegia and pulmonary preservative solutions have both been given. The heart is elevated and the pericardium incised posteriorly below the inferior pulmonary veins joining right and left pleural spaces. It is now possible to elevate the heart, the back of the left atrium and both hila, dividing the connective tissue between these structures and

the descending aorta and oesophagus and vertebral column posteriorly. As the surgeon proceeds up the descending aorta the ligamentum arteriosum is encountered and divided. On the righthand side, the divided azygos vein is seen as dissection proceeds in a cephalad direction. At this point the heart–lung bloc is placed back in the chest and attention turned to the aorta, which is divided below the cross-clamp. The anaesthetist is now asked to withdraw the endotracheal tube into the upper trachea whilst still ventilating. A clamp can now be placed across the trachea below the endotracheal tube and the trachea divided above. All that remains is to divide the connective tissue behind the ascending aorta and trachea and remove the entire heart–lung bloc. The trachea is stapled to allow removal of the clamp whilst leaving the lungs inflated for transfer.

If the lungs are to be sent to a different destination from the heart, it is now necessary to split the bloc. This is performed by incising the left atrium anterior to the hilum on each side to separate pulmonary veins from the left atrium. It is important to leave a small cuff of left atrium on the pulmonary veins to facilitate implantation in the lung recipient. The pulmonary artery is divided at its bifurcation leaving a good length of pulmonary artery attached to each lung. All that remains now is to separate the ascending aorta and heart from the pulmonary arteries on each side and from loose connective tissue connecting it to the carina posteriorly. Lungs and heart can now be transported separately to different destinations as required.

SINGLE LUNG IMPLANTATION

Anaesthesia is established with a double-lumen endotracheal tube to permit ventilation of the native lung whilst implantation proceeds. A pulmonary artery flotation catheter is often used to monitor pulmonary artery pressure during implantation and full arterial and venous monitoring is established. Facilities for cardiopulmonary bypass are made available but are used only if unacceptable desaturation during implantation occurs or if systemic hypotension or pulmonary hypertension develop.

A lateral thoracotomy is performed and the native lung is excised with ligation of inferior and superior pulmonary veins and pulmonary artery. The bronchus is divided and the native organ removed. Care is taken not to contaminate the pleural space with endobronchial secretions. Meticulous haemostasis at the hilum is established. The pericardium is now incised adjacent to the pulmonary veins and these are mobilised to develop a cuff of left atrium. The pulmonary artery is mobilised in a similar fashion. The donor lung is now prepared by trimming the left atrial cuff, cutting the pulmonary artery to length and excising the stapled end of the bronchus to deflate the lung.

Implantation commences with the bronchial anastomosis. The membranous part of the bronchus is anastomosed with a continuous 4/0 Prolene suture. A series of figure-of-eight interrupted sutures is now placed on the anterior cartilaginous part of the bronchus to complete the anastomosis. Loose connective tissue at the hilum of donor lung can now be used to cover the anastomosis. A long side-biting clamp is next placed across the native left atrial cuff, which encompasses the pulmonary veins; the cuff is then opened longitudinally. The left atrial anastomosis is now performed with a continuous 4/0 Prolene suture and the clamp is left applied. The pulmonary artery anastomosis is performed in the same fashion and the donor organ is now de-aired by partially releasing the clamp from the pulmonary artery and de-airing through the left atrial anastomosis. The left atrial clamp can now be removed. Ventilation of the new lung commences (**Fig. 11.4**).

Apical and basal chest drains are now inserted. The thoracotomy is closed and the patient is returned to the intensive care unit for further monitoring and care. It is usually possible to extubate the stable patient after the insertion of an epidural analgesic catheter. Typically the patient will return to the ward after approximately 24–48 hours.

BILATERAL SEQUENTIAL LUNG IMPLANTATION

Single-lumen intubation for anaesthesia is performed. At many centres, this procedure is undertaken as sequential single lung transplants to avoid the perceived increase in acute lung injury postoperatively that is said to accompany extracorporeal perfusion. At our institution and others, cardio-

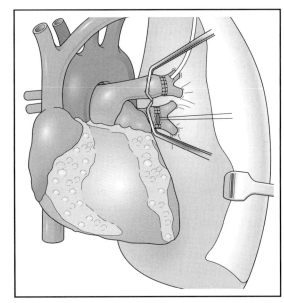

Figure 11.4 • The technique of vascular anastomosis in lung transplantation.

pulmonary bypass is routinely used and seems to have little impact on lung function following surgery.[50] The operation is approached through a submammary 'clam shell' incision that divides the sternum transversely. A median sternotomy is a less painful incision that can be used in some cases although access can sometimes be more of a challenge.

The patient is fully heparinised, the pericardium is opened and the patient is placed on cardiopulmonary bypass with an ascending aortic inflow cannula and venous drainage from individual cannulation of the caval veins. Excision of each lung now proceeds with electrocautery division of adhesions. Care is taken to preserve the phrenic nerve while mobilising structures at each hilum, especially in patients with septic lung disease where large lymph nodes and dense hilar adhesions make excision of the lung difficult. Excision of each lung proceeds in turn, and in cases of pulmonary sepsis the pleural cavities are irrigated thoroughly with the antiseptic Taurolin. Implantation of the donor lungs is performed in exactly the fashion described for single lung transplantation, the right side being anastomosed first. The patient is usually cooled to 32°C during implantation, the heart being allowed to continue to beat and eject in sinus rhythm. After implantation, de-airing and reperfusion are performed and ventilation is recommenced. At normothermia cardiopulmonary bypass can be weaned.

It is important that the pulmonary artery (PA) pressure at reperfusion is controlled. A number of experimental studies have shown reduced lung reperfusion injury when this is the case, and even a short period of controlled pressure reperfusion is beneficial.

We keep the mean PA pressure at less than 20 mmHg for at least 10 minutes while reperfusing a lung transplant.

Each thoracic cavity is drained with basal and apical drains and the wound is closed. The patient is then returned to the intensive care unit for further monitoring and can usually be extubated at 8–12 hours postoperatively. Epidural analgesia is essential following the 'clam shell' incision. Return to the ward is usually at about 24 to 48 hours.

PERI- AND POSTOPERATIVE CARE FOR LUNG TRANSPLANTS

On notification of a possible donor the selected recipient is admitted and reassessed for deterioration or unexpected infection.

Infection and colonisation of the airway and lung is a major feature of lung transplant and a leading cause of morbidity and mortality in the postoperative period. Antibiotic prophylaxis is largely directed by the known flora of the recipient but flucloxacillin is used for Gram-positive cover and metronidazole for Gram-negative cover in the absence of other positive cultures. Colomycin is administered by nebuliser in the immediate postoperative period. Antibiotic therapy is modified in the first few days after transplant as the results of perioperative donor and recipient bronchoalveolar lavages become available. In the absence of infection, antibacterial agents are stopped after the first routine bronchoscopy and biopsy at 1 week provided airway anastomoses appear healthy. Aciclovir, antifungal agents and pneumocystis prophylaxis are used routinely as in cardiac transplantation.[51]

Immunosuppression, as in heart transplantation, commences preoperatively with the administration of azathioprine and ciclosporin A. Methyl-prednisolone is administered at reperfusion and continued intravenously for 24 hours, after which oral steroids may be commenced. However, since many pulmonary recipients have malabsorption and early ciclosporin levels may be erratic, antithymocyte globulin (ATG) is administered routinely for the first 3 days as induction therapy, with dosage and timing being regulated by daily flow cytometry lymphocyte counts. With this exception, immunosuppression is managed in an identical fashion with the same dosage regimens as in cardiac transplantation.

In recent years, other immunosuppressants have been put forward for use in postoperative immunosuppressive regimens. In particular the use of induction therapy with ATG has been questioned due to concerns over increased rates of infection and of post-transplant lymphoma, though this is very controversial. Tacrolimus, mycophenolate mofetil (MMF) and rapamycin have been investigated but so far no conclusive advantages have been demonstrated although side effect profiles may be subject to some improvements.[52]

If any lung injury is present in the immediate postoperative period, ventilation can present great difficulties. Such reperfusion injury results from the sequestration of neutrophils in the lung parenchyma with release of injurious enzymes and oxygen free radicals. Lungs may be oedematous or infected, with poor gas exchange. Meticulous control of fluid balance, optimisation of ventilation and microbiological control are needed in this situation.

Nitric oxide administration has many benefits in reperfusion injury and is distributed preferentially to ventilated areas of the lung. It improves ventilation–perfusion matching and lowers pulmonary artery pressures. It reduces the adhesion of neutrophils to the endothelium and so alleviates reperfusion injury.[53,54]

A number of other interventions (controlled pressure reperfusion, pentoxifylline, extracorporeal filters, adhesion molecule modulators) affecting neutrophil sequestration in the lung have been put forward to try to combat this problem postoperatively but have not been widely evaluated in clinical practice.[55]

In the case of the single lung transplant for emphysema, the residual overcompliant lung can inflate excessively with air-trapping and resultant mediastinal shift if the expiratory period of ventilation is insufficient. Modification of the ventilatory cycle can help but sometimes independent ventilation of each lung through a double-lumen endotracheal tube is needed. When the time comes to wean the recipient from the ventilator an epidural catheter to administer analgesics is essential. Epidural infusions can be continued for some days after extubation to assist expectoration of secretions.

Transbronchial biopsy and bronchoalveolar lavage with a flexible bronchoscope under sedation are performed at 1 week, 1 month and then every 3 months before reverting to annual biopsies to detect rejection and direct antimicrobial intervention. Additional biopsies are taken if rejection is suspected on the grounds of unexplained fever, symptomatic deterioration with arterial desaturation or a fall in pulmonary function tests including spirometry and transfer factor.

Rejection grading in lung transplants is summarised in **Box 11.4**. Treatment is by augmentation of steroid therapy – 3 days of intravenous methylprednisolone (500 mg) and subsequent augmentation

Box 11.4 • Grading of pulmonary allograft rejection

A	Acute rejection
0	None
1	Minimal – scattered mononuclear infiltrates
2	Mild – frequent infiltrates of activated lymphocytes: 'endotheliatis'
3	Moderate – vascular cuffing, alveolar macrophages, extension of infiltrate into perivascular and air spaces
4	Severe – intra-alveolar necrosis, hyaline membrane, haemorrhage

With or without:

B	Airway inflammation
0–4	According to severity

C	Chronic airway rejection
A	Active
B	Inactive

D	Chronic vascular rejection

of oral steroids. Treatment is required for grades 3 and 4 and for grade 2 if there is clinical concern.

OUTCOMES AND COMPLICATIONS OF LUNG TRANSPLANTATION

Generally, the 30-day survival is approximately 85%, with 75% surviving to 1 year. At 5 years, 45% remain alive, and 25% after a decade. Survival curves for bilateral lung transplantation are a little better than for unilateral procedures. The early decline in survival mirrors that seen in heart transplantation and reflects operative mortality and donor organ dysfunction. The causes of perioperative mortality are similar to those seen in cardiac transplantation, and include unsuspected donor lung injury (infection, oedema, embolic disease or poor preservation) and reperfusion injury. Specific technical difficulties include anastomotic stenoses with pulmonary oligaemia (pulmonary arterial obstruction) or pulmonary oedema (venous stenosis)[56] and airway ischaemia and dehiscence with resultant mediastinitis.

The vascular supply of bronchial and tracheal anastomoses is compromised and early dehiscence with ischaemia is a life-threatening complication with prolonged air leak and mediastinitis. Attention to detail when the anastomosis is performed, with care not to denude the airway, minimises this risk. It is no longer thought necessary to wrap the anastomosis in a vascularised pedicle or omentum. Concurrent steroid therapy (once considered a contraindication to lung transplantation) may even reduce dehiscence as development of capillaries at the anastomosis is enhanced. Some early in-hospital deaths result from infection and acute rejection episodes.

Quality of life is significantly improved by transplantation for pulmonary failure.

Studies in lung transplant patient groups consistently show improvements in functional status and the perception of symptoms, irrespective of the type of transplant performed or the primary pathology.[57]

The diagnosis and treatment of acute rejection have been discussed. Diagnosis is often made more difficult by concurrent infection, and the decision to treat can also be problematic because of the fear of resulting uncontrollable sepsis. As in cardiac grafts, persistent or repeated episodes of rejection are managed with cytolytic therapy (ATG), monoclonal therapy or a change in immunosuppressive agent, perhaps to one of the newer agents such as tacrolimus or MMF.

Fungal and viral infections are seen commonly in the early postoperative period (*Aspergillus* and CMV) and carry a significant morbidity. *Pseudomonas* colonisation is common in the cystic population. If preoperative data suggest that multiresistant pseudomonads are present antibacterial therapy is kept to a minimum to allow growth of sensitive organisms.

CMV infection can be a major clinical problem. Diagnosis is by immunofluorescence at lavage, by transbronchial biopsy, estimation of antigenaemia and culture on bronchoalveolar lavage samples. Recently quantitative CMV-PCR (polymerase chain reaction) has been performed on a weekly basis to estimate viral load and identify those requiring treatment. Infection is common in all except the donor-negative/recipient-negative transplants (see Chapter 12). Lymphoproliferative disease and other malignancies are seen as in cardiac transplantation although lymphomas are more common (one series reports an incidence of 3.4% in heart recipients and 7.9% in lung recipients). Mortality is significantly higher in lymphomas appearing after the first year after transplantation. Reduction in immunosuppression can be highly effective in early disease but later conventional chemotherapy may be required.

Longer-term airway complications can arise with overgrowth of granulation tissue at the anastomosis, especially in the presence of chronic infection, or fibrotic stricture formation, which is usually ischaemic in origin. Treatment is local with laser therapy, sometimes augmented with expandable stenting devices.

Chronic rejection in lung transplantation manifests itself as obliterative bronchiolitis or vascular atherosclerosis, the former being the greatest cause of long-term morbidity and mortality in recipients. Gradual deterioration in exercise tolerance and lung function arouse suspicion. Characteristic appearances are seen on the chest radiograph and CT scan, and the diagnosis is confirmed by transbronchial biopsy. Predisposing factors may include the occurrence of reperfusion injury and multiple episodes of acute rejection in the postoperative period, and CMV infection may be an aetiological factor. Treatment is directed towards decreased intensity of immunosuppression and total lymphoid irradiation may also help in some cases.

RECENT ADVANCES AND CONTROVERSIES

Most recent changes in practice in lung transplantation are driven by a need to optimise the donor pool. To this end, donation has been considered from both older and more marginal donors and in attempting to prolong the permissible ischaemic time. Encouraging results have been obtained and expansion of the donor pool through these methods can be expected in due course.[58]

Developments have been directed by a shortage of donor organs. Living-related donation of lungs by blood relatives of patients needing pulmonary transplantation has been performed with encouraging results. This technique is most applicable to paediatric transplantation for cystic fibrosis, where lobar donation by relatives alone may provide sufficient lung tissue to fill the recipient chest. Early reports show good results although recipients are often critically ill,[59] but donor morbidity can also be significant and this raises difficult ethical dilemmas.

A resurgence of interest in lung reduction surgery for symptomatic, non-prognostic emphysematous disease has diverted away from transplant lists some patients who might otherwise have been transplanted on the grounds of symptomatic restriction. Lung reduction surgery selectively excises the overexpanded, underventilated and underperfused areas of emphysematous lung. The reduction in lung volume permits better aeration of remaining lung and improves the ventilatory performance of the thoracic cavity by normalising its previously overexpanded volume and improving ventilation–perfusion matching.

 Unfortunately, initial enthusiasm has been tempered by major questions regarding the optimal surgical approach, safety, selection criteria and confirmation of long-term benefits.[60]

There has been a recent focus both in the laboratory and in limited clinical practice to utilise lungs from ventilated non-heart-beating donors. Clearly the practice raises difficult ethical and logistic problems with regard to organ retrieval, but good lung function has been reported in large animal experimental models. The optimal criteria for retrieval and the preservation technique used are still under investigation but the procedure has some potential for further expanding the donor pool.[61]

Key points

- Heart transplantation improves survival and quality of life for selected patients with end-stage heart failure.
- Heart transplantation is most beneficial in patients with greatest risk of dying.
- More specific immunosuppression agents continue to decrease the impact of acute and chronic rejection and immunosuppression-related side effects.
- Lung transplantation provides good survival and functional improvement in many forms of end-stage lung disease.
- Single or bilateral lung transplantation is possible depending on the underlying pathology.
- Colonisation with *Burkholderia cepacia* in cystic fibrosis patients is an important adverse prognostic marker.
- Reperfusion injury is a major challenge postoperatively but nitric oxide administration has the potential to limit this in clinical practice.

REFERENCES

1. Taylor DO, Edwards LB, Mohacsi PJ et al. The registry of the International Society for Heart and Lung Transplantation: twentieth official adult heart transplant report – 2003. J Heart Lung Transplant 2003; 22(6):616–24.

2. McMurray JJ, Stewart S. Epidemiology, aetiology, and prognosis of heart failure. Heart 2000; 83(5): 596–602.

3. Stevenson LW, Tillisch JH, Hamilton M et al. Importance of hemodynamic response to therapy in predicting survival with ejection fraction less than or equal to 20% secondary to ischemic or nonischemic dilated cardiomyopathy. Am J Cardiol 1990; 66(19):1348–54.

4. Figulla HR, Rahlf G, Nieger M et al. Spontaneous hemodynamic improvement or stabilization and associated biopsy findings in patients with congestive cardiomyopathy. Circulation 1985; 71(6):1095–104.

5. Matitiau A, Perez-Atayde A, Sanders SP et al. Infantile dilated cardiomyopathy. Relation of outcome to left ventricular mechanics, hemodynamics, and histology at the time of presentation. Circulation 1994; 90(3):1310–18.

6. Mancini DM, Eisen H, Kussmaul W et al. Value of peak exercise oxygen consumption for optimal timing of cardiac transplantation in ambulatory patients with heart failure. Circulation 1991; 83(3):778–86.

   This clinical study nicely demonstrated the value of measurement of peak oxygen consumption during maximal exercise testing and has brought some objectivity in assessment of patients for heart transplantation.

7. Aaronson KD, Schwartz JS, Chery TM et al. Development and prospective validation of a clinical index to predict survival in ambulatory patients referred for cardiac transplant evaluation. Circulation 1997; 95(12):2660–7.

8. Deng MC, De Meeste JM, Smits JM et al. Effect of receiving a heart transplant: analysis of a national cohort entering a waiting list, stratified by heart failure severity. Comparative Outcome Clinical Profiles in Transplantation (COCPIT) Study Group. BMJ 2000 (Sept 2); 321(7260):540–5.

   This paper is mandatory reading for anyone interested in cardiac transplantation. It challenges the current role of cardiac transplantation in heart failure management.

9. Khaghani A, Santini F, Dyke CM et al. Heterotopic cardiac transplantation in infants and children. J Thorac Cardiovasc Surg 1997; 113(6):1042–8; discussion 1048–9.

10. Olbrisch ME, Levenson JL. Psychosocial evaluation of heart transplant candidates: an international survey of process, criteria, and outcomes. J Heart Lung Transplant 1991; 10(6):948–55.

11. Alonso C, Leclercq C, Victory F et al. Electrocardiographic predictive factors of long-term clinical improvement with multisite biventricular pacing in advanced heart failure. Am J Cardiol 1999; 84(12):1417–21.

12. Batista RJ, Santos JL, Takeshita N et al. Partial left ventriculectomy to improve left ventricular function in end-stage heart disease. J Card Surg 1996; 11(2):96–7; discussion 98.

13. Franco-Cereceda A, McCarthy PM, Blackstone EH et al. Partial left ventriculectomy for dilated cardiomyopathy: is this an alternative to transplantation? J Thorac Cardiovasc Surg 2001; 121(5):879–93.

14. Marelli D, Laks H, Bresson S et al. Results after transplantation using donor hearts with preexisting coronary artery disease. J Thorac Cardiovasc Surg 2003; 126(3):821–5.

15. Young JB, Naftel DC, Bourge RC et al. Matching the heart donor and heart transplant recipient. Clues for successful expansion of the donor pool: a multivariable, multiinstitutional report. The Cardiac Transplant Research Database Group. J Heart Lung Transplant 1994; 13(3):353–64; discussion 364–5.

16. Potapov EV, Ivanitskaia EA, Loebe M et al. Value of cardiac troponin I and T for selection of heart donors and as predictors of early graft failure. Transplantation 2001; 71(10):1394–400.

17. Sethi GK, Lanause P, Rosado LJ et al. Clinical significance of weight difference between donor and recipient in heart transplantation. J Thorac Cardiovasc Surg 1993. 106(3):444–8.

18. West LJ, Pollock-Barziv SM, Dipchard AI et al. ABO-incompatible heart transplantation in infants. N Engl J Med 2001; 344(11):793–800.

19. Loh E, Bergin JD, Couper GS et al. Role of panel-reactive antibody cross-reactivity in predicting survival after orthotopic heart transplantation. J Heart Lung Transplant 1994; 13(2):194–201.

   This is the first report of successful heart transplantation with ABO-incompatible donors in children. It has already made a major impact in expanding the donor pool for this group of patients.

20. Wheeldon DR, Potter CD, Odano A et al. Transforming the 'unacceptable' donor: outcomes from the adoption of a standardized donor management technique. J Heart Lung Transplant 1995; 14(4):734–42.

21. Lower RR, Stofer RC, Shumway NE. Homovital transplantation of the heart. J Thorac Cardiovasc Surg 1961; 41:196–204.

22. Aziz TM, Burgess AI, Rahman A et al. Risk factors for tricuspid valve regurgitation after orthotopic heart transplantation. Ann Thorac Surg 1999; 68(4):1247–51.

23. Hasan A, Au J, Hamilton JR et al. Orthotopic heart transplantation for congenital heart disease. Technical considerations. Eur J Cardiothorac Surg 1993; 7(2):65–70.

24. Bleasdale RA, Bannen NR, Anyanwu AC et al. Determinants of outcome after heterotopic heart transplantation. J Heart Lung Transplant 2002; 21(8):867–73.

25. Miller LW, Naftal DC, Bourge RC et al. Infection after heart transplantaion: a multiinstitutional study. Cardiac Transplant Research Database Group. J Heart Lung Transplant 1994; 13(3):381–92; discussion 393.

26. Johnson DE, Gao SZ, Schroeden JS et al. The spectrum of coronary artery pathologic findings in human cardiac allografts. J Heart Transplant 1989; 8(5):349–59.

27. Deng MC, Plenz G, Erren M et al. Transplant vasculopathy: a model for coronary artery disease? Herz 2000; 25(2):95–9.

28. St Goar FG, Pinto FJ, Alderman EL et al. Detection of coronary atherosclerosis in young adult hearts using intravascular ultrasound. Circulation 1992; 86(3):756–63.

29. Spes CH, Klauss V, Mudra H et al. Diagnostic and prognostic value of serial dobutamine stress echocardiography for noninvasive assessment of cardiac allograft vasculopathy: a comparison with coronary angiography and intravascular ultrasound. Circulation 1999; 100(5):509–15.

30. Wenke K, Meiser B, Thiery J et al. Simvastatin reduces graft vessel disease and mortality after heart transplantation: a four-year randomized trial. Circulation 1997; 96(5):1398–402.

31. Schroeder JS, Gao SZ, Alderman EL et al. A preliminary study of diltiazem in the prevention of coronary artery disease in heart-transplant recipients. N Engl J Med 1993; 328(3):164–70.

32. Eisen HJ, Tuzai EM, Dorent R et al. Everolimus for the prevention of allograft rejection and vasculopathy in cardiac-transplant recipients. N Engl J Med 2003; 349(9):847–58.

   This study of a randomised, double-blind clinical trial comparing everolimus and azathioprine may turn out to be a significant breakthrough in reducing the incidence of cardiac allograft vasculopathy.

33. Penn I. Tumors after renal and cardiac transplantation. Hematol Oncol Clin North Am 1993; 7(2):431–45.

34. Zilz ND, Olson LJ, McGregor CG. Treatment of post-transplant lymphoproliferative disorder with monoclonal CD20 antibody (rituximab) after heart transplantation. J Heart Lung Transplant 2001; 20(7):770–2.

35. Corcos T, Tamburino C, Leger P et al. Early and late hemodynamic evaluation after cardiac transplantation: a study of 28 cases. J Am Coll Cardiol 1988; 11(2):264–9.

36. Ojo AO, Held PJ, Port FK et al. Chronic renal failure after transplantation of a nonrenal organ. N Engl J Med 2003; 349(10):931–40.

37. Brozena SC, Johnson MR, Ventura H et al. Effectiveness and safety of diltiazem or lisinopril in treatment of hypertension after heart transplantation. Results of a prospective, randomized multicenter trail. J Am Coll Cardiol 1996; 27(7):1707–12.

38. Trulock EP, Edwards LB, Taylor DO et al. The Registry of the International Society for Heart and Lung Transplantation. Twentieth official adult lung and heart-lung transplant report – 2003. J Heart Lung Transplant 2003; 22(6):625–35.

39. D'Alonzo GE, Barst RJ, Ayres SM et al. Survival in patients with primary pulmonary hypertension. Results from a national prospective registry. Ann Intern Med 1991; 115(5):343–9.

40. Cooper DK. Clinical xenotransplantation – how close are we? Lancet 2003; 362(9383):557–9.

41. Cooper DK, Keogh AM, Brink J et al. Report of the Xenotransplantation Advisory Committee of the International Society for Heart and Lung Transplantation. The present status of xenotransplantation and its potential role in the treatment of end-stage cardiac and pulmonary diseases. J Heart Lung Transplant 2000; 19(12):1125–65.

42. Hardy JD, Alican F. Lung transplantation. Adv Surg 1966; 2:235–64.

43. Bando K, Armitage J, Paradis IL et al. Indications for and results of single, bilateral, and heart-lung transplantation for pulmonary hypertension. J Thorac Cardiovasc Surg 1994; 108(6):1056–65.

44. Anyanwu AC, Banner NR, Radley-Smith R et al. Long-term results of cardiac transplantation from live donors: the domino heart transplant. J Heart Lung Transplant 2002; 21(9):971–5.

45. Kadikar A, Maurer J, Kesten S. The six-minute walk test: a guide to assessment for lung transplantation. J Heart Lung Transplant 1997; 16(3):313–19.

46. Aris RM, Routh JC, Lipuma JJ et al. Lung transplantation for cystic fibrosis patients with Burkholderia cepacia complex. Survival linked to genomovar type. Am J Respir Crit Care Med 2001; 164(11):2102–6.

This is an important paper demonstrating the influence of colonisation with *B. cepacia*. The mortality rate was 33% in those infected compared to 12% in the control group. Moreover genomovar III patients were at the highest risk of death.

47. Flume PA, Egan TM, Westerman JH et al. Lung transplantation for mechanically ventilated patients. J Heart Lung Transplant 1994; 13(1):15–21; discussion 22–3.

48. Aziz TM, El-Gamel A, Saad RA et al. Pulmonary vein gas analysis for assessing donor lung function. Ann Thorac Surg 2002; 73(5):1599–604; discussion 1604–5.

Radial artery blood gas evaluation is the standard method for assessing donor lungs. The use of individual pulmonary vein gases is investigated in this paper, which is of important clinical significance to maximise the number of donor lungs deemed suitable for transplantation.

49. Rabanal JM, Ibaanez AM, Mons R et al. Influence of preservation solution on early lung function (Euro-Collins vs Perfadex). Transplant Proc 2003; 35(5):1938–9.

This clinical study compared Perfadex and Euro-Collins lung preservation solutions prospectively demonstrating the superiority of the former in terms of postoperative graft function.

50. Szeto WY, Kreisel D, Karakousis GC et al. Cardiopulmonary bypass for bilateral sequential lung transplantation in patients with chronic obstructive pulmonary disease without adverse effect on lung function or clinical outcome. J Thorac Cardiovasc Surg 2002; 124(2):241–9.

51. Chan KM, Allen SA. Infectious pulmonary complications in lung transplant recipients. Semin Respir Infect 2002; 17(4):291–302.

52. Lama R, Santos F, Algar FJ et al. Lung transplants with tacrolimus and mycophenolate mofetil: a review. Transplant Proc 2003; 35(5):1968–73.

53. Adatia I, Lillemei C, Arnolds JH et al. Inhaled nitric oxide in the treatment of postoperative graft dysfunction after lung transplantation. Ann Thorac Surg 1994; 57(5):1311–18.

This clinical study illustrates the beneficial effects of nitric oxide administration in postoperative lung transplantation. Improvements in oxygenation and pulmonary artery pressure are shown without the development of major side effects.

54. Bacha EA, Hervae P, Murakami S et al. Lasting beneficial effect of short-term inhaled nitric oxide on graft function after lung transplantation. Paris-Sud University Lung Transplantation Group. J Thorac Cardiovasc Surg 1996; 112(3):590–8.

55. Clark SC, Sudarshan CD, Dark JH et al. Controlled reperfusion and pentoxifylline modulate reperfusion injury after single lung transplantation. J Thorac Cardiovasc Surg 1998; 115(6):1335–41.

56. Clark SC, Levine AJ, Hasan A et al. Vascular complications of lung transplantation. Ann Thorac Surg 1996; 61(4):1079–82.

57. Charman SC, Sharples LD, McNeil AD et al. Assessment of survival benefit after lung transplantation by patient diagnosis. J Heart Lung Transplant 2002; 21(2):226–32.

This review of 653 patients undergoing lung transplantation used Cox regression analysis to demonstrate the survival advantages of postoperative patients irrespective of their primary pathology. There was no survival difference between patients having single or bilateral lung transplantation.

58. Meyer DM, Bennett LE, Novick RJ et al. Effect of donor age and ischemic time on intermediate survival and morbidity after lung transplantation. Chest 2000; 118(5):1255–62.

59. Starnes VA, Barr ML, Cohen RG. Lobar transplantation. Indications, technique, and outcome. J Thorac Cardiovasc Surg 1994; 108(3):403–10; discussion 410–11.

60. Koebe HG, Kugler C, Dienemann H. Evidence-based medicine: lung volume reduction surgery (LVRS). Thorac Cardiovasc Surg 2002; 50(5):315–22.

61. Corris PA. Non-heart beating lung donation: aspects for the future. Thorax 2002; 57: II53–II56.

Twelve

Cytomegalovirus and Epstein-Barr virus following solid-organ transplantation

Charles G. Newstead

CYTOMEGALOVIRUS

Cytomegalovirus (CMV) is one of the herpes group of viruses, which are widely distributed among mammals. The various strains are species-specific and produce a cytopathic effect resulting in greatly enlarged (cytomegalic) cells containing cytoplasmic and intranuclear inclusions. As is typical for the herpes class of viruses, primary infection results in the most severe disease. After primary CMV infection the viral genome enters leucocytes and remains latent. Reinfection with a different human strain can occur, as can reactivation of the latent viral infection. Reactivation is typically provoked by immunosuppression due to another disease, such as advanced carcinoma or AIDS, or treatment with immunosuppressive drugs or chemotherapy.

The incidence of antibody indicating previous infection increases with age in all human populations that have been studied. In the developed world the percentage of the population that is seropositive increases linearly with age; it is approximately 25% at age 20 and 80% at age 60.[1]

Transmission occurs via direct person-to-person contact. As the virus is labile, intimate exposure to saliva, urine, breast milk, genital secretions, stools and blood has to occur, with the result that the risk of transmission to healthcare workers is very low. Although congenital and perinatal CMV infection only rarely leads to typical disease (hepatitis, microcephaly, purpura, prematurity and haemolysis) it is an important healthcare burden, particularly in developing countries. In the immunocompetent child or adult most commonly the primary infection is subclinical. Malaise, fever and myalgia are the most frequent symptoms, with biochemical hepatitis and atypical lymphocytes found on investigations.

Tests for the diagnosis of CMV infection and disease

In the past it has been difficult to discriminate between latent CMV infection and CMV disease in transplant recipients. Given the primary infection/ latent infection reactivation cycle seen with herpesvirus this is not surprising. The detection of the classical large cells in culture takes several weeks, making this test of little practical use. As well as the symptoms detailed in the section 'CMV infection in transplant recipients' (see below) routine blood tests may detect bone marrow suppression, especially of the white cell series, as well as biochemical hepatitis. After a primary infection an individual would be expected to mount IgM and later an IgG response against CMV. It is the presence of the latter that is used to determine prior exposure of both donors and recipients to CMV infection. In immunosuppressed patients the antibody rise may be delayed or absent, and this delay in a serological change makes these tests at best only of use for retrospective diagnosis. A new recombinant antigen-based cytomegalovirus immunoglobulin M immunoassay has been reported. The new assay was sensitive for CMV-specific IgM, but in a group of liver transplant recipients the IgM was only found before detection of the virus when the recipient was seropositive prior to transplantation. Therefore in this setting the assay had a very low positive predictive value.[2]

Direct early antigen fluorescent fixation tests rely on the detection of CMV-generated antigen in cells from urine or alveolar macrophages obtained by direct lavage. As with all fluorescein techniques, subjective interpretation is a problem as well as the fact that the test is positive in a proportion of patients with latent infection but no CMV disease.[3] CMV p65 antigen in circulating polymorphonuclear leucocytes in the buffy coat may discriminate between infection and disease, but again subjective interpretation and poorly reproducible results are problems, particularly if delay occurs in the processing of specimens.[4] The rapid detection of CMV infection was first made possible using the shell viral assay. Unfortunately, a significant proportion of patients with viraemia are missed.[5] Tests based on the polymerase chain reaction (PCR) carried out on plasma or whole blood as well as leucocytes are much more sensitive. Contamination and inhibition are technical problems, as is the lack of standardisation between laboratories.[6] Experience and the availability of commercial assays have allowed PCR-based diagnosis to be offered on a routine basis.[7,8] The hybrid capture CMV DNA assay test should offer the advantages of objective CMV DNA detection and quantification without the technical hazards of PCR. In a study using two such commercial molecular assays the sensitivity for disease detection was 100%, with disease predicted approximately 12 days before the onset of symptoms.[9] **Figure 12.1**, taken from this paper, shows the relationship between viral load and probability of disease. **Figure 12.2** shows the viral load in patients with either disease or infection. The sensitivity of this assay may allow it to be used to monitor the response to therapy. Others have used similar assays to reliably predict CMV disease in kidney/pancreas[10] and other solid-organ recipients.[11,12]

On occasions it is necessary to prove CMV organ-specific dysfunction by obtaining a biopsy. This can be especially useful if coinfection with another organism is possible or if another cause of allograft

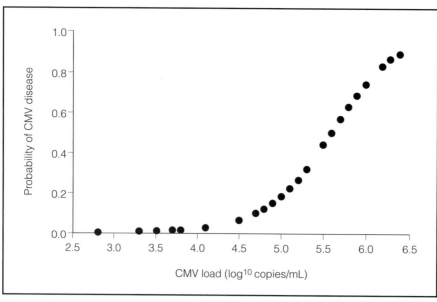

Figure 12.1 • Probability of acquiring CMV disease with increasing viral load.

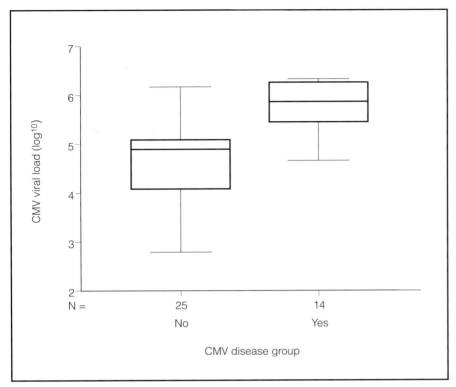

Figure 12.2 • Box-and-whisker plot to show the relationship between viral load and CMV disease. Yes: 14 victims with CMV disease; No: 25 victims without CMV disease.

dysfunction, such as rejection, is within the differential diagnosis. Liver (both native and allograft), bone marrow, lung, renal allograft and gastrointestinal biopsies can be diagnostic. The usual clinical approach is to choose to biopsy the most severely affected organ; CMV is a systemic infection and histological diagnosis may be achieved from unlikely sites.[13]

CMV infection in transplant recipients

The clinical consequences of CMV infection will be determined by a number of factors, but one of the most important is the degree of immunosuppressive treatment that the patient receives. Various authors have reported that serotherapy with T-cell antibodies derived from animals is associated with an increased risk of disease. This is illustrated by collating data from several studies and plotting the frequency of CMV disease against the frequency of antilymphocyte globulin (ALG) usage (**Fig. 12.3**).[14]

The risk to the seronegative recipient of a seropositive organ after treatment with antithymocyte globulin (ATG) can be estimated from analysis of the literature in the era before prophylaxis was available; mortality rates of 30% were not exceptional.[22]

Primary infection with CMV typically occurs 6 weeks post-transplantation in a seronegative individual who receives an organ from a seropositive donor. The symptoms due to primary disease may occur as early as 20 days and rarely more than 50 days post-transplantation. This is well illustrated from inspecting the time of onset of CMV disease in the placebo arm of a study of ganciclovir prophylaxis in liver transplantation, which is shown as **Fig. 12.4**.[23] Many symptoms, such as fever, night sweats, fatigue and myalgia, are non-specific. Retinitis can be pathognomonic, but it is relatively rarely seen in the transplant population. Respiratory distress, noticed at first on exercise, is a sinister symptom and measurement of oxygen saturation and blood gas analysis (the former at both rest and

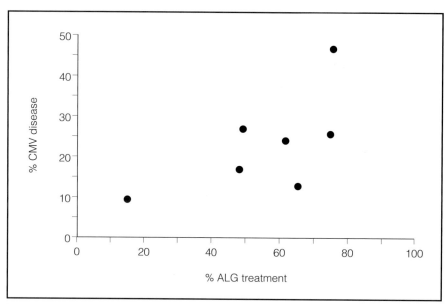

Figure 12.3 • Percentage of patients who were diagnosed as suffering from CMV disease plotted against the percentage of patients who received antilymphocyte globulin (ALG) (total of 522 patients). Original data from refs 15–21.

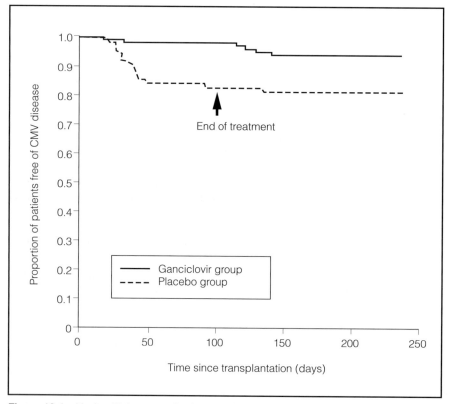

Figure 12.4 • Kaplan–Meier curves for the cumulative probability of freedom from CMV disease with time after transplantation.

exercise) can give an early clue to pulmonary involvement. Gastrointestinal disease, with dysphagia, diarrhoea, abdominal pain and nausea, is relatively frequent. One group has suggested that epigastric pain that decreases in the supine position is a clinical entity unique to CMV gastritis.[24] Symptomatic adrenal insufficiency is most unusual, probably because transplant recipients usually receive supraphysiological doses of corticosteroids. Allograft dysfunction due to CMV disease, although not rare, is usually not so severe as to cause direct symptoms.

The potential morbidity due to CMV disease is illustrated in an audit for one calendar year carried out in a renal transplant programme in the UK where, at the time, no prophylactic strategy was employed.[14] The distribution of CMV disease by donor and recipient serology is shown in **Table 12.1**. Of the 17 patients in the high-risk group, two had fever and neutropenia managed as outpatients; the rest required inpatient care for 5–31 (average 6.7) days and seven received intravenous ganciclovir. One patient received full support in the intensive therapy unit (ITU) but died despite this. A retrospective study from Canada examined 11 renal transplant recipients with organ-specific CMV disease and compared the resource utilisation and costs for the first year with a control group of recipients without CMV disease. The patients with CMV disease averaged 59 inpatient days in the first year post-transplantation compared with 22 in the control group. Overall, the cost of care was 2.5 times higher in the group with CMV disease.[25]

Because of the multiple human strains of CMV, seropositive organ recipients are at risk of primary disease when receiving a graft from a seropositive donor with a different strain of virus. In this situation the clinical syndrome is usually less severe than the consequences of primary infection in a seronegative recipient and disease onset is delayed to approximately 3 months post-transplantation.[26] Seropositive recipients of seronegative grafts (and blood products) can develop CMV disease due to reactivation of latent virus. Again, this is usually mild compared with primary infection and is often delayed to approximately 3 months post-transplantation. Leucodepleted blood or properly filtered whole blood has a very low risk for transmission of CMV disease.[27]

Since effective prophylactic strategies (as discussed below) have become available the pattern of disease seen in clinical practice has changed. Important from a clinical perspective is that prophylactic treatment can delay the onset of primary CMV disease, and this diagnosis must now be considered for 2 to 3 months after the end of prophylactic treatment, whereas before the era of prophylactic therapies primary CMV disease was very rarely diagnosed more than 3 months post-transplantation.

CMV infection may decrease cell-mediated immunity, reducing the T-helper to suppressor cell ratio as well as the ability of T cells to produce interferon gamma (IFN-γ). This may allow coincident infection with other viral, bacterial, protozoal or fungal organisms. CMV infection can also be immunostimulatory, which is possibly of importance in autoimmune disorders. It has been implicated in idiopathic thrombotic thrombocytopenic purpura as well as in systemic lupus erythematosus (SLE) where seropositivity is 14 times more prevalent in affected compared with control patients.[28] Cross-reactivity

Table 12.1 • Results of an audit on the incidence of CMV disease during one calendar year at the Manchester Royal Infirmary

Donor	Recipient	N	No. CMV disease	Deaths (all)
+	−	31	17	1
+	+	34	1	1
−	+	26	1	2
−	−	23	0	0
Unknown		2	0	0
Total		116	19	4

between autoimmune targets in lupus and CMV RNA has been demonstrated, indicating that molecular mimicry or an influence on gene expression may be possible disease-promoting mechanisms.[29] Despite the immunosuppressive effects of acute CMV disease it has long been recognised that CMV infection can be coincident with acute allograft rejection. CMV increases the expression of major histocompatibility (MHC) class I and II molecules on both vascular endothelial cells and tubular epithelial cells, which are the targets for renal allograft rejection. CMV infection has also been linked to the production of IFN-γ by T cells[30,31] as well as the increased expression of MHC molecules. Another mechanism of enhanced rejection may be the fact that CMV encodes for a molecule similar to MHC class I antigens and there is some homology between the immediate early-region protein of CMV and some class II antigens. These effects would be expected to enhance alloantigen-dependent rejection. CMV infection would be expected to enhance the alloantigen-independent pathway of rejection by increasing co-stimulatory molecules on antigen-presenting cells, vascular endothelial cells, tubular epithelial cells and T lymphocytes.[32,33] There has been considerable recent interest regarding the potential role of CMV infection in both native coronary and cardiac allograft atherosclerosis. In 60 histological specimens of re-stenoses after native coronary angioplasty, 38% were found to have accumulated a high amount of the tumour suppressor protein p53, and this correlated with the presence of CMV in the lesions. Furthermore, smooth muscle cells from the re-stenoses grew a CMV protein IE84, which in cell culture inhibited p53 function, and the authors suggest this mechanism may have contributed to the relapse.[34] It has been known for some while that in the rat aortic allograft model (of chronic vascular rejection) early infection with rat CMV doubled the rate of smooth muscle proliferation and arteriosclerotic alterations in the intima. Late infection had almost no effect.[35] In this model immunosuppression had a protective (rather than detrimental) effect on vascular wall histology.[36] In a whole organ model in the rat, CMV significantly enhanced the development of renal chronic allograft rejection.[37] In other experiments, again in the rat allograft model, treatment with ganciclovir blocked the early adventitial inflammation and reduced

smooth-muscle cell proliferation.[38] With this background there has been considerable interest in a post hoc analysis of a subset from a randomised placebo-controlled study that reviewed 149 consecutive heart transplant patients who received either intravenous ganciclovir or placebo for the initial 28 days after transplantation.[39] The patients underwent annual arteriography. Twenty-eight could not be evaluated, mostly because of early death. The rest had a mean follow-up of 4.7 years. The actuarial incidence of transplant coronary artery disease was 43% vs. 60% in the ganciclovir-treated vs. control group. One of the independent risk factors for coronary artery disease was no ganciclovir treatment (relative risk 2.1, confidence interval 1.1–5.3, $P = 0.04$). The report has considerable limitations: as the authors emphasise, it was not designed to address the specific question explored in this paper. Despite the intriguing animal in vivo and human data, there is other in vitro work showing that the induction of cell-surface adhesion molecules after CMV infection is not influenced by ganciclovir.[40] A study of 60 liver transplant recipients who had at least four blood specimens for PCR analyses showed that acute infection with CMV and HHV6 was associated with acute graft rejection.[41]

Also in a liver transplant population of 33 patients who received 57 transplants, persistent CMV infection detected by serial PCR measurements was significantly associated with graft loss through chronic rejection. However, there was no significant correlation between primary infection or symptomatic disease and chronic rejection, although the sample size was small.[42]

An attempt was made to separate the impact of acute rejection and CMV disease on long-term graft survival in a single-centre study of 1339 renal transplant recipients. Multivariate analysis showed that CMV disease appeared to influence long-term graft survival but only when coupled with the occurrence of acute rejection.[43]

Interesting and contradictory data with regard to the incidence of CMV infection on long-term outcome come from a series of 1545 cadaveric renal transplant recipients divided into two groups on the basis of availability of ganciclovir. In the early group, the survival of the D+R− patients was significantly poorer.[44] However, close inspection of the survival curves shows no change in late graft survival before and after the use of universal antiviral prophylaxis, arguing against a role for CMV infection causing late graft loss in renal transplantation.

Large registry data, as well as single-centre studies, demonstrate a reduced graft and patient survival, both in individuals who experience CMV disease and those who are at highest risk of primary infection. In the UNOS database, which includes over 47 000 patients, the renal graft survival disadvantage if the donor is CMV-positive compared with seronegative donors was of the order of 4% at 3 years.[45] Some single centres have reported even more deleterious outcome,[46] but others have shown no such effects.[47]

Clearly this area of the potential impact of acute CMV disease on chronic rejection needs to be addressed by prospective studies.

Prevention of CMV disease

The management of CMV disease post-transplantation has been comprehensively reviewed (see, e.g., ref. 48). Guidelines were published in 1998 focusing on adult patients undergoing renal transplantation.[49] More current are guidelines regarding post-renal transplant care published by the European Dialysis and Transplant Association, which include the management of CMV disease[50] as well as guidelines published by the British Transplantation Society.[51]

CMV matching to avoid transplanting a seronegative individual with a seropositive organ is an option. Given the life-sustaining nature of successful heart, lung and liver transplantation it is rarely practised in these settings. In renal, pancreas or small-bowel transplantation it is an option that could be exercised in a situation where there is more than one equally good candidate for a single organ. Widespread adoption of CMV matching would disadvantage younger recipients as they are more likely to be CMV-negative and could compromise HLA matching or other criteria that are currently used to determine allocation.

 CMV disease has been reported in 8% of renal, 29% of liver, 25% of heart and 39% of heart/lung transplant recipients.[52]

Because of this frequency and the associated morbidity and mortality risk there has been considerable interest in developing an effective prophylactic strategy. Such strategies in transplantation have been reviewed,[52,53] but this area has recently undergone rapid change.

One difficulty when comparing the results of trials using different prophylactic regimens has been the variable degree of immunosuppression used, as well as the fact that the definition of CMV disease has varied from trial to trial. To some extent this problem can be overcome by ignoring the actual rate of CMV disease that is seen in either the treated or placebo arm (as this is greatly influenced by immunosuppression) and rather concentrating on the ratio of disease seen in the two groups. This approach would allow, for example, a treatment that reduced the frequency of CMV disease (however diagnosed or defined) to a tenth in the treatment arm to be declared as better than one which only reduced the frequency of disease to one half.

VACCINATION

One attractive option for prophylaxis would be vaccination. Early attempts using the Towne virus strain in renal transplant recipients were unsuccessful: 9 of the 37 seronegative patients failed to produce antibodies. In those transplanted in the placebo group 71% developed disease compared with 56% in the vaccinated cohort.[54] There have been other studies, when the rate of CMV disease was reduced from approximately 50 to 37% and severe disease from 29 to 5% in the vaccinated patients.[55,56]

The heterogeneity of strains has limited the success of vaccination as a prophylactic strategy. Vaccines directed against envelope glycoproteins have generated renewed interest, as these are well conserved between strains. The biggest public health return would be achieved by vaccinating young women prior to reproductive age.

CMV GLOBULIN

CMV hyperimmune globulin, which is obtained from multiple donors with high-titre IgG, was the first treatment shown to offer worthwhile prophylaxis to seronegative recipients of renal transplants from seropositive donors.[57] Of four studies enrolling between 28 and 76 patients only one was placebo-controlled, the rate of CMV disease being roughly halved by prophylaxis with hyperimmune globulin.[58] The number of patients enrolled who were in the high-risk donor-positive/recipient-negative group was either very small (at two) or not stated. A randomised placebo-controlled study was conducted in seven centres in the British Isles sponsored by Alpha-Therapeutics. Seronegative recipients of seropositive renal transplants from seropositive donors were studied. Forty-three patients were in the treated and 36 in the placebo groups. An intention-to-treat analysis showed a halving of the incidence of CMV disease (from 42% to 21%, $P = 0.03$), the need to use ganciclovir (from 36% to 19%, $P = 0.04$) and episodes of hospital admission to manage CMV (from 39% to 19%, $P = 0.02$). Another study with a placebo arm, this time in liver transplants, randomised 141 patients, a third of whom received OKT3. The hyperimmune globulin provided significant overall protection from severe disease. However, no protection in the recipient-negative/donor-seropositive subgroup was seen.[59] Intravenous treatment is generally less convenient for the patient or healthcare provider, but it does have the advantage of allowing compliance to be documented and on occasions this may have significant advantages. The treatment carries the theoretical risk of transmitting blood-borne viruses (or variant CJD in the UK).

INTERFERON

Interferon was shown to reduce CMV excretion in pilot studies, but unfortunately with little clinical benefit in renal transplant recipients.[60,61] In a formal, blinded, placebo-controlled study in renal transplant recipients a similar result was obtained.[62]

ACICLOVIR AND VALACICLOVIR

Aciclovir was shown to reduce CMV disease by about two-thirds, from 28% to 8% in a prospective, placebo-controlled, randomised clinical trial in renal transplantation with approximately 50 patients in each arm.[63]

In liver transplantation, results have been contradictory, with some or no benefit seen.[64,65] Others have shown no benefit in renal transplantation if ATG/OKT3 was used.[66] Aciclovir will probably only provide significant protection in less high-risk recipients such as seropositive recipients of sero-positive organs or where the degree of initial immunosuppression is relatively modest, for example in that small percentage of renal recipients who receive ciclosporin A monotherapy.

In a randomised prospective controlled trial in renal transplant recipients, aciclovir versus ganciclovir prophylaxis was compared. The patients received quadruple immunosuppression including OKT3. In the D+/R– subgroup, 5 of 13 receiving aciclovir but 0 of 14 receiving ganciclovir experienced CMV disease during the 12-week period of prophylaxis. However, post-prophylaxis three patients in the ganciclovir group developed evidence of infection.[67]

Valaciclovir, which has a three- to five-fold improved oral bioavailability compared with aciclovir, will greatly influence the use of aciclovir in this setting.

Valaciclovir has been shown to offer nearly complete protection against CMV disease for 90 days in a prospective, double-blind, placebo-controlled, randomised clinical trial involving 616 renal transplant recipients treated for 90 days.[68] The frequency of CMV disease in the control group was low, probably because those recruited included all serotype combinations with the exception of both donor- and recipient-negative. A retrospective study compared 60 renal transplant recipients who had received oral ganciclovir with 70 who had received valaciclovir. There was no difference in the incidence of CMV infection in the two groups: 6.9% vs. 5.4%.[69]

GANCICLOVIR

A variety of regimens using intravenous ganciclovir have been used,[70,71] but this approach has been largely superseded by the use of oral ganciclovir.

Despite its extremely poor bioavailability (in the order of 5% of the oral dose) a prospective, double-blind, placebo-controlled, randomised clinical trial in liver transplant recipients (only excluding donor and recipient seronegative) showed that the drug reduced morbidity due to CMV disease to about a quarter of that seen in the placebo group. Total CMV disease was reduced from 19% to 5% ($P < 0.001$), CMV syndrome from 12% to 4% ($P = 0.006$) and tissue-invasive CMV disease from 9% to 1% ($P < 0.001$).[23] Others have shown similar results in renal transplants.[72] Despite these results in recipients of renal and liver allografts it is important to emphasise that where the degree of immunosuppression is more intense, as is typical in cardiac transplantation, intravenous ganciclovir for 28 days has been shown in placebo-controlled, randomised trials to significantly reduce the incidence of CMV disease, but there was no impact on the highest risk (D+R–) subgroup.[54] In this situation other strategies may be necessary, such as the combination of antiviral drugs and CMV hyperimmune globulin or perhaps more protracted intravenous drug therapy.

A variety of new antiviral drugs have been studied for efficacy against CMV disease, most usually in the HIV-positive population. Some, such as cidofovir, have unwelcome side effects such as nephrotoxicity. However, in the setting of ganciclovir resistance the agent clearly may be of considerable value.[73]

VALGANCICLOVIR

Valganciclovir, which offers with oral therapy similar blood levels to those achieved by intravenous dosing of ganciclovir, is likely to represent a significant advance in both treatment and prophylaxis. The key data come from a randomised, double-blind, multicentre study that recruited 364 adult CMV-negative recipients of CMV-positive solid-organ transplants. The recipients were randomised 2:1 to valganciclovir or ganciclovir prophylaxis. The randomisation was stratified among the organ types, with 177 liver, 120 kidney, 11 kidney/pancreas and 56 heart transplant recipients recruited. Treatment started within 10 days of transplantation and continued until 100 days post-surgery. The frequency of CMV disease in the first 6 months was 17.2% in the valganciclovir-treated group compared with 18.4% in the ganciclovir-treated group. After 6 months CMV disease occurred in 5% in the valganciclovir group and 3.2% in the ganciclovir group.[74] The frequency of detectable viral load[75] and drug-associated side effects was similar. At the end of the prophylactic period 198 valganciclovir-treated and 103 ganciclovir-treated patients were assessed for the presence of ganciclovir-resistant CMV strains. The incidence was 0% for the valganciclovir patients and 1.9% in patients who had received ganciclovir.[76]

Another strategy is to use CMV hyperimmune globulin in combination with antiviral drugs; this has been done in an uncontrolled study and it is difficult to assess the utility of this approach.[77]

With all prophylactic strategies there are disadvantages. To be effective they rely on good patient compliance. The treatments add to the cost of the procedure and are likely to be unnecessary for a proportion of individuals who receive them. The agents have a side effect profile that must be balanced against the advantages of therapy. Although viral resistance has been rarely reported in the transplant literature,[78–81] this may reflect under-reporting. When PCR was used, 22% of 45 AIDS patients receiving long-term ganciclovir developed resistance,[82] and a figure of 20% has been reported for solid-organ transplant recipients.[83] The duration of therapy is likely to be important.[84] Ganciclovir resistance is shown in about 8% of patients with AIDS after 3 months of treatment;[85] this rises to 11% with resistant blood or urine CMV isolates at 6 months, and 28% at 9 months.[86]

PRE-EMPTIVE PROPHYLAXIS

Finally, blanket prophylactic therapy has the potential to delay the onset, but not necessarily reduce the frequency of CMV disease. This is a particular problem in heavily immunosuppressed patient groups. An abstract reported that 3 months of ganciclovir treatment in a renal transplant population (70% of whom had received ALG) delayed the onset of CMV disease until on average 164 days post-transplantation, but by the end of 1 year nearly half of the patients who received ganciclovir had experienced CMV disease.[87]

Because of the disadvantages of universal prophylaxis there has been considerable interest in pre-emptive prophylactic strategies. In this approach patients are regularly surveyed, and when judged to be at high risk of developing CMV disease, are treated, in the past with intravenous ganciclovir and more recently with oral valganciclovir. Clearly, for this to be a successful approach, a reliable predictor of imminent disease is required. A variety of markers for predicting future CMV disease have been described; these include the shell viral assay, PCR in serum, PCR from peripheral blood mononuclear cells, PCR from whole blood and antigenaemia. These have sensitivities varying from 57% to approximately 85% and specificities ranging from about 35% to 90%. The absolute levels of viraemia that are recommended as the threshold to start pre-emptive therapy will depend upon the assay used. Most real-time PCR assays (which are popular because of simplicity and high level of automation) report lower levels of viraemia compared to the hybrid capture assay. Clearly the proportion of individuals who receive 'unnecessary' pre-emptive treatment versus those who develop CMV disease because they are not offered pre-emptive therapy will depend on where the threshold is set. In a study of 52 asymptomatic renal transplant recipients, 23 (44%) had positive CMV PCR tests on at least one occasion. However, only two (8.6%) developed CMV disease. This study suggests that in this population with this assay a treatment strategy based on positive PCR alone would treat a large fraction of patients who did not necessarily require it. The authors reassuringly noted that none of the 29 patients who were continuously negative for CMV PCR developed CMV disease. However, as a guide to treatment in this setting it seems somewhat limited.[88]

In a study of 71 liver transplant recipients, CMV antigenaemia occurred in 22 and these patients were randomised into two groups. One received intravenous ganciclovir for 7 days and the other oral ganciclovir for 10 weeks. Although of low power because of the sample size, it is striking that CMV disease was only seen in one patient (in the intravenous treatment arm).[89] Two different strategies were adopted in a study of renal transplant recipients who were CMV seropositive at the time of transplantation. In one centre patients received oral ganciclovir for 12 weeks or until antigen-negative for two consecutive weeks, whereas in the other centre the regimen consisted of intravenous ganciclovir for 2 weeks and then oral treatment until antigen-negative for two consecutive weeks. Of 192 patients who met the study criteria 90 were treated. All patients cleared antigen and there were no relapses. The single case of tissue-invasive CMV disease occurred in the intravenous treatment group.[90]

A retrospective study of 39 renal, 28 liver and 23 heart transplant recipients noted 26 episodes of infection managed according to a pre-emptive strategy; 4 of these developed CMV disease but there were no deaths.[91] However, there were also 21 episodes 'not managed according to the programme'

where 12 individuals developed CMV disease and there were two deaths possibly related to CMV infection. This emphasises that when a pre-emptive strategy is put in place it is most important that all the elements for monitoring it appropriately are available.

A randomised, placebo-controlled trial in 69 liver transplant patients gave 8 weeks of oral ganciclovir therapy when CMV DNA was detected by PCR.[92] CMV disease developed in 12% of recipients receiving placebo compared with 0% of those receiving ganciclovir. This trial provides the strong evidence base for using pre-emptive therapy to control CMV disease in recipients of liver transplants.

In a study of renal transplant recipients, 38 patients were evaluable from a group randomised to be monitored by CMV pp65 antigen tests; if a positive test was demonstrated the patients received oral ganciclovir, and these were compared with a control group of 38 who received treatment if they developed disease. No patients in the pre-emptive group but nine in the control group developed CMV disease.[93]

The duration of pre-emptive antiviral therapy is important, although the optimum length has not been formally tested. Some authors have recommended a minimum period of 4 weeks.[93] It would be logical to be guided by serial measurements of the viral load, and others have recommended that treatment continue for 2–4 weeks after the patient has tested negative for viral replication.[94]

The authors of a recent review, when discussing prophylaxis for CMV and solid-organ transplantation, pointed out that 'conventional prophylactic therapy has a large body of supportive controlled clinical studies demonstrating efficacy and cost-effectiveness. The strategy also has the advantage of preventing other herpes viruses. There is some information to suggest that prophylactic therapy may benefit by reducing rejection'.[95] The authors contrast pre-emptive therapy, pointing out 'it is limited by reliance on intensive surveillance with significant logistic difficulties and requiring good patient compliance. There is ambiguity about the best surveillance method and at the present time purported benefits of pre-emptive therapy, such as decreased cost, fewer adverse medication effects and less antiviral resistance have not been proven in head to head clinical studies'. However, in the counterpoint article published side by side, the problems of prophylaxis were discussed.[96] These include preventing antigen presentation to the immune system so that patients are at risk of developing disease once the drug is stopped, and the encouragement of drug resistance. It is clear that either approach can be adopted and both require close collaboration between the clinical team and laboratory-based specialists.

Treatment

It is important to recognise early CMV disease and consider prompt reduction of immunosuppression. This option is clearly easier for renal rather than life-sustaining transplants. In the situation where there is fever and a white blood count greater than 3.0, withdrawal of azathioprine or mycophenolate from a triple-drug regime may be all that is required. If the patient is unwell (as opposed to merely uncomfortable) or there is evidence of organ dysfunction, most commonly with marrow suppression, hepatitis, gastrointestinal ulceration or pneumonitis, it is appropriate to reduce (to about a half) the dose of calcineurin inhibitor and treat with intravenous ganciclovir. Early concerns about neutropenia coincident with ganciclovir have become less of an anxiety with increased use and the appreciation that marrow suppression due to CMV disease can be treated by the drug. A common clinical problem is deciding on the duration of intravenous treatment after resolution of clinical signs. The author's practice has been to continue to treat with intravenous ganciclovir for 5 days after the patient becomes afebrile. In the future DNA PCR may offer an objective measure of the degree of viraemia and may help to decide the duration of treatment. Very high doses of intravenous hyperimmune globulin (0.5 g/kg body weight) have been used for treatment but with the advent of effective antiviral drugs this approach is now rarely used.[97–99] An important clinical point is the fact that infection with other co-pathogens in an immunosuppressed patient with CMV is common, and another infection in addition to CMV disease should always be ruled out by repeated clinical examination and special investigations. In one subgroup analysis of a randomised controlled trial in cardiac transplant recipients, intravenous ganciclovir was shown to decrease the incidence of fungal infections.[100]

 Following successful treatment of CMV disease there is a significant risk of relapse with recurrent CMV disease, as has been reported for a variety of organ recipients.[101–106]

In one study on kidney and kidney/pancreas recipients relapse was seen in approximately one-third of patients after treatment of the initial episode with ganciclovir.[107] Foscarnet is reserved as second-line therapy partly because of significant risk of nephrotoxicity and electrolyte disturbances especially an acute reduction in ionised calcium. There is a smaller risk of neurotoxicity particularly grand mal convulsions. However, there is extensive clinical experience of the agent, mostly for treating patients with AIDS. The drug remains a valuable option in the presence of virus resistant to ganciclovir.[109,109]

Cidofovir is also reserved as second-line therapy, particularly in the presence of renal impairment. The drug is an option in the presence of virus resistant to other agents.[73]

EPSTEIN–BARR VIRUS

Background

Epstein–Barr virus (EBV) is a gamma human herpesvirus widespread in all populations. There are two types, although no difference in disease syndromes can be attributed to infection with either strain. The virus attaches to the C3d complement component receptor so that effects are confined to cells carrying this receptor. These include squamous epithelial cells of the oropharynx and genital tract and, most critically for the immunocompromised, B lymphocytes. The main target of EBV is CD21+ B cells, and after infecting these cells the virus circularises and then equilibrates into one of several types of latent infection. In this latent state the virus and cell differ in the expression of a variety of latency-associated proteins like LMP-1, LMP-2a and LMP-2b, and EBNA 1, 2, 3a, 3b, 3c and LP. The latency-associated proteins protect the target B cell from cell death and cause proliferation, which is normally controlled by the mammal's T-cell response. LMP-1 is thought to be the main onco-genic protein of EBV but it is not clear what triggers the cellular activation seen in post-transplant lymphoproliferative disorder (PTLD). Also in latency form, EBV early RNAs (EBERs) are expressed. The function of these EBERs is not known.

Convention states that infection of squamous epithelial cells results in lysis with cell death and viral shedding. It has proved very difficult to unequivocally confirm squamous cell infection and it is possible primary infection occurs in B lymphocytes that are 'traversing' the oropharyngeal mucosa. In B lympho-cytes a latent infection occurs and the virus has the capability of transforming these cells into con-tinuously growing immortalised lymphoblastoid lines. The latent infection can be transformed into a lytic phase in cell culture by agents that provoke B-cell differentiation. Most commonly subclinical infection occurs in early childhood, followed by a lifelong carrier state. Antibodies develop, as do EBV-specific CD8-cytotoxic T lymphocytes. The neutralising antibodies may be especially important to prevent re-infection. Latent infection of some circulating B cells can be detected and an ongoing lytic infection of the squamous epithelium of the oropharynx, and to a lesser extent the genital tract, may release virus. Virus in buccal fluid provides the main route for transmission via droplets or direct contamination. In students sequential salivary samples for EBV-specific IgG and IgA were obtained before, during and after two important examinations. In these asymptomatic individuals a statistically significant increase in the EBV antibody titre was detected. This suggests, as with other latent viruses, that the individual is in a perpetual state of fluctuating suppression of the virus.[110]

In developing countries almost all children are infected in the first 5 years of life. In the developed world roughly 50% of young adults may be sero-negative. The seronegative adults are commonly infected when they become sexually active; again a large fraction of infections are subclinical but in the rest fever, anorexia, headache, fatigue and a sore throat with inflammation of the oropharynx may be accompanied by generalised lymphadenopathy, particularly of the cervical region. Hepato-splenomegaly may be present. The disease duration is variable but most patients recover to resume normal activities within 2 weeks.

Endemic Burkitt's lymphoma is confined to parts of Africa and Papua New Guinea where the tem-perature is always over 16°C and rainfall in excess of 55 cm per year. It is probable that Epstein–Barr virus infection in conjunction with an alteration in immunological control due to hyperendemic malaria results in the B-cell proliferation. The tumour is usually multifocal, most commonly in the area of the jaw, and symptoms are due to local mass effects. Cytotoxic chemotherapy is the treatment of choice, and sustained remission is common, although success is at least in part dependent on the tumour load at presentation.

Undifferentiated nasopharyngeal carcinoma, which has a marked predominance in the Southern Chinese and some other ethnic groups, always carries the Epstein–Barr virus genome in affected cells, and individuals with this tumour show a specific pattern of antibody response to Epstein–Barr virus antigen. It is accepted that the virus has a major role in causing the tumour, but that a cofactor, probably acquired from either the diet or snuff, is also necessary for its development. In early disease radio-therapy can result in prolonged remission.

The precise role of Epstein–Barr virus infection in Hodgkin's disease and other T-cell lymphomas has not been elucidated but there is strong epidemiological evidence that primary infection with the virus outside childhood is a major risk factor for the development of tumour in a subgroup of patients with lymphomas. In B-cell neoplasms, T-cell lymphomas, undifferentiated nasopharyngeal carcinomas and gastric cancers there are multiple extra chromosomal copies of the circular EBV genome in the tumour cells and expression of EBV-encoded latent genes. There is considerable interest in understanding the contribution of EBV infection to the malignant phenotype and the hope that such understanding will allow innovative alternative therapeutic approaches.[111]

In patients with HIV infection, usually prior to the development of AIDS, hairy leucoplakia manifests most usually as white patches on the tongue. The squamous epithelial cells contain large amounts of replicating Epstein–Barr virus and the condition can be arrested by continuous treatment with aciclovir.

Patients with AIDS can develop Burkitt's lymphoma as well as a large-cell lymphoma; the latter is often atypical with many extranodal sites involved. There is a strong association of these lymphomas with Epstein–Barr virus, which is close to 100% in patients with cerebral lymphoma. Radiotherapy and chemotherapy can be used but results are usually disappointing, in part due to the significant comorbid disease burden.

Post-transplant lymphoproliferative disorder (PTLD)

RISK FACTORS AND BASIC BIOLOGY

It has long been recognised that solid-organ transplant recipients are at a greatly increased risk of lymphoproliferative tumours. New approaches to the diagnosis and management of PTLD have been reviewed recently.[112–114]

The majority were noted to be of B-cell origin and subsequently shown to contain the Epstein–Barr virus genome and express viral proteins on the cell surface.[115–117]

The incidence of PTLD in renal transplant recipients is of the order of 1%,[118] a risk of lymphoma approximately 20 times greater than that seen in the general population. In adults CMV disease increases the risk of subsequent PTLD approximately seven-fold. An incidence ranging from 6% to 11% for early lymphomas has been reported in heart and heart–lung allograft recipients.[118–121] In small-bowel transplantation PTLD has occurred in 10% of patients reported to the International Registry, and at the University of Pittsburgh 5 years' experience showed a significant age-related risk at 9% in adults and 27% in paediatric recipients.[122]

In a single renal transplant centre a univariate analysis showed that the only significant risk factor for late-onset PTLD in 20 cases in a population of 928 patients was EBV seronegative status at the time of grafting.[123] The risk ratio showed approximately a seven-fold increased risk. This strongly suggests that at least a proportion of late-onset PTLD follows primary infection, most probably acquired from social contact.

Immunoglobulin sequencing of stored tissue from 13 cases of PTLD in recipients of a variety of solid-organ and stem-cell transplants showed 11 tumours that were monoclonal or biclonal.[124] The majority showed randomly mutated or sterile mutations, which would normally be incompatible with B-cell survival. These PTLD tumours are therefore genotypically (as well as phenotypically) different from the mature antigen-selected B cells that arise from EBV infection in vitro and are presumably similar to the circulating EBV-infected B cells seen in vivo. The iatrogenic interference with natural T-cell function therefore not only allows an increase in EBV-infected B cells but permits the expansion of subsets of malignant B cells that would normally not survive.

The major risk factor for PTLD in solid-organ transplantation has long been thought to be the degree of immunosuppression. A spectacularly high incidence of PTLD was seen following the introduction of ciclosporin A but was greatly reduced after drug-level monitoring became widespread and doses were reduced to about one-fifth of that initially used.[125,126] The incidence of PTLD with tacrolimus is probably comparable to that seen with ciclosporin A, at least in the adult population.[127,128] In recipients of heart transplants the major risk factor is multiple courses of OKT3, an antibody that profoundly depletes circulating CD3+ T lymphocytes.[129] In a registry of 50 000 renal and heart transplant recipients the incidence of PTLD was 0.15% in patients not receiving OKT3/ATG against approximately 0.50% in patients receiving these agents.[118] In a comprehensive Australasian registry, among nearly 8000 renal transplant recipients the incidence of lymphoma was 1.21% in those given serotherapy and 0.9% in those who had not.[130] This increased risk following antibody treatment has been confirmed by several series.[118,130–133] That the degree or intensity of any particular immunosuppressive agent is principally responsible for PTLD has been challenged by others, at least in a renal transplant population. In a single centre in a careful retrospective study all 22 cases of PTLD seen (in 866 transplants) in the period 1969–2002 were reviewed. When comparing patients treated using prednisolone and azathioprine with those on ciclosporin monotherapy there was no difference in incidence of PTLD. Also the routine introduction of OKT3 and polyclonal anti-T-cell globulin did not lead to a significant change. The numbers at risk are, however, relatively small and the incidence of

PTLD low. The study therefore may have little power to detect a difference in incidence. In more recent data, where a protective effect of treatment with mycophenolate mofetil is postulated, it is difficult to interpret as the duration of follow-up must be small (and is obviously unequal) to allow adequate assessment.[134] The therapeutic suppression of natural cytotoxic T-cell activity is likely to be the cause of uncontrolled EBV-driven proliferation of B cells.[135,136] Initially, a polyclonal expansion would be expected, but single clones with a growth advantage will predominate as time passes.

In another setting, chronic antigen stimulation by infection can provoke lymphoma. The example is the association of longstanding gastritis with *Helicobacter pylori* infection and subsequent mucosa-associated lymphoid tissue lymphoma of the stomach.[137] In this example, eradication of the *H. pylori* (and so, presumably, removal of the antigenic challenge) has been associated with cure.[138,139] Others have suggested that the degree of chronic antigen stimulation from the solid organ transplant is a possible oncogenic factor in PTLD.[140]

The incidence of PTLD is influenced by several variables. Besides the intensity of immuno-suppression – particularly T-cell depleting – these include age, with children more at risk compared with adults; also, those who experience a primary infection are more at risk compared with those at risk of reactivation; moreover, the type of allograft also influences the degree of risk. Recipients of T-cell-depleted bone marrow grafts are at the highest risk, then recipients of intestinal grafts, then heart–lung transplants and then recipients of kidney or liver transplants.[141]

The experience of PTLD in intestinal transplantation is clearly different from that in the general solid-organ transplant population. Authors from the Pittsburgh centre have emphasised both the very high frequency, at nearly one-third of children with an intestinal transplant, and that the risk did not relate to recipient serostatus prior to transplantation. This is different from that seen in most other solid-organ transplants, where the seronegative recipient of the seropositive organ is at most risk.[142] In addition, the simultaneous occurrence of PTLD and rejection of the small bowel is a particular problem and contrasts with that seen in solid-organ transplants, where rejection is rare until regression of tumour (coincident with reduction in immuno-

suppression) is seen.[143] The phenomenon of acute rejection and PTLD may explain the very high mortality rate of 50% in small-bowel recipients, which is worse than is typically seen in this condition when it is complicating liver, renal or cardiac transplants.[144] The experience in bone marrow transplantation is instructive, as PTLD is uncommon (less than 1%[145]) in a situation where immunosuppression is intense. However, if there has been treatment with OKT3 or T-cell depletion of donor marrow, the incidence doubles from approximately 12 to 24%.[146,147] All these clinical observations emphasise that potent T-cell immuno-suppression is an important modifiable risk factor for PTLD.

The primary infection that is seen in a sero-negative recipient of a graft from a seropositive donor is an important risk factor for PTLD, with a 76-fold increase in the risk ratio in this situation.[148,149] In the paediatric transplant recipient population this is a particular problem, partly because of the high proportion who are seronegative and partly because more initial immunosuppression is used.[127, 148,150]

CLINICAL PRESENTATION OF PTLD

PTLD is heterogeneous, but most cases can be divided into one of four syndromes:

1. An acute infectious mononucleosis-like disease with marked constitutional upset and rapid enlargement of tonsils and cervical nodes. This is the most typical pattern in the first year post-transplantation.[151]
2. A fulminant presentation, which can occur within weeks of transplantation and presents with widespread infiltrative disease and multiorgan involvement. This has a grave prognosis.[121,152]

   The above two presentations are more common in young recipients who are seronegative and receive a seropositive organ.
3. Isolated or multiple tumours (the latter often involving the allograft and on occasions being mistaken for rejection) is the usual pattern more than 1 year post-grafting. The presentation is usually of indolent disease and visceral, nodal and extranodal tumours are the rule. Gastrointestinal involvement is relatively common, as are pulmonary nodules; the lung may be the only site involved.[153,154]

4. EBV-negative B-cell PTLD occurs in approximately 10% of cases. This is usually of late onset and clinically resembles non-Hodgkin's lymphoma. No associated virus has yet been identified.[153,154]

Aggressive EBV-negative T-cell lymphomas have a poor prognosis and occur late at a median of 15 years following transplantation.[155] In solid-organ transplantation approximately 80% of PTLD is due to recipient B-cell expansion (unlike that seen in bone marrow transplants). Donor B-cell-associated PTLD tends to be allograft-limited and may have a better prognosis.

Clinical features do not correlate with the histological classification. At the present time the histological division is into hyperplastic, polymorphic and lymphomatous PTLD.[156–158] It may be that recipients of different solid-organ transplants experience different morbidity from PTLD. In a review of 400 lung transplant recipients there were ten cases of PTLD in contrast to what is seen in liver, renal and orthotopic liver transplantation where only one patient responded to immunosuppressive withdrawal alone. Radiotherapy and rituximab resulted in 'a favourable response' but both patients treated with chemotherapy died.[159]

As more sensitive techniques have been employed it has been appreciated that tissue found to be polyclonal by immunophenotyping contains monoclonal subpopulations.[157,158] Similarly, as techniques have improved, the percentage of tumours shown to contain EBV has increased. The pathology and classification have been reviewed and summarised.[153,160]

PREVENTION OF PTLD

In children receiving orthotopic liver transplants reactivation of EBV may be coincident with PTLD.[161] However, a large proportion, perhaps as much as 90%, of PTLD in the first year is triggered by a primary EBV infection that occurs within 4 months of a seronegative recipient receiving a graft from a seropositive donor.[162,163] Where practicable, avoiding such mismatches, especially in particularly high-risk groups, is a sensible tactic.

There has been progress towards creating a vaccine directed against an envelope glycoprotein (gp340)[164,165] and a latent membrane protein.[166]

This approach would be of value in several areas of medicine. It has been pointed out that the best prospects for a vaccine against EBV-related human disease is one to prevent infectious mononucleosis. The prospects for immunotherapy against nasopharyngeal carcinoma are poor. The commercial prospects for a vaccine that protects against nasopharyngeal carcinoma are less promising compared with those for one that protects against Hodgkin's disease.[167]

TREATMENT OF PTLD

Immunosuppression reduction

The mainstay of management is the drastic reduction or cessation of immunosuppressive treatment.[121,168] This is clearly easier in kidney transplantation, where dialysis treatment is an option, compared with life-sustaining transplants. Such a strategy allows the recovery of the recipient's cytotoxic T-cell-directed EBV surveillance mechanism. When the tumour is life threatening, rapid and near complete withdrawal of immunosuppression is usually practised. The likelihood of response appears to be related to the interval since the transplant. In one series of heart transplant recipients, 80% of patients presenting less than 1 year post-transplantation responded to a reduction in immunosuppression, whereas no patients presenting more than 1 year post-transplantation responded.[120] Despite attempts to predict from histology or clinical features, there is as yet no reliable way of determining which tumours will respond to immunosuppressive dose reduction.[151,155,158] In the event of remission the immunosuppressive therapy will need to be restarted, preferably prior to graft rejection. It is usual to restart immunosuppression at reduced dosage and it is reassuring that recurrent disease is relatively rare.[169]

The speed and degree of immunosuppression reduction is difficult to judge. In renal transplantation, withdrawal of azathioprine or mycophenolate is advised, as is reduction of prednisolone to approximately 10 mg/day. Ciclosporin A or tacrolimus can be reduced in a stepwise fashion by about one-fifth every 2 weeks. The patients are closely monitored, for evidence both of graft rejection and of tumour growth or regression. It is common to stop ciclosporin A or tacrolimus dose reduction when approximately 30% of the initial dose is reached.

EBV viral load estimation

In the recent past there have been considerable efforts directed towards estimating viral load and using this measure to direct prophylaxis and treatment strategies. Oropharyngeal shedding of Epstein–Barr virus was prospectively measured in a cohort of renal and heart transplant recipients. Higher levels, which were inhibited by intravenous ganciclovir and aciclovir, were found in patients with PTLD.[170] However, salivary viral loads do not correlate with the amount of EBV in peripheral blood lymphocytes.[171] Various authors have used semiquantitative PCRs to evaluate EBV viral load in different transplant recipient groups.[172–174] Although in general an increased load was found in patients with PTLD there is overlap of the measurements between affected and unaffected individuals. The EBV viral load can be more accurately measured using quantitative competitive PCR,[175] and there appears to be a cut-off that discriminates between recipients who do and those who do not have PTLD. Because of technical considerations there is interest in quantifying EBV DNA in serum rather than peripheral blood lymphocytes, and a sensitivity of 83% and specificity of 100% for one such test has been reported.[176] One potential use for such a measure, as well as diagnosis, is to monitor the response to therapy. There have been reports of such serum monitoring in only 19 patients after reduction of immunosuppression.[143,177] Generally a fall in viral load is seen and this correlates with clinical resolution. The utility of this approach for fine adjustment of immunosuppressive medication is yet to be determined. In particular, the authors point out that rebound of the viral load is common but relapse of PTLD relatively rare at less than 10%;[143,177] therefore measurement of viral load after recovery from PTLD is not recommended. At least in allogenic stem cell transplantation the value of circulating EBV DNA load is unproven in patients at relatively low risk of PTLD. One week prior to the development of PTLD EBV load was low and the same as levels seen in patients who did not develop the disease.[178]

EBV DNA loads can be measured in whole blood, plasma and peripheral blood lymphocytes (PBLs) by competitive PCR. There appears to be a good correlation between whole blood and PBL loads ($R^2 > 0.9$) but poor correlation between plasma and PBL load ($R^2 = 0.5$).[179]

In a patient (post-bone marrow transplantation) with multiple CNS lesions that at biopsy were proven to be PTLD, no circulating EBV DNA was detected until 6 weeks after the initial presentation. This suggests that isolated CNS involvement may well not be excluded by negative circulating EBV DNA.[180]

In a study of 96 cardiothoracic transplant recipients EBV DNA and viral mRNA transcripts in peripheral blood mononuclear cells (PBMs) were measured serially for a median of 268 days post-transplant.[181] Although overall post-transplant levels were significantly higher than those seen pre-transplant in healthy controls, EBV DNA levels in non-immunosuppressed patients with infectious mononucleosis and in patients with PTLD were significantly higher than those seen in healthy controls. Importantly, however, 12 individuals post-transplant had isolated readings equal in magnitude to those seen in PTLD. Single measurements are therefore not predictive of PTLD development. The range of values seen is well illustrated by **Fig. 12.5**.

In an important study 45 children post-liver transplantation were followed. Twenty-eight patients experienced primary EBV infection and some of these went on to develop PTLD. The primary EBV infection was detected soon after transplantation at a median of 6 weeks.[182] Importantly, the peak viral load measured in the 4 weeks following primary infection could not discriminate between the seven individuals who went on to develop PTLD and those who had an uncomplicated course (**Fig. 12.6**). The authors point out that in healthy subjects during primary EBV infection there is a rapid development of cellular immunity principally by CD8+ cytotoxic T cells targeted against EBV antigens.[183,184] The authors, as well as measuring the viral load, for the first time in solid-organ transplant recipients measured specific anti-EBV T lymphocytes. All seven patients with PTLD had both high viral load and low levels of anti-EBV-specific T lymphocytes. No patients developed PTLD, irrespective of the viral load, when the number of anti-EBV-specific T lymphocytes was above a certain low threshold. **Figure 12.7** shows three scenarios. In the first (**Fig. 12.7a**) a recipient who is EBV positive at the time of grafting has a moderate viral load and low levels of anti-EBV T lymphocytes. In the second (**Fig. 12.7b**) an uncomplicated primary EBV infection shows a rapid and simultaneous rise in

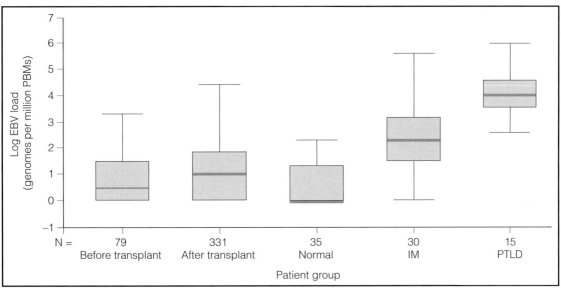

Figure 12.5 • EBV genome copy number in peripheral blood of control groups and transplant recipients. Boxes represent interquartile range containing 50% of values. Lines extending from the boxes represent the highest and lowest values (excluding outlines). Bold lines in each box represent the median. IM, infectious mononucleosis. From Transplantation 2002; 74:197, with permission.

circulating virus and EBV T lymphocytes. The third scenario (**Fig. 12.7c–f**) is where individuals develop PTLD with a rise in circulating virus to a high level without a rise in anti-EBV T lymphocytes. This paper emphasised strongly the regulatory function of cytotoxic T lymphocytes.[182]

Given that the rise in EBV viral load can be detected by serial measurements prior to PTLD,[172–174] there is interest in monitoring to allow pre-emptive prophylaxis to avoid PTLD. Unfortunately, the optimal prophylactic strategy is far from clear. In a study of 40 paediatric liver transplant recipients, 14 were high risk (donor EBV-positive/recipient seronegative) and the rest (all combinations) were assigned as low risk. The high-risk group received 100 days of intravenous ganciclovir and the other group 2 weeks of intravenous ganciclovir, and then both groups had 2 years of oral aciclovir treatment. Asymptomatic patients with a high viral load received intravenous ganciclovir (or continued on it) and adjustment of tacrolimus trough level to 2–5 ng/mL. The overall incidence of PTLD was 5% and this compared favourably to a historical experience of 10% in this centre with a tacrolimus-based immunosuppressive regimen.[143] It is not possible to separate the effect of the antiviral drugs and the reduction in immunosuppression on the

outcome. Serial viral load monitoring in the hands of experts who follow a particular high-risk group of patients may be most useful for predicting those at low risk of developing disease. In 30 children followed with serial measurements, 12 with a median follow-up of approximately 16 months who had persistent low values did not develop PTLD.[185] As with other reports, however, a high viral load did not reliably predict PTLD. In this series 5 out of 18 children with a high viral load on at least one occasion developed PTLD.

In bone marrow transplant recipients it is striking that the viral load as assessed by the number of genome copies per peripheral blood mononuclear cells (PBMCs) of individuals who were disease free after treatment of PTLD overlapped with healthy seropositive controls. Most important for understanding the pathology is the observation that the patients treated with rituximab showed an immediate and dramatic decline in viral loads. This confirms the localisation of viral genomes in PBMCs to B cells. However, the rapid decline in circulating viral load post-rituximab occurred even in those patients in whom PTLD progressed. The number of genome copies per PBMC is similar to that seen in healthy controls. So the increase in viral load in PTLD is due to an increase in circulating

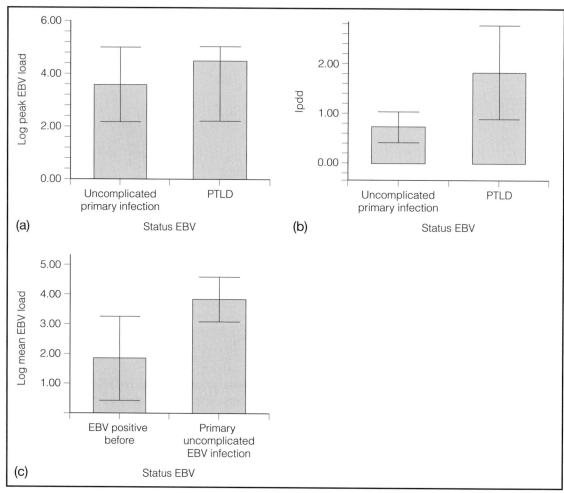

Figure 12.6 • Because post-transplant lymphoproliferative disease (PTLD) is related mainly to primary Epstein–Barr virus (EBV) infection and because the aim was to determine an early marker of PTLD risk, data analysis focused on the month after primary EBV infection detection. **(a)** In patients with primary EBV infection post-transplant for whom two or three consecutive elispot and simultaneous viral load were available in the 2 or 4 weeks after the first sign of infection, respectively, we compared the maximal viral loads (peak EBV load) measured in this period. No significant difference was observed between the ten patients with uncomplicated primary EBV infection and the seven patients with (PTLD) on follow-up ($P = 0.085$). Respective geographic means are 5505 and 29 977 EBV copies/µg DNA. **(b)** For the same period and patients, increase of the EBV load and simultaneous increase of the anti-EBV-specific T lymphocytes (EBV-TL) were compared as numerator/denominator of an index, the I_{ptld}. The I_{ptld} was statistically higher in patients with subsequent PTLD, illustrating a defect of the specific cellular immune response in this condition. Respective means are 0.73 and 1.83 in patients with primary uncomplicated EBV infection and with PTLD respectively ($P < 0.001$). **(c)** Finally, we compared long-term viral load between ten patients who were EBV positive before transplant and 16 patients with primary uncomplicated EBV infection post-transplant. A mean viral load was calculated for each patient. In patients who had primary infection post-graft, the mean included only viral loads measured from 6 months post-acute infection, after viral load stabilization. Patients with previous immunity had a significantly lower viral load than those with primary infection. Respective geographic means are 72 and 7244 EBV copies/µg DNA ($P < 0.001$). From Transplantation 2002; 73:1609, with permission.

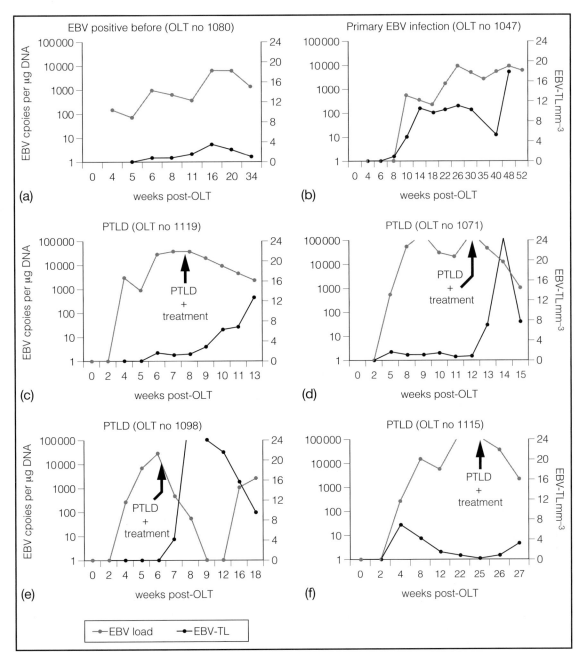

Figure 12.7 • Patients' follow-up included regular determination of the EBV load in peripheral blood mononuclear cells (PBMC) by real-time quantitative PCR and of the anti-EBV-specific T lymphocytes (EBV-TL) level by elispot detection of IFN-γ-secreting PBMC after 22 h stimulation with the autologous LCL. Clinical symptoms, lymphoproliferation occurrence, and response to treatment were correlated to these parameters. Representative follow-up of patients is illustrated by **(a)** one patient with EBV immunity before transplant; **(b)** one patient with uncomplicated primary EBV infection post-transplant; and **(c–f)** four patients with post-transplant lymphoproliferative disease (PTLD) after primary EBV infection (c–e, early onset; f, late onset). From Transplantation 2002; 73:1606, with permission.

B lymphocytes. That the disease can progress despite falling viral load (due to the disappearance of circulating B lymphocytes) after rituximab emphasises the clinical difference in behaviour between EBV-infected PBMCs and neoplastic cells in PTLD.[186]

INTERFERON ALPHA

Remission has been achieved with interferon alpha in a number of cases,[187,188] but as the treatment regimens are complicated and the number of patients treated is small it is difficult to be sure of the value of this approach, although it does appear to be well tolerated.

ANTIVIRAL THERAPY

Although intravenous ganciclovir or aciclovir will inhibit the lytic phase and decrease the degree of oropharyngeal shedding of virus,[170] the number of EBV-infected cells in peripheral blood is not altered by aciclovir treatment.[189] The problem is that the antiviral drugs only inhibit lytic activity and typically only about 1% of the cells infected are in a lytic phase. Antiviral drugs would not be expected to influence the malignant B cells, which are responsible for the PTLD syndrome. Consistent with this is the observation of several authors that viral loads increase while patients are receiving aciclovir or ganciclovir.[143,144,173,189] However, it is possible but unproven that inhibiting the lytic phase may influence progression of PTLD. Aciclovir, valaciclovir and ganciclovir have only weak in vitro activity against Epstein–Barr virus, whereas the activity of foscarnet is good, and that of cidofovir is high. Antiviral drugs that are active against CMV may have some effect in PTLD as CMV will produce B-cell-stimulating cytokines. But antiviral agents have been generally disappointing for both prophylaxis and treatment of PTLD. Aciclovir and ganciclovir are not likely to be effective because in EBV-associated lymphoid tissue the viral thymidine kinase enzyme is not reliably encoded. In contrast foscarnet is directed against viral DNA independent of the presence of viral thymidine kinase. Remission following treatment with foscarnet has been reported.[190]

Despite the theoretical lack of efficacy of oral antiviral drugs on EBV it is possible that prophylaxis may protect because of effects on herpesviruses, whose replication could contribute by increased immunosuppression to EBV-derived B-cell proliferation. In lung transplant recipients PTLD is a particular problem. In a single centre none of 15 recent EBV-seronegative recipients who received either aciclovir, valaciclovir or ganciclovir developed PTLD. This compares favourably with an overall rate of PTLD of 4.2% (7 of 167) in a historical group. The data are difficult to interpret, however, as induction antibody treatment was stopped more or less coincident with the oral antiviral prophylaxis, the duration of follow-up was different, and the analysis also ignored early fatalities.[191]

Cidofovir is an acyclic nucleoside phosphonate analogue that may exert an antiproliferative activity in some human virus-related tumours. In cell lines infected with EBV cidofovir significantly reduced oncogene expression and enhanced radiation-induced apoptosis.[192] This may offer a novel anticancer strategy.

PASSIVE IMMUNISATION

Another approach is to use passive immunisation with anti-EBV antibody.[193] The influence of intravenous immunoglobulin in conjunction with treatment with intravenous ganciclovir as well as a 'when possible' reduction in immunosuppression in paediatric intestinal transplant recipients has been reported in a preliminary fashion.[194] Thirteen of 18 children with elevated viral loads were successfully managed. However, five patients developed PTLD and three of these had received the pre-emptive prophylaxis. The incidence of five cases of PTLD in 30 patients followed with the pre-emptive protocol should be compared with an incidence of 12 in 30 recipients who received their transplants prior to the initiation of the protocol. The development of trials to assess properly the value of this and other approaches will not be easy given the small number of patients involved. But they are probably necessary before the widespread adoption of any particular strategy. There are various ways of measuring EBV viral load in blood and a need to standardise methodology.[195]

SURGERY

Unlike non-Hodgkin's lymphoma in general, PTLD can be cured by surgical excision or irradiation of strictly localised lesions. This approach should be considered in circumstances where this situation arises.[120,152,194]

CHEMOTHERAPY

Conventional chemotherapy, which is usually employed after failure of immunosuppressive dose reduction and the use of antiviral drugs to influence the progression of PTLD, has a poor reputation in the transplant community. A mortality rate of 70% has been reported for patients treated more than 1 year after transplantation.[120,196] Refractory tumour or sepsis are major problems.[121,196,197] There are issues peculiar to particular grafts with regard to chemotherapy. The cardiac allograft appears to be especially sensitive to doxorubicin cardiomyopathy, and the lung allograft to injury following treatments that include bleomycin. In cardiac recipients somewhat more encouraging was a mortality rate of 25% with remission in the rest at a median follow-up of 64 months using a cytotoxic regimen that was principally ProMACE-CytaBOM.[152] Preliminary findings of the combination of cyclophosphamide, prednisolone and rituximab in six solid-organ transplant recipients have been reported. At median follow-up of 1 year there were five patients in complete remission and one who showed an initial partial response but then subsequently died of progressive disease.[198] From this report it is difficult to recommend this approach at this time.

ANTI-CD20 MONOCLONAL ANTIBODIES

Anti-B-cell monoclonal antibodies are an attractive treatment option and were found to be successful in a European multicentre trial.[197,199,200] They are not immunosuppressive; the antigens targeted are such that they deplete the EBV-infected cell pool; they are lysed by antibody-dependent cellular cytotoxicity. The original European studies used anti-CD21 and anti-CD24, which are no longer commercially available. They were well tolerated with a transient fever and reduction in polymorphonuclear cells. A reduction in immunoglobulin was the only important haematological side effect noted. Approximately 50% of patients developed antimouse antibody and this presumably will limit efficacy in the medium term. More recently, a CD20 antibody has undergone commercial development for use in indolent B-cell lymphomas.[201] This is an attractive therapeutic option in part because it is extremely well tolerated. There have now been several reports of its use in the setting of solid-organ transplants. Although many reports suggest a good outcome there is always the problem of publication bias. Clinicians are less likely to report therapeutic failures. It is rare for rituximab to be used as the single approach and most patients also have an alteration in their immunosuppressive therapy making it difficult to separate the relative contribution of the various strategies.[202,203]

Prophylactic rituximab has been employed in 49 patients following stem-cell transplantation.[204] In this report patients were regularly monitored for circulating EBV by PCR. Seventeen patients who showed an elevated level (defined on viral reactivation) received a single infusion of rituximab. It is only possible to compare with historical controls and the numbers are small, but the incidence of lymphoproliferative disorder decreased from 18% to 4%. The mortality rate due to PTLD in those who developed PTLD fell from 26% to 0%. Whether this approach will be useful in solid-organ transplant recipients is unclear.

CYTOTOXIC T LYMPHOCYTES

Given the incomplete efficacy and side effect profile of antiviral agents, monoclonal antibodies, radiotherapy and chemotherapy, and the risk of graft loss associated with immunosuppressive reduction, it is appealing to attempt to treat PTLD with immunotherapy. The optimal approach would be to augment the EBV-directed cytotoxic T lymphocytes. In bone marrow transplantation, where the tumorous cells are of donor origin, CD4 and CD8 T-lymphocyte clones can be expanded in vitro with cytokines and repetitive infusion offers good prophylaxis, although the role in treatment remains unclear.[205] The utility of this approach in bone marrow recipients has been reviewed.[206–208] In bone marrow recipients PTLD has been controlled by the infusion of peripheral blood leucocytes from the donor.[209] Unfortunately, this is less likely to be of significant use for recipients of solid-organ transplants because the T-cell response is MHC-limited. In addition, the majority of PTLDs arise from B cells of recipient (rather than donor) origin. Of more interest to the solid-organ situation has been the experience of four patients with EBV-associated PTLD who were treated by autologous lymphokine-activated killer cells expanded ex vivo by interleukin-2,[210] an approach that at present is experimental. The use of recipient cytotoxic T lymphocytes, which are stimulated in the same way as used for the bone marrow donors,[205] is in its early stages. For practical reasons peripheral white blood cells taken at the time of the diagnosis of PTLD are used and after approximately 30 days of cell culture and purification are available for infusion. The dose schedule and efficacy have yet to be reported. A further approach is to use a bank of blood donors of known HLA type and generate cell lines of cytotoxic T lymphocytes. The idea would be to try to match the HLA type of a recipient with PTLD to the bank and select a cell line that achieved good killing of the tumour cells but little (non-specific) killing of the patient's white blood cells.[193,211] In a child with EBV-positive PTLD following intestinal and liver transplantation one infusion of partially HLA-matched EBV-specific cytotoxic T lymphocytes grown ex vivo from an EBV-positive blood donor was administered. The infusion was well tolerated and there was no evidence of graft vs. host disease. There were no detectable EBV-specific cytotoxic T lymphocytes prior to the infusion but high numbers 24 hours post-infusion. There was rapid clinical resolution and the patient remains in complete remission 2 years later.[212]

CENTRAL NERVOUS SYSTEM INVOLVEMENT

PTLD with CNS involvement is particularly difficult to treat. There have now been a few cases treated with rituximab. In a recipient of a haemopoietic stem cell transplant with symptomatic peripheral lymphoma and CNS involvement the combination of rituximab and cidofovir was associated with complete remission, and this combination should be considered for solid-organ transplant recipients with rare but difficult to treat CNS involvement.[213]

RE-TRANSPLANTATION

The issue of re-transplantation has been explored in only a few publications. In life-sustaining transplants, such as the liver, this must be a rare event.[214,215] The largest series is possibly that of five individuals who underwent renal re-transplantation.

In this series no relapse or de novo PTLD was reported.[216] It is likely, however, that the number of cases are under-reported.

Key points

- CMV is one of the most important opportunistic infections seen in the first year post-transplantation.
- Prophylactic or pre-emptive treatments to reduce the incidence of disease are available and popular, especially in seropositive-donor/seronegative-recipient cases.
- The mainstay of treatment for CMV disease is intravenous ganciclovir and reduction of immunosuppression. Coinfection with other pathogens is common.
- Molecular biological techniques are making the discrimination of CMV disease from latent infection easier.
- CMV disease (or even infection) may have a role in chronic transplant dysfunction.
- The majority of PTLDs in solid-organ transplantation are due to EBV-driven recipient B-lymphocyte proliferation.
- The risk is increased in seronegative recipients of seropositive organs, children, recipients receiving anti-T-cell serotherapy and recipients of intestinal grafts.
- The measurement of viral load alone appears to be of little use in predicting disease. But the measurement of both viral load and anti-EBV cytotoxic T cells shows considerable promise.
- The mainstay of treatment is immunosuppressive dose reduction. Antiviral drug therapy has so far shown very limited benefit and there are theoretical reasons why it may be ineffective.
- Monoclonal antibody therapy directed against cells expressing CD20 is safe and a promising treatment strategy.
- Cytotoxic T cells are at present in development and may be of significant clinical use in the future.

REFERENCES

1. Wentworth BB, Alexander ER. Sero epidemiology of infections due to members of the herpes virus group. Am J Epidemiol 1971; 94(6):496–507.

2. Halling VW, Maine GT, Groettum CM et al. Clinical evaluation of a new recombinant antigen-based cytomegalovirus immunoglobulin M immunoassay in liver transplant recipients. Transplantation 2001; 71(3):395–7.

3. Evans PC, Gray JJ, Wreghitt TG et al. Comparison of three PCR techniques for detecting cytomegalovirus (CMV) DNA in serum, detection of early antigen fluorescent foci and culture for the diagnosis of CMV infection. J Med Microbiol 1999; 48(11):1029–35.

4. Landry ML, Ferguson S, Cohen K et al. Effect of delayed specimen processing on cytomegalovirus antigenemia test result. J Clin Microbiol 1995; 33:257–9.

5. Pillay D, Charman H, Lok K et al. Detection of cytomegalovirus by a rapid culture system: a comparison of monoclonal antibodies in a clinical setting. J Virol Methods 1992; 40:219–24.

6. Grundy JE, Ehrnst A, Einsele H et al. A three-center European external quality control study of PCR for detection of cytomegalovirus DNA in blood. J Clin Microbiol 1996; 34:1166–70.

7. Einsele H, Ehninger G, Hebart H et al. Polymerase chain reaction monitoring reduces the incidence of cytomegalovirus disease and the duration and side effects of antiviral therapy after bone marrow transplantation. Blood 1995; 86: 2815–20.

8. Emery VC, Sabin CA, Cope AV et al. Application of viral-load kinetics to identify patients who develop cytomegalovirus disease after transplantation. Lancet 2000; 355:2032–6.

9. Aitken C, Barrett-Muir W, Millar C et al. Use of molecular assays in diagnosis and monitoring of cytomegalovirus disease following renal transplantation. J Clin Microbiol 1999; 37(9):2804–7.

10. Imbert-Marcille BM, Cantarovich D, Ferre-Aubineau V et al. Usefulness of DNA viral load quantification for cytomegalovirus disease monitoring in renal and pancreas/renal transplant recipients. Transplantation 1997; 63(10):1476–81.

11. Rautenberg P, Lubbert C, Weers W et al. Evaluation of the AmpliSensor PCR and the SHARP signal detection system for the early prediction of symptomatic CMV infection in solid transplant recipients. J Clin Virol 1999; 13(1–2):81–94.

12. Abecassis MM, Koffron AJ, Kaplan B et al. The role of PCR in the diagnosis and management of CMV in solid organ recipients: what is the predictive value for the development of disease and should PCR be used to guide antiviral therapy? Transplantation 1997; 63(2):275–9.

13. Shutze WP, Kirklin JK, Cummings OW et al. Cytomegalovirus hemorrhoiditis in cardiac allograft recipients. Transplantation 1991; 51:918–22.

14. Newstead CG. Cytomegalovirus disease in renal transplantation. Nephrol Dial Transplant 1995; 10(1):68–73.

15. Pass RF, Whitley RJ, Diethelm AG et al. Cytomegalovirus infection in patients with renal transplants: potentiation by antithymocyte globulin and an incompatible graft. J Infect Dis 1980; 142:9–17.

16. Bia MJ, Andiman W, Gaudio K et al. Effect of treatment with Cyclosporin versus Azathioprine on incidence and severity of cytomegalovirus infection post transplantation. Transplantation 1985; 40: 610–14.

17. Rubin RH, Cosmi AB, Hirsch MS et al. Effects of antithymocyte globulin on cytomegalovirus infection in renal transplant recipients. Transplantation 1981; 31:143–5.

18. Hoitsra AJ, Wetzels JF, Berden JH et al. Anti-rejection treatment with antithymocyte globulin in renal transplant recipients treated with Cyclosporin as basic immunosuppression. Transplant Proc 1988; 20(5 suppl. 6):12–13.

19. Metselaar HJ, Rothbarth PH, Wenting GJ et al. Mononuclear subsets during cytomegalovirus disease in renal transplant recipients treated with Cyclosporin and rabbit antithymocyte globulin. J Med Virol 1986; 19:95–100.

20. Weir MR, Irwin BC, Maters AW et al. Incidence of cytomegalovirus disease in cyclosporine-treated renal transplant recipients based on donor/recipient pretransplant immunity. Transplantation 1987; 43:187.

21. Snydman DR, Werner BG, Heinze-Lacey B et al. Use of cytomegalovirus immune globulin to prevent cytomegalovirus disease in renal-transplant recipients. N Engl J Med 1987; 317(17):1049–54.

22. Snydman DR, Werner BG, Tilney NL et al. Final analysis of primary cytomegalovirus disease prevention in renal transplant recipients with a cytomegalovirus immune globulin: comparison of the randomized and open-label trials. Transplant Proc 1991; 22:1357–60.

23. Gane E, Saliba F, Valdecasas GJ et al. Randomised trial of efficacy and safety of oral ganciclovir in the prevention of cytomegalovirus disease in liver-transplant recipients. The Oral Ganciclovir International Transplant Study Group. Lancet 1997; 350(9093):1729–33.

24. Giladi M, Lembo A, Johnson BL Jr. Postural epigastric pain: a unique symptom of primary cytomegalovirus gastritis? Infection 1998; 26(4):234–5.

25. McCarthy JM, Karim MA, Krueger H et al. The cost impact of cytomegalovirus disease in renal transplant recipients. Transplantation 1993; 55(6):1277–82.

26. Grundy JE, Lui SF, Super M et al. Symptomatic cytomegalovirus infection in seropositive kidney recipients: reinfection with donor virus rather than reactivation of recipient virus. Lancet 1988; 2(8603):132–5.

27. Sayers MH, Anderson KC, Goodnough LT et al. Reducing the risk for transfusion-transmitted cytomegalovirus infections. Ann Intern Med 1992; 116:55.

28. Rider JR, Ollier WE, Lock RJ et al. Human cytomegalovirus infection and systemic lupus erythematosus. Clin Exp Rheumatol 1997; 15(4): 405–9.

29. Lord PC, Rothschild CB, DeRose RT et al. Human cytomegalovirus RNAs immunoprecipitated by multiple systemic lupus erythematosus antisera. J Gen Virol 1989; 70(9):2383–96.

30. Arbustini E, Morbini P, Grasso M et al. Human cytomegalovirus early infection, acute rejection, and major histocompatibility class II expression in transplanted lung. Molecular, immunocytochemical, and histopathologic investigations. Transplantation 1996; 61(3):418–27.

31. Tuder RM, Weinberg A, Panajotopoulos N et al. Cytomegalovirus infection amplifies class I major histocompatibility complex expression on cultured human endothelial cells. J Heart Lung Transplant 1994; 13:129–38.

32. Yilmaz S, Koskinen PK, Kallio E et al. Cytomegalovirus infection-enhanced chronic kidney allograft rejection is linked with intercellular adhesion molecule-1 expression. Kidney Int 1996; 50(2):526–37.

33. Ito M, Watanabe M, Kamiya H et al. Changes of adhesion molecule (LFA-1, ICAM-1) expression on memory T cells activated with cytomegalovirus antigen. Cell Immunol 1995; 160(1):8–13.

34. Speir E, Modali R, Huang E et al. Potential role of human cytomegalovirus and p53 interaction in coronary restenosis. Science 1994; 265:391–4.

35. Lemstrom KB, Bruning JH, Bruggeman CA et al. Cytomegalovirus infection enhances smooth muscle cell proliferation and intimal thickening of rat aortic allografts. J Clin Invest 1993; 92(2):549–58.

36. Lemstrom KB, Bruning JH, Bruggeman CA et al. Triple drug immunosuppression significantly reduces immune activation and allograft arteriosclerosis in cytomegalovirus-infected rat aortic allografts and induces early latency of viral infection. Am J Pathol 1994; 144(6):1334–47.

37. Koskinen PK, Yilmaz S, Kallio E et al. Rat cytomegalovirus infection and chronic kidney allograft rejection. Transplant Int 1996; 9(suppl. 1):S3–S4.

38. Lemstrom KB, Bruning JH, Bruggeman CA et al. Cytomegalovirus infection-enhanced allograft arteriosclerosis is prevented by DHPG prophylaxis in the rat. Circulation 1994; 90:1969–78.

39. Valantine HA, Gao SZ, Menon SG et al. Impact of prophylactic immediate posttransplant ganciclovir on development of transplant atherosclerosis. Circulation 1999; 100:61–6.

40. Craigen JL, Grundy JE. Cytomegalovirus induced up-regulation of LFA-3 (CD58) and ICAM-1 (CD54) is a direct viral effect that is not prevented by ganciclovir or foscarnet treatment. Transplantation 1996; 62:1102–8.

41. Griffiths PD, Ait-Khaled M, Bearcroft CP et al. Human herpesviruses 6 and 7 as potential pathogens after liver transplant: prospective comparison with the effect of cytomegalovirus. J Med Virol 1999; 59(4):496–501.

42. Evans PC, Soin A, Wreghitt TG et al. An association between cytomegalovirus infection and chronic rejection after liver transplantation. Transplantation 2000; 69 (1):30–5.

43. Humar A, Gillingham KJ, Payne WD et al. Association between cytomegalovirus disease and chronic rejection in kidney transplant recipients. Transplantation 1999; 68(12):1879–83.

44. Schneeberger H, Aydemir S, Muller R et al. Hyper-immunoglobulin prophylaxis, monitoring and preemptive ganciclovir treatment eliminate the risk of CMV infection to improve patient and renal allograft survival. Transplant Int 2000; 13(suppl. 1): S354–8.

45. Hirata M, Terasaki PI, Cho YW. Cytomegalovirus antibody status and renal transplantation: 1987–94. Transplantation 1996; 62(1):34–7.

46. Ranjan D, Burke G, Exquenazi V et al. Factors affecting the ten-year outcome of human renal allografts. Transplantation 1991; 51(1):113–17.

47. Martin S, Morris D, Dyer PA et al. The association between cytomegalovirus-specific antibodies, lymphocytotoxic antibodies, HLA-DR phenotype and graft outcome in renal transplant recipients. Transplantation 1991; 51:1303–5.

48. Patel R, Snydman DR, Rubin RH et al. Cytomegalovirus prophylaxis in solid organ transplant recipients. Transplantation 1996; 61(9):1279–89.

49. Jassal SV, Roscoe JM, Zaltzman JS et al. Clinical practice guidelines: prevention of cytomegalovirus disease after renal transplantation. J Am Soc Nephrol 1998; 3:1697–708.

50. Berthous F, Abramowicz D, Bradley B et al. European best practice guidelines for renal transplantation (Part 1). Nephrol Dial Transplant 2000; 15(suppl. 7):71–4.

51. Newstead CG, Griffiths P, O'Grady J et al. Guidelines for the prevention and management of cytomegalovirus disease after solid organ

transplantation 2nd edn. British Transplantation Society, 2004.

52. Patel R, Snydman DR, Rubin RH et al. Cytomegalovirus prophylaxis in solid organ transplant recipients. Transplantation 1996; 61(9):1279–89.

53. Jassal SV, Roscoe JM, Zaltzman JS et al. Clinical practice guidelines: prevention of cytomegalovirus disease after renal transplantation. J Am Soc Nephrol 1998; 3:1697–708.

54. Plotkin SA, Friedman HM, Fleisher GR et al. Towne-vaccine-induced prevention of cytomegalovirus disease after renal transplants. Lancet 1984:i:528–530.

55. Plotkin SA, Higgins R, Kurtz JB et al. Multicenter trial of Towne strain attenuated virus vaccine in seronegative renal transplant recipients. Transplantation 1994; 58(11):1176–8.

56. Plotkin SA, Starr SE, Friedman HM et al. Effect of Towne live virus vaccine on cytomegalovirus disease after renal transplant. A controlled trial. Ann Intern Med 1991; 114(7):525–31.

57. Snydman DR, Werner BG, Heinze-Lacey B et al. Use of cytomegalovirus immune globulin to prevent cytomegalovirus disease in renal-transplant recipients. N Engl J Med 1987; 317(17):1049–54.

58. Snydman DR, Werner BG, Tilney NL et al. Final analysis of primary cytomegalovirus disease prevention in renal transplant recipients with a cytomegalovirus-immune globulin: comparison of the randomized and open-label trials. Transplant Proc 1991; 23(1 Pt 2):1357–60.

59. Snydman DR, Werner BG, Dougherty NN et al. Cytomegalovirus immune globulin prophylaxis in liver transplantation. Ann Intern Med 1993; 119(10):985.

60. Hirsch MS, Schooley RT, Cosimi AB et al. Effects of interferon-alpha on cytomegalovirus reactivation syndromes in renal-transplant recipients. N Engl J Med 1983; 308:1489–93.

61. Cheeseman SH, Rubin RH, Stewart JA et al. Controlled clinical trial of prophylactic human-leukocyte interferon in renal transplantation: effects on cytomegalovirus and herpes simplex virus infections. N Engl J Med 1979; 300:1234–49.

62. Lui SF, Ali AA, Grundy JE et al. Double-blind, placebo-controlled trial of human lymphoblastoid interferon prophylaxis of cytomegalovirus infection in renal transplant recipients. Nephrol Dial Transplant 1992; 7:1230–7.

63. Balfour HH Jr, Chace BA, Stapleton JT et al. A randomized, placebo-controlled trial of oral Acyclovir for the prevention of cytomegalovirus disease in recipients of renal allografts. N Engl J Med 1989; 320(21):1381–7.

64. Green M, Reyes J, Nour B et al. Randomized trial of ganciclovir followed by high-dose oral acyclovir vs ganciclovir alone in the prevention of cytomegalovirus disease in pediatric liver transplant recipients: preliminary analysis. Transplant Proc 1994; 26(1):173–4.

65. Saliba F, Eyraud D, Smauel D et al. Randomized controlled trial of acyclovir for the prevention of cytomegalovirus infection and disease in liver transplant recipients. Transplant Proc 1993; 25(1 Pt 2):1444–5.

66. Frey DN, Matas AJ, Gillingham KJ et al. Sequential therapy – a prospective randomized trial of MALG versus OKT3 for prophylactic immunosuppression in cadaver renal allograft recipients. Transplantation 1992; 54(1):50–6.

67. Rubin RH, Kemmerly SA, Conti D et al. Prevention of primary cytomegalovirus disease in organ transplant recipient oral ganciclovir or oral acyclovir prophylaxis. Transplant Infect Dis 2000; 2(3):112–17.

68. Nicol DL, MacDonald AS, Belitsky P et al. Reduction by combination prophylactic therapy with CMV hyperimmune globulin and Acyclovir of the risk of primary CMV disease in renal transplant recipients. Transplantation 1993; 55(4):841–6.

69. Yango A, Zanabli A, Morrisey P et al. A comparative study of prophylactic oral gancyclovir and valacyclovir in high-risk kidney transplant recipients. J Am Soc Transplant 2001; abstract 202.

70. Lowance D, Neumayer HH, Legendre CM et al. Valacyclovir for the prevention of cytomegalovirus disease after renal transplantation. International Valacyclovir Cytomegalovirus Prophylaxis Transplantation Study Group. N Engl J Med 1999; 340(19):1462–70.

71. Merigan TC, Renlund DG, Keay S et al. A controlled trial of ganciclovir to prevent cytomegalovirus disease after heart transplantation. N Engl J Med 1992; 326(18):1182–6.

72. Rondeau E, Bourgeon B, Peraldi MN et al. Effect of prophylactic ganciclovir on cytomegalovirus infection in renal transplant recipients. Nephrol Dial Transplant 1993; 3:858–62.

73. Chou SW. Cytomegalovirus drug resistance and clinical implications. Transplant Infect Dis 2001: 3(suppl. 2):20–4.

74. Pescovitz MD, Paya C, Humar A et al. Valganciclovir for prevention of CMV disease: 12 month follow up of a randomized trial of 364 D+/R− transplant recipients. Am J Transplant 2003; 3(suppl. 5):299.

75. Humar A, Paya C, Pescovitz MD et al. CMV virologic outcomes in D+/R− solid organ transplant recipients receiving valganciclovir vs ganciclovir prophylaxis. Am J Transplant 2003: 3(suppl. 5):430.

76. Boivin G, Goyette N, Gilbert C et al. Valganciclovir prophylaxis is not associated with the emergence of

cytomegalovirus UL97 and UL54 resistance mutations in solid organ transplant recipients: results from a multicenter trial. Am J Transplant 2003: 3(suppl. 5):431.

77. Brennan DC, Garlock KA, Singer GG et al. Prophylactic oral ganciclovir compared with deferred therapy for control of cytomegalovirus in renal transplant recipients. Transplantation 1997; 64(12):1843–6.

78. Knox KK, Drobyski WR, Carrigan DR. Cytomegalovirus isolate resistant to Ganciclovir and Foscarnet from a marrow transplant patient (letter). Lancet 1991; 337:1292–3.

79. Boivin G, Erice A, Crane DD et al. Ganciclovir susceptibilities of cytomegalovirus (CMV) isolates from solid organ transplant recipients with CMV viraemia after antiviral prophylaxis. J Infect Dis 1993; 168:332–5.

80. Slavin MA, Bindra RR, Gleaves CA et al. Ganciclovir sensitivity of cytomegalovirus at diagnosis and during treatment of cytomegalovirus pneumonia in marrow transplant recipients. Antimicrob Agents Chemother 1993; 36(6):1360–3.

81. Bhorade SM, Lurain NS, Jordan A et al. Emergence of ganciclovir-resistant cytomegalovirus in lung transplant recipients. J Heart Lung Transplant 2002; 21(12):1274–82.

82. Bowen EF, Emery VC, Wilson P et al. CMV PCR viraemia in patients receiving ganciclovir maintenance therapy for retinitis: correlation with disease in other organs, progression of retinitis and appearance of resistance. AIDS 1998; 12:605–11.

83. Limaye AP, Corey L, Koelle DM et al. Emergence of ganciclovir-resistant cytomegalovirus disease among recipients of solid-organ transplants. Lancet 2000; 356(9230):645–9.

84. Emery VC, Griffiths PD. Prediction of cytomegalovirus load and resistance patterns after antiviral chemotherapy. Proc Natl Acad Sci USA. 2000; 97:8039–44.

85. Drew WL, Miner RC, Busch DR et al. Prevalence of resistance in patients receiving ganciclovir for serious cytomegalovirus infection. J Infect Dis 1991; 163(4):716–19.

86. Jabs DA, Enger C, Dunn JP et al. Cytomegalovirus retinitis and viral resistance: ganciclovir resistance. CMV Retinitis and Viral Resistance Study Group. J Infect Dis 1998; 177(3):770–3.

87. Olyaei AJ, Wahba IM, Norman DJ et al. Incidence of CMV-disease beyond 90 days after gancyclovir prophylaxis: results from a cohort of high-risk renal transplant recipients. J Am Soc Nephrol 1999; 10:763A.

88. Benedetti E, Mihalov M, Asolati M et al. A prospective study of the predictive value of polymerase chain reaction assay for cytomegalovirus in asymptomatic kidney transplant recipients. Clin Transplant 1998; 12(5):391–5.

89. Singh N, Paterson DL, Gayowski T et al. Cytomegalovirus antigenemia directed pre-emptive prophylaxis with oral versus IV ganciclovir for the prevention of cytomegalovirus disease in liver transplant recipients. Transplantation 2000; 70:717–22.

90. Tinckam K, Djurdjev O, Stephens G et al. The efficacy of oral versus intravenously administered ganciclovir in the pre-emptive treatment of cytomegalovirus antigenemia in renal transplant recipients. American Society of Transplant Surgeons/American Society of Transplantation 2001.

91. Kunzle N, Petignat C, Francioli P et al. Preemptive treatment approach to cytomegalovirus (CMV) infection in solid organ transplant patients: relationship between compliance with the guidelines and prevention of CMV morbidity. Transplant Infect Dis 2000; 2:118–26.

92. Paya CV, Wilson JA, Espy MJ et al. Preemptive use of oral ganciclovir to prevent cytomegalovirus infection in liver transplant patients: a randomised, placebo-controlled trial. J Infect Dis 2002: 185(7):854–60.

93. Sagedal S, Nordal KP, Hartmann A et al. Preemptive therapy of CMV pp65 antigen positive renal transplant recipients with oral ganciclovir: a randomized, comparative study. Nephrol Dial Transplant 2003; 18:1899–908.

94. Ketteler M, Kunter U, Floege J. An update on herpes virus infection in graft recipients. Nephrol Dial Transplant 2003; 18:1703–6.

95. Hart GD, Paya CV. Prophylaxis for CMV should now replace pre-emptive therapy in solid organ transplantation. Rev Med Virol 2001; 11(2):73–81.

96. Emery VC. Prophylaxis for CMV should not now replace pre-emptive therapy in solid organ transplantation. Rev Med Virol 2001; 11:83–6.

97. Reed EC. Treatment of cytomegalovirus pneumonia in transplant patients. Transplant Proc 1991; 23(suppl. 1):8–12.

98. Emanuel D, Cunningham I, Jules-Elysee K et al. Cytomegalovirus pneumonia after bone marrow transplantation successfully treated with the combination of Ganciclovir and high dose intravenous immunoglobulin. Ann Intern Med 1988; 109: 777–82.

99. Crumpacker C, Marlowe S, Zhang JL et al. and the Ganciclovir Bone Marrow Transplant Treatment Group. Treatment of cytomegalovirus pneumonia. Rev Infect Dis 1998; 10(suppl. 3):538–46.

100. Wagner JA, Ross H, Hunt S et al. Prophylactic ganciclovir treatment reduces fungal as well as cytomegalovirus infections after heart transplantation. Transplantation 1995; 60(12):1473–7.

101. Falgas ME, Snydman DR, Griffith J et al. Clinical and epidemiological predictors of recurrent cytomegalovirus disease in orthotopic liver transplant recipients. Clin Infect Dis 1997; 25:314.

102. Van den Berg AP, Van Son WJ, Haagsma EB et al. Prediction of recurrent cytomegalovirus disease after treatment with ganciclovir in solid-organ transplant recipients. Transplantation 1993; 55:847.

103. Gould FK, Freeman R, Taylor CE et al. Prophylaxis and management of cytomegalovirus pneumonitis after lung transplantation: a review of experience in one center. J Heart Lung Transplant 1993; 12:695.

104. Kirklin JK, Naftel DC, Levine TB et al. Cytomegalovirus after heart transplantation. Risk factors for infection and death: a multiinstitutional study. J Heart Lung Transplant 1994; 13:394.

105. Manez R, Kusne G, Green M et al. Incidence and risk factors associated with the development of cytomegalovirus disease after intestinal transplantation. Transplantation 1995; 59:1010.

106. Sawyer MD, Mayoral JL, Gillingham KJ et al. Treatment of recurrent cytomegalovirus disease in patients receiving solid organ transplants. Arch Surg 1993; 128:165.

107. Humar A, Uknis M, Carlone-Jambor C et al. Cytomegalovirus disease recurrence after ganciclovir treatment in kidney and kidney-pancreas transplant recipients. Transplantation 1999; 67(1):94–7.

108. Erice A. Resistance of human cytomegalovirus to antiviral drugs. Clin Microbiol Rev 1999; 12:286–97.

109. Rubin RH. Prevention and treatment of cytomegalovirus disease in heart transplant patients. J Heart Lung Transplant 2000; 19:731–5.

110. Sarid O, Anson O, Yaari A et al. Epstein–Barr virus specific salivary antibodies as related to stress caused by examinations. J Med Virol 2001; 64(2):149–56.

111. Murray PG, Young LS. Epstein–Barr virus infection: basis of malignancy and potential for therapy. Expert Rev Mol Med 2001; 3:1–20.

112. Ambinder RF. Posttransplant lymphoproliferative disease: pathogenesis, monitoring and therapy. Curr Oncol Rep 2003; 5(5):359–63.

113. Green M. Management of Epstein–Barr virus-induced post-transplant lymphoproliferative disease in recipients on solid organ transplantation. Am J Transplant 2001; 1(2):103–8.

114. Loren AW, Porter DL, Stadtmauer EA et al. Post-transplant lymphoproliferative disorder: a review. Bone Marrow Transplant 2003; 31(3):145–55.

115. Randhawa PS, Jaffe R, Demetris AJ et al. Expression of Epstein–Barr virus-encoded small RNA (by the EBER-1 gene) in liver specimens from transplant recipients with post-transplantation lymphoproliferative disease. N Engl J Med 1992; 327:1710–14.

116. Hanto DW, Frizzera G, Purtilo DT et al. Clinical spectrum of lymphoproliferative disorders in renal transplant recipients and evidence for the role of Epstein–Barr virus. Cancer Res 1981; 41:4253–61.

117. Young L, Alfiere C, Hennessy K et al. Expression of Epstein–Barr virus transformation-associated genes in tissues of patients with EBV lymphoproliferative disease. N Engl J Med 1989; 321:1080–5.

118. Opelz G, Henderson R. Incidence of non-Hodgkin lymphoma in kidney and heart transplant recipients. Lancet 1993; 342:1514–16.

119. Swinnen LJ, Costanzo-Nordin MR, Fisher SG et al. Increased incidence of lymphoproliferative disorder after immunosuppression with the monoclonal antibody OKT3 in cardiac-transplant recipients. N Engl J Med 1990; 323:1723–8.

120. Armitage JM, Kormos RL, Stuart RS et al. Post-transplant lymphoproliferative disease in thoracic organ transplant patients: ten years of cyclosporine-based immunosuppression. J Heart Lung Transplant 1991; 10:877–86.

121. Nalesnik MA, Makowka L, Starzl TE. The diagnosis and treatment of posttransplant lymphoproliferative disorders. Curr Probl Surg 1988; 25:367–472.

122. Reyes J, Green M, Bueno J et al. Epstein Barr virus associated posttransplant lymphoproliferative disease after intestinal transplantation. Transplant Proc 1996; 28:2768–9.

123. Shahinian VB, Muirhead N, Jevnikar AM et al. Epstein–Barr virus seronegativity is a risk factor for late-onset posttransplant lymphoproliferative disorder in adult renal allograft recipients. Transplantation 2003; 75(6):851–6.

124. Timms JM, Bell A, Flavell JR et al. Target cells of Epstein–Barr virus (EBV)-positive post-transplant lymphoproliferative disease: similarities to EBV-positive Hodgkin's lymphoma. Lancet 2003; 361:217–23.

125. Starzl TE, Nalesnik MA, Porter KA et al. Reversibility of lymphomas and lymphoproliferative lesions developing under cyclosporin steroid therapy. Lancet 1984; 1:583–7.

126. Beveridge T, Krupp P, McKibbin C. Lymphomas and lymphoproliferative lesions developing under cyclosporin therapy (letter). Lancet 1984; 1:788.

127. Armitage JM, Fricker FJ, Del Nido P et al. A decade (1982 to 1992) of pediatric cardiac transplantation and the impact of FK 506 immunosuppression. J Thorac Cardiovasc Surg 1993; 105:464–72.

128. Deschler DG, Osorio R, Ascher NL et al. Post-transplantation lymphoproliferative disorder in patients under primary tacrolimus (FK 506)

immunosuppression. Arch Otolaryngol Head Neck Surg 1995; 121:1037–41.

129. Szczech LA, Berlin JA, Aradhye S et al. Effect of anti-lymphocyte induction therapy on renal allograft survival: a meta-analysis. J Am Soc Nephrol 1997; 8:1771–7.

130. Hibberd AD, Trevillian PR, Wlodarzcyk JH et al. Cancer risk associated with ATG/OKT3 in renal transplantation. Transplant Proc 1999; 31:1271–2.

131. Swinnen LJ, Costanzo-Nordin MR, Fisher SG et al. Increased incidence of lymphoproliferative disorder after immunosuppression with the monoclonal antibody OKT3 in cardiac-transplant recipients. N Engl J Med 1990; 323:1723–8.

132. Walker RC, Marshall WF, Strickler JG et al. Pretransplantation assessment of the risk of lymphoproliferative disorder. Clin Infect Dis 1995; 20:1346–53.

133. Penn I. The changing pattern of posttransplant malignancies. Transplant Proc 1991; 23:1101–3.

134. Birkeland SA, Hamilton-Dutoit S. Is posttransplant lymphoproliferative disorder (PTLD) caused by any specific immunosuppressive drug or by the transplantation per se? Transplantation 2003; 76(6):984–8.

135. Purtilo DT. Epstein–Barr-virus-induced oncogenesis in immune-deficient individuals. Lancet 1980; 1:300–3.

136. Klein G. Lymphoma development in mice and humans: diversity of initiation is followed by convergent cytogenetic evolution. Proc Natl Acad Sci USA. 1979; 76:2442–6.

137. Zucca E, Bertoni F, Roggero E et al. Molecular analysis of the progression from Helicobacter pylori-associated chronic gastritis to mucosa-associated lymphoid-tissue lymphoma of the stomach. N Engl J Med 1998; 338(12):804–10.

138. Wotherspoon AC, Doglioni C, Diss TC et al. Regression of primary low-grade B-cell gastric lymphoma of mucosa-associated lymphoid tissue type after eradication of Helicobacter pylori. Lancet 1993; 342(8871):575–7.

139. Bayerdorffer E, Neubauer A, Rudolph B et al. Regression of primary gastric lymphoma of mucosa-associated lymphoid tissue type after cure of Helicobacter pylori infection. MALT Lymphoma Study Group. Lancet 1995; 345(8965):1591–4.

140. Birkeland SA. Chronic antigenic stimulation from the graft as a possible oncogenic factor after renal transplant. Scand J Urol Nephrol 1983; 17(3):355–9.

141. Nalesni KM, Demetris AJ, John J et al. Posttransplantation lymphoproliferative disorders. Transplantation Clinical Management 2000; vol. 4. http://www.medscape.com/px/urlinfo.

142. Green M, Reyes J, Rowe D. New strategies in the prevention and management of Epstein–Barr virus infection and posttransplant lymphoproliferative disease following solid organ transplantation. Curr Opin Organ Transplant 1998; 3:143–7.

143. Green M, Reyes J, Webber S et al. The role of viral load in the diagnosis, management and possible prevention of Epstein–Barr virus-associated posttransplant lymphoproliferative disease following solid organ transplantation. Curr Opin Organ Transplant 1999; 4:292–6.

144. McDiarmid SV, Jordan S, Geoffrey SL et al. Prevention and preemptive therapy of posttransplant lymphoproliferative disease in pediatric liver recipients. Transplantation 1998; 66:1604–11.

145. Zutter MM, Martin PJ, Sale GE et al. Epstein–Barr virus lymphoproliferation after bone marrow transplantation. Blood 1998; 72:520–9.

146. Witherspoon RP, Fisher LD, Schoch G et al. Secondary cancers after bone marrow transplantation for leukemia or aplastic anemia. N Engl J Med 1989; 321:784–9.

147. Shapiro RS, McClain K, Frizzera G et al. Epstein–Barr virus associated B cell lymphoproliferative disorders following bone marrow transplantation. Blood 1988; 71:1234–43.

148. Ho M, Jaffe R, Miller G et al. The frequency of Epstein–Barr virus infection and associated lymphoproliferative syndrome after transplantation and its manifestations in children. Transplantation 1988; 45:719–27.

149. Walker RC, Paya CV, Marshall WF et al. Pretransplantation seronegative Epstein–Barr virus status is the primary risk factor for posttransplantation lymphoproliferative disorder in adult heart, lung, and other solid organ transplantations. J Heart Lung Transplant 1995; 14:214–21.

150. Boyle GJ, Michaels MG, Webber SA et al. Posttransplantation lymphoproliferative disorders in pediatric thoracic organ recipients. J Pediatr 1997; 131:309–13.

151. Knowles DM, Cesarman E, Chadburn A et al. Correlative morphologic and molecular genetic analysis demonstrates three distinct categories of posttransplantation lymphoproliferative disorders. Blood 1995; 85:552–65.

152. Swinnen LJ, Mullen GM, Carr TJ et al. Aggressive treatment for postcardiac transplant lymphoproliferation. Blood 1995; 86:3333–40.

153. Harris NL, Ferry JA, Swerdlow SH. Posttransplant lymphoproliferative disorders: summary of Society for Hematopathology Workshop. Semin Diagn Pathol 1997; 14:8–14.

154. Hanson MN, Morrison VA, Peterson BA et al. Posttransplant T-cell lymphoproliferative disorders – an

aggressive, late complication of solid-organ transplantation. Blood 1996; 88:3626–33.

155. Frizzera G, Hanto DW, Gajl-Peczalska KJ et al. Polymorphic diffuse B-cell hyperplasias and lymphomas in renal transplant recipients. Cancer Res 1981; 41:4262–79.

156. Nalesnik MA, Jaffe R, Starzl TE et al. The pathology of posttransplant lymphoproliferative disorders occurring in the setting of cyclosporine A-prednisone immunosuppression. Am J Pathol 1988; 133:173–92.

157. Cleary ML, Warnke R, Sklar J. Monoclonality of lymphoproliferative lesions in cardiac-transplant recipients. Clonal analysis based on immunoglobulin-gene rearrangements. N Engl J Med 1984; 310: 477–82.

158. Hanto DW, Birkenbach M, Frizzera G et al. Confirmation of the heterogeneity of posttransplant Epstein–Barr virus-associated B cell proliferations by immunoglobulin gene rearrangement analyses. Transplantation 1989; 47:458–64.

159. Reams BD, McAdams HP, Howell DN et al. Post-transplant lymphoproliferative disorder: incidence, presentation, and response to treatment in lung transplant recipients. Chest 2003; 124(4):1242–9.

160. Swerdlow SH. Classification of the posttransplant lymphoproliferative disorders: from the past to the present (review). Semin Diagn Pathol 1997; 14:2–7.

161. Breinig MK, Zitelli B, Starzl TE. Epstein–Barr virus, cytomegalovirus, and other viral infection in children after liver transplantation. J Infect Dis 1987; 156:273.

162. Ho M, Jaffe R, Miller G et al. The frequency of Epstein–Barr virus infection and associated lymphoproliferative syndrome after transplantation and its manifestations in children. Transplantation 1988; 45:719.

163. Ho M, Miller G, Atchison RW et al. Epstein–Barr virus infections and DNA hybridization studies in posttransplantation lymphoma and lymphoproliferative lesions: the role of primary infection. J Infect Dis 1985; 152:876.

164. Stewart JP, Micali N, Usherwood EJ et al. Murine gamma-herpesvirus 68 glycoprotein 150 protects against virus-induced mononucleosis: a model system for gamma-herpesvirus vaccination. Vaccine 1999; 17(2):152–7.

165. Wilson AD, Lovgren-Bengtsson K, Villacres-Ericsson M et al. The major Epstein–Barr virus (EBV) envelope glycoprotein gp340 when incorporated into Iscoms primes cytotoxic T-cell responses directed against EBV lymphoblastoid cell lines. Vaccine 1999; 17(9–10):1282–90.

166. Ranieri E, Herr W, Gambotto A et al. Dendritic cells transduced with an adenovirus vector encoding Epstein–Barr virus latent membrane protein 2B: a new modality for vaccination. J Virol 1999; 73(12):10416–25.

167. Moss DJ, Khanna R, Bharadwaj M. Will a vaccine to nasopharyngeal carcinoma retain orphan status? Dev Biol 2002; 110:67–71.

168. Starzl TE, Nalesnik M, Porter KA et al. Reversibility of lymphomas and lymphoproliferative lesions developing under cyclosporin-steroid therapy. Lancet 1984; 1:583.

169. Wu TT, Swerdlow S, Locker J et al. Pathologic analysis of recurrent posttransplant lymphoproliferative disorders. Transplant Proc 1995; 27:1193–4.

170. Preiksatis JK, Diaz-Mitoma F, Mirzayans F et al. Quantitative oropharyngeal Epstein–Barr virus shedding in renal and cardiac transplant recipients: relationships to immunosuppressive therapy, serologic responses and the risk of post-transplant lymphoproliferative disorder. J Infect Dis 1992; 166:986–94.

171. Savoie A, Perpete C, Carpentier L et al. Direct correlation between the load of Epstein–Barr virus-infected lymphocytes in the peripheral blood of pediatric transplant patients and risk of lymphoproliferative disease. Blood 1994; 83:2715–22.

172. Riddler SA, Breinig MC, McKnight JLC. Increased levels of circulating Epstein–Barr virus-infected lymphocytes and decreased EBV nuclear antigen antibody responses are associated with the development of post-transplant lymphoproliferative disease in solid-organ transplant recipients. Blood 1994; 84:972–84.

173. Kenagy DN, Schlesinger Y, Weck K et al. Epstein–Barr virus DNA in peripheral blood leukocytes of patients with posttransplant lymphoproliferative disease. Transplantation 1995; 60:547–54.

174. Rooney CM, Loftin SK, Holladay MS et al. Early identification of Epstein–Barr virus-associated post-transplant lymphoproliferative disease. Br J Haematol 1995; 89:98–103.

175. Rowe DT, Qu L, Reyes J et al. Use of quantitative competitive PCR to measure Epstein–Barr virus genome load in peripheral blood of pediatric transplant recipients with lymphoproliferative disorders. J Clin Microbiol 1997; 35:1612–15.

176. Limaye AP, Huang ML, Athneza E et al. Detection of Epstein–Barr virus DNA in sera from transplant recipients with lymphoproliferative disorders. J Clin Microbiol 1999; 37:1113–16.

177. Wu TT, Swerdlow SH, Locker J et al. Recurrent Epstein–Barr virus-associated lesions in organ transplant recipients. Hum Pathol 1996; 27:157–64.

178. Gartner BC, Schafer H, Marggraff K et al. Evaluation of use of Epstein–Barr viral load in

patients after allogeneic stem cell transplantation to diagnose and monitor posttransplant lymphoproliferative disease. J Clin Microbiol 2002; 40(2):351–8.

179. Wadowsky RM, Laus S, Green M et al. Measurement of Epstein–Barr virus DNA loads in whole blood and plasma by TaqMan PCR and in peripheral blood lymphocytes by competitive PCR. J Clin Microbiol 2003; 41(11):5245–9.

180. Terasawa T, Ohashi H, Tsushita K. Failure to detect Epstein–Barr virus (EBV) DNA in plasma by real-time PCR in a case of EBV-associated posttransplantation lymphoproliferative disorder confined to the central nervous system. Int J Hematol 2002; 75(4):416–20.

181. Hopwood PA, Brooks L, Parratt R et al. Persistent Epstein–Barr virus infection: unrestricted latent and lytic viral gene expression in healthy immunosuppressed transplant recipients. Transplantation 2002; 74(2):194–202.

182. Smets F, Latinne D, Bazin H et al. Ratio between Epstein–Barr viral load and anti-Epstein–Barr virus specific T-cell response as a predictive marker of posttransplant lymphoproliferative disease. Transplantation 2002; 73(10):1603–10.

183. Rickinson AB, Moss DJ. Human cytotoxic T lymphocyte responses to Epstein–Barr virus infection. Annu Rev Immunol 1997; 15:405–31.

184. Hoshino Y, Morishima T, Kimura H et al. Antigen-driven expansion and contraction of CD8+-activated T cells in primary EBV infection. J Immunol 1999; 163(10):5735–40.

185. Green M, Bueno J, Rowe D et al. Predictive negative value of persistent low Epstein–Barr virus viral load after intestinal transplantation in children. Transplantation 2000; 70(4):593–6.

186. Yang J, Tao Q, Flinn IW et al. Characterization of Epstein–Barr virus-infected B cells in patients with posttransplantation lymphoproliferative disease: disappearance after rituximab therapy does not predict clinical response. Blood 2000; 96(13): 4055–63.

187. Shapiro RS, Chauvenet A, McGuire W et al. Treatment of B-cell lymphoproliferative disorders with interferon alfa and intravenous gamma globulin (letter). N Engl J Med 1988; 318:1334.

188. Filipovich AH, Mathur A, Kamat D et al. Lymphoproliferative disorders and other tumours complicating immunodeficiencies. Immunodeficiency 1994; 5:91–112.

189. Yao QY, Ogan P, Rowe M et al. Epstein–Barr virus-infected B cells persist in the circulation of acyclovir treated carriers. Int J Cancer 1989; 43:67–71.

190. Oertel SH, Riess H. Antiviral treatment of Epstein–Barr virus-associated lymphoproliferations. Recent results. Cancer Res 2002; 159:89–95.

191. Malouf MA, Chhajed PN, Hopkins P et al. Antiviral prophylaxis reduces the incidence of lymphoproliferative disease in lung transplant recipients. J Heart Lung Transplant 2002; 21(5):547–54.

192. Abdulkarim B, Sabri S, Zelenika D et al. Antiviral agent cidofovir decreases Epstein–Barr virus (EBV) oncoproteins and enhances the radiosensitivity in EBV-related malignancies. Oncogene 2003; 22(15): 2260–71.

193. Haque T, Crawford DH. The role of adoptive immunotherapy in the prevention and treatment of lymphoproliferative disease following transplantation. Br J Haematol 1999; 106(2):309–16.

194. Dror Y, Greenberg M, Taylor G et al. Lymphoproliferative disorders after organ transplantation in children. Transplantation 1999; 67:990–8.

195. Stevens SJ, Verschuuren EA, Verkuijlen SA et al. Role of Epstein–Barr virus DNA load monitoring in prevention and early detection of post-transplant lymphoproliferative disease. Leuk Lymphoma 2002; 43:831–40.

196. Morrison VA, Dunn DL, Manivel JC et al. Clinical characteristics of post-transplant lymphoproliferative disorders. Am J Med 1994; 97:14–24.

197. Leblond V, Sutton L, Dorent R et al. Lymphoproliferative disorders after organ transplantation: a report of 24 cases observed in a single center. J Clin Oncol 1995; 13:961–8.

198. Orjuela M, Gross TG, Cheung YK et al. A pilot study of chemoimmunotherapy (cyclophosphamide, prednisone, and rituximab) in patients with post-transplant lymphoproliferative disorder following solid organ transplantation. Clin Cancer Res 2003; 9(10 Pt 2):3945S–52S.

199. Fischer A, Blanche S, Le Bidois J et al. Anti-B-cell monoclonal antibodies in the treatment of severe B-cell lymphoproliferative syndrome following bone marrow and organ transplantation. N Engl J Med 1991; 324(21):1451–6.

200. Benkerrou M, Jais JP, Leblond V et al. Anti-B-cell monoclonal antibody treatment of severe post-transplant B-lymphoproliferative disorder: prognostic factors and long-term outcome. Blood 1998; 92(9):3137–47.

201. Maloney DG. Preclinical and phase I and II trials of rituximab. Semin Oncol 1999; 26(5 suppl. 14): 74–8.

202. Ganne V, Siddiqi N, Kamalath B et al. Humanized anti-CD20 monoclonal antibody (Rituximab) treatment for post-transplant lymphoproliferative disorder. Clin Transplant 2003; 17(5):417–22.

203. Cook RC, Connors JM, Gascoyne RD et al. Treatment of post-transplant lymphoproliferative disease with rituximab monoclonal antibody after lung transplantation. Lancet 1999; 354(9191):1698–9.

204. van Esser JW, Niesters HG, van der Holt B et al. Prevention of Epstein–Barr virus-lymphoproliferative disease by molecular monitoring and preemptive rituximab in high-risk patients after allogeneic stem cell transplantation. Blood 2002; 99(12):4364–9.

205. Rooney CM, Smith CA, Ng CY et al. Use of gene-modified virus-specific T lymphocytes to control Epstein–Barr-virus-related lymphoproliferation. Lancet 1995; 345:9–13.

206. Heslop HE, Ng CY, Li C et al. Long-term restoration of immunity against Epstein–Barr virus infection by adoptive transfer of gene-modified virus-specific T lymphocytes. Nature Med 1996; 2:551–5.

207. O'Reilly RJ, Small TN, Papadopoulos E et al. Biology and adoptive cell therapy of Epstein–Barr virus-associated lymphoproliferative disorders in recipients of marrow allografts. Immunol Rev 1997; 157:195–216.

208. Heslop HE, Rooney CM. Adoptive cellular immunotherapy for EBV lymphoproliferative disease. Immunol Rev 1997; 157:217–22.

209. Papadopoulos EB, Ladanyi M, Emanuel D et al. Infusions of donor leukocytes to treat Epstein–Barr virus-associated lymphoproliferative disorders after allogenic bone marrow transplantation. N Engl J Med 1994; 330:1185–91.

210. Nalesnik MA, Rao AS, Furukawa H et al. Autologous lymphokine-activated killer cell therapy of Epstein–Barr virus-positive and -negative lymphoproliferative disorders arising in organ transplant recipients. Transplantation 1997; 63:1200–5.

211. Taylor GS. T cell-based therapies for EBV-associated malignancies. Expert Opin Biol Ther 2004; 4(1):11–21.

212. Haque T, Taylor C, Wilkie GM et al. Complete regression of posttransplant lymphoproliferative disease using partially HLA-matched Epstein Barr virus-specific cytotoxic T cells. Transplantation 2001; 72(8):1399–402.

213. Hanel M, Fiedler F, Thorns C. Anti-CD20 monoclonal antibody (Rituximab) and Cidofovir as successful treatment of an EBV-associated lymphoma with CNS involvement. Onkologie 2001; 24(5):491–4.

214. Chachap P, Carone Filho E, Porta G et al. Post-transplant lymphoproliferative disease of the liver successfully treated by retransplantation. Transplantation 1991; 52(4):736–7.

215. Glez-Chamorro A, Jimenez C, Moreno-Glez E et al. Management and outcome of liver recipients with post-transplant lymphoproliferative disease. Hepatogastroenterology 2000; 47(31):211–19.

216. Birkeland SA, Hamilton-Dutoit S, Bendtzen K. Long-term follow-up of kidney transplant patients with posttransplant lymphoproliferative disorder: duration of posttransplant lymphoproliferative disorder-induced operational graft tolerance, interleukin-18 course, and results of retransplantation. Transplantation 2003; 76(1):153–8.

CHAPTER Thirteen
Chronic transplant dysfunction

Keith P. Graetz and
Keith M. Rigg

INTRODUCTION

In recent years, a consistent improvement in 1-year graft survival rates has been achieved throughout the field of solid-organ transplantation.[1] This is due to advances in immunosuppressive agents and improved donor and recipient care. Unfortunately there has not been a corresponding improvement in long-term graft survival. The graft attrition rate after the first year post-transplantation has remained relatively constant since the late 1960s, with 4–5% of grafts lost per annum[1] (**Fig. 13.1**).

The 1-year graft survival rate is currently 80–90% for kidney, liver, heart and lung transplantation, and consequently more attention has been focused on the causes of late graft loss. In particular, attention has been directed towards the problem of 'chronic rejection', which is a misleading term. The word 'chronic' fails to reflect the fact that the initiating factors of the condition may occur in the peritransplant period. Also, the word 'rejection' suggests that the aetiology of the disease is predominantly immune-mediated, whereas non-immune factors also have an important role to play. As a generic term, 'chronic transplant dysfunction' is more descriptive than 'chronic rejection' and will therefore be used throughout the rest of this chapter, although the literature varies in the usage of these terms. However, each organ has a specific clinico-pathological entity representing the generic condition, such as chronic allograft nephropathy in kidney transplantation.

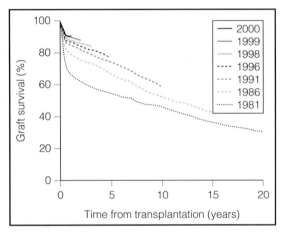

Figure 13.1 • First cadaveric kidney transplant survival according to year of transplantation. Reproduced with permission of UK Transplant. Statistics from UK Transplant from the National Transplant Database, maintained on behalf of transplant services in the UK.

Chronic transplant dysfunction (CTD) is charac-terised clinically by a progressive deterioration in graft function occurring months to years after trans-plantation and it is associated with typical histo-logical changes of graft arteriosclerosis and fibrosis. By the time the diagnosis has been made irreversible changes have usually occurred in the organ. The process has an insidious onset but once established it is irreversible and will ultimately lead to graft loss. For the majority of solid organs transplanted, CTD represents the leading cause of graft loss after the first year. At 5 years post-transplantation, 30–50%

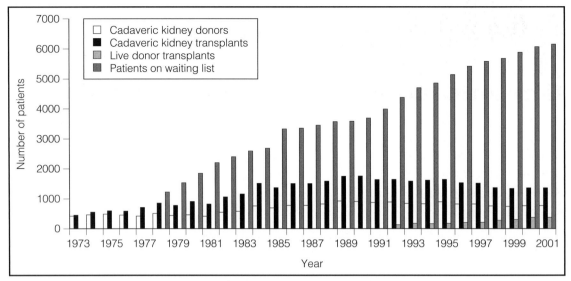

Figure 13.2 • The supply and demand for kidney transplantation. Reproduced with permission of UK Transplant. Statistics from UK Transplant from the National Transplant Database, maintained on behalf of transplant services in the UK.

of kidney, heart, lung and pancreas allografts, and 5–20% of liver allografts demonstrate typical morphological changes. The combination of the ongoing shortage of organs for transplantation and the increasing demand (**Fig. 13.2**) has emphasised the need to study and understand the mechanisms underlying CTD in an attempt to identify therapeutic targets for its prevention and treatment.

This chapter will discuss the problems associated with defining CTD clinically and histopathologically. The histopathological features common to all organs will be presented, and organ-specific changes highlighted. Both the aetiology and pathophysiology will be considered in detail with a review of the clinical and experimental evidence gained to date. The main area of development since the last edition of this book has been the promising use of some of the newer immunosuppressive agents in prolonging graft survival in patients with established CTD. This will be expanded more fully in the section on therapeutic options.

WHAT IS CHRONIC TRANSPLANT DYSFUNCTION?

Clinically, CTD is manifested by a progressive decline in organ function in the absence of any other diagnosed cause for this deterioration, such as

an acute rejection episode, drug nephrotoxicity or recurrence of the original disease. Some of these factors may have played an initiating role in the development of CTD. Transplant biopsy remains the gold standard for establishing a definitive diagnosis of CTD and is usually performed once other relevant non-invasive tests have been completed. The histological features of CTD common to all organ types are graft vessel arteriosclerosis, perivascular inflammation and organ fibrosis. In addition the heart, kidney, liver, lung and pancreas have organ-specific histological findings.

Heart

CTD in transplanted hearts remains the most common cause of graft loss after the first post-transplant year. It is manifested as accelerated cardiac allograft arteriosclerosis or cardiac allograft vasculopathy (CAV).

Transplanted organs are denervated at the time of retrieval and therefore patients do not present with angina pectoris when the cardiac allograft is deteriorating. Patients will have cardiac arrhythmias and ventricular dysfunction and will therefore present with either sudden cardiac death or symptoms and signs of cardiac failure.

Cross-sections of affected vessels in biopsy specimens are difficult to obtain, thus grading of the primary histological feature is also problematic. The diagnosis of CAV in heart transplant recipients relies on the clinical and radiographic features of arteriosclerosis, which is the cause of patient presentation. Clinical evaluation of the extent of disease using coronary angiography often underestimates the histological findings later demonstrated at autopsy.[2] The concentric nature of the arteriosclerotic lesions is thought to be the cause of this underestimation. Studies where angiography has been used have estimated its prevalence as 10–18% at 1 year and 50% at 5 years.[3] Intravascular ultrasound is gaining acceptance as a method of evaluating concentric lesions by being able to assess both intimal thickening and lumen narrowing. Its usefulness in assessing the length of lesions is less clear. When results are compared against conventional coronary angiography, it would appear that lesions have been underrated with an intimal thickening prevalence of 50% at 1 year.[4] Patients with significant intimal thickening at 1 year (>5 mm) have now been shown to be more likely to develop accelerated arteriosclerotic lesions and therefore have a worse prognosis.[5]

The pathognomonic lesion of CAV in heart allografts is concentric intimal thickening affecting the coronary vessels, particularly the smaller distal intramyocardial vessels. The internal elastic lamina is often intact but may have small breaks in its circumference. The media is usually preserved but there is often an associated low-grade perivasculitis. The disease can affect the whole vessel but more typically demonstrates a heterogeneous distribution without a predilection for the extramyocardial or intramyocardial branches. This is in contrast to the process of atherosclerosis, where the extramyocardial portions of the coronary vasculature are predominantly affected.[6]

Diagnostic criteria for CAV were presented in the consensus document of 1993 from the fourth Alexis Carrel Conference.[7]

The document proposed the following guidelines:

1. Histological diagnosis should be based on the presence of tubular myointimal hyperplasia with an intact elastic lamina containing few breaks. There should be little or no calcification.
2. The histopathological diagnosis should be made on explanted transplants or at autopsy, recognising that endomyocardial biopsies rarely contain arteries.
3. The clinical diagnosis should be made on angiography and reported according to categories described by the Stanford group.[3]
   a. Type A lesions: discrete stenoses in the proximal, middle or distal segment branches.
   b. Type B lesions: diffuse concentric narrowing arising in the mid- to distal arteries.
   c. Type C lesions: narrowed irregular vessels with occluded side branches.

Type A changes in the proximal arteries are likely to represent prior coronary artery disease or new-onset atherosclerosis typical of that found in native hearts.

Kidney

Chronic allograft nephropathy (CAN) represents the leading cause of graft loss after the first year post-transplantation in kidney transplant recipients.[8] Initial deterioration in graft function is usually only manifested as a biochemical deterioration (usually assessed by an increasing serum creatinine caused by a decreasing glomerular filtration rate). Only when nephron reserve is exhausted will the patient potentially become symptomatic with symptoms and signs of uraemia. There is associated proteinuria, worsening hypertension and a reduced creatinine clearance. Other causes of graft deterioration should be excluded before performing a transplant biopsy to confirm the diagnosis of CAN. Differential diagnoses include.

- urinary obstruction;
- recurrent disease;
- renal artery stenosis;
- drug nephrotoxicity (mainly caused by calcineurin inhibitors);
- BK (polyoma virus) nephropathy;
- urinary tract infection.

The typical histopathological features of CAN were first described in 1955 and include arteriosclerosis, tubular atrophy, glomerulopathy and interstitial fibrosis. Myointimal thickening occurs in the same way as in cardiac allografts as a consequence of smooth muscle cell proliferation (Fig. 13.3). Glomeruli are lost as the basement membranes

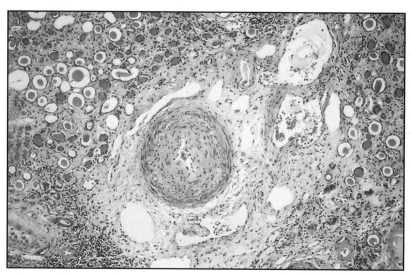

Figure 13.3 • The typical vascular lesion of chronic allograft nephropathy.

undergo reduplication ultimately resulting in glomerulosclerosis. Tubular atrophy follows as a consequence with infiltration of the interstitium by myofibroblasts leading to interstitial fibrosis.

In 1986, a group from Helsinki analysed protocol core biopsies taken at 2 years post-transplantation from 128 patients involved in a trial of immuno-suppressive agents.[9] They found that even in grafts with stable function, histopathological changes consistent with those of chronic rejection could be seen. The group proposed the concept of 'chronic allograft damage index' (CADI) to allow com-parison of the biopsy findings between each of the treatment groups. The CADI was calculated as the sum of the scores of six histopathological changes identified as being associated with decreasing graft function in the study. In a subsequent publication, at 6 years of follow-up, they demonstrated that the CADI score at 2 years could be used to predict reliably those grafts that would go on to develop chronic rejection.[10] The CADI score was also found to correlate significantly with transplant function at this time point.

It was recognised that there was little standard-isation in the histological diagnosis and reporting of the histological findings of rejection between transplant centres. A working group therefore met at Banff, Canada, in 1991 to 'develop a schema for the international standardisation of nomenclature and criteria for the histological diagnosis of renal allograft rejection'.[11] The Banff schema covered all the recognised types of renal allograft rejection, with chronic rejection falling into a category entitled 'chronic allograft nephropathy'. Within this category the process of chronic rejection overlapped histo-pathologically with at least three other causes of chronic graft dysfunction, namely chronic ciclosporin toxicity, hypertensive vascular disease and chronic infection with or without reflux. The chronic changes were separated into four main structural components (vascular, interstitial, glomerular and tubular) and were graded individually on a scale of 1 to 3. In cases where new-onset fibrous intimal thickening was prominent, it was suggested that this entity was likely to represent 'chronic rejection' as opposed to the other causes of chronic allograft damage. Likewise, hyaline arteriolar thickening was deemed to be more indicative of ciclosporin nephrotoxicity and less so of 'chronic rejection'.

The Banff 97 classification for renal allograft pathology was subsequently published.[12] Within the chronic/sclerosing allograft nephropathy group, no changes were recommended for grading of chronic interstitial fibrosis and tubular atrophy. However, modifications were made for glomerular and vascular changes. Glomerular changes of 'double contours' in capillary loops and, to a lesser extent an increase in mesangial matrix are more specific for chronic transplant glomerulopathy. Specific vascular changes that are consistent with chronic allograft nephropathy include disruption of the elastica and inflammatory cell in the fibrotic intima, whilst myofibroblast proliferation in the intima and formation of a second 'neointima' are also useful features.

A consensus document was published in 1993 following the fourth Alexis Carrel Conference.[7] The document was designed to provide a working definition of chronic rejection in heart and kidney transplants, thereby facilitating clinical studies and the assessment of interventions. It supported the Banff recommendations for the histological diagnosis of chronic rejection but in addition placed emphasis on the requirement to demonstrate progression of loss of function within the graft. This recommendation was based on the fact that a percentage of grafts develop proteinuria and show the typical histopathological changes of chronic rejection but do not proceed to graft loss within 5 years.

The following working definition was proposed for the diagnosis of chronic renal transplant rejection.

1. Graft histology should be consistent with chronic rejection and reported according to the Banff schema.
2. The regression of the reciprocal of plasma creatinine over time is significantly different from zero (requires a minimum of ten consecutive creatinine values or the use of creatinine values over a 3-month interval to perform the regression).
3. Patients should be at least 3 months post-transplantation.
4. Other causes of graft dysfunction must be excluded.

Liver

Chronic liver rejection is again one of the most common causes of late graft loss, but it occurs far less frequently than in other solid organ transplants. The overall incidence of chronic transplant dysfunction is between 5 and 20% of all liver transplants.[13–15]

The liver is immunologically privileged, with all forms of rejection being less common. Specifically, CTD is becoming less common,[16] with graft loss more likely from recurrent disease, late acute rejection or non-compliance, but it is still a major indication for re-transplantation.[17]

A cholestatic picture with abnormal liver function tests and cholestasis is the usual presentation. The onset is insidious and usually without warning. Patients rarely present with cirrhotic complications from progressive allograft fibrosis. The differential diagnosis includes late acute rejection, viral hepatitis, recurrence of primary disease and late technical complications such as a biliary stricture. It is important that these are excluded first as chronic liver rejection is inevitably progressive and irreversible.

Histological diagnosis is also essential, with liver cell dropout, vanishing bile duct syndrome and obliterative vasculopathy being the cardinal features.[18] 'Vanishing bile duct syndrome' when diagnosed on biopsy is a good indicator for severe chronic allograft damage. It is a uniform loss of small bile ducts (<75 µm) throughout the liver[19] without replacement by fibrosis. Ductule proliferation does not occur as in other cholestatic conditions, that is, primary biliary cirrhosis. When seen in biopsy specimens, large and medium-sized arteries have a foam cell and macrophage-laden intima as is found in other allografted organs.

Lung

Bronchiolitis obliterans syndrome (BOS) is the clinical manifestation of CTD in the lung, and the typical histopathological features are referred to as obliterative bronchiolitis. BOS accounts for over one-third of late graft losses and the prevalence of BOS in patients greater than 3 months post-transplantation may be as high as 68%.[20] The mortality rate is 50% once the diagnosis of BOS has been made, with few patients coming for re-transplantation.[21] In common with the disease process in other organs, BOS is progressive and has no effective treatment at present. Clinically it presents with slowly progressing dyspnoea on exertion. Worsening airflow obstruction follows as a consequence of deteriorating graft function.[22] Physiologically there is a mixed picture of airflow obstruction and restrictive pulmonary disease.[22]

The diagnosis of BOS can only be made when other causes of graft function have been excluded and is done using spirometry.[23] Sequential spirometry confirms the gradual decline in pulmonary function.[23] Hyperinflation may be seen on the chest radiograph. High-resolution computed tomography (CT) is more predictive with bronchiectasis and ground-glass opacities on expiration, indicative of air trapping.[24] Transbronchial biopsy material can be obtained during bronchoscopy performed to exclude other diagnoses. A confirmatory histological diagnosis is necessary and the term 'obliterative bronchiolitis' should be reserved for when this has been done.

Histologically there is inflammation and fibrosis of the cartilaginous airways and particularly within the smaller airways. Bronchioles usually demonstrate areas of inflammation and fibrosis in the lamina propria and luminal surfaces whilst the larger bronchi show peribronchial fibrosis and bronchiectasis. Airway narrowing follows, accounting for the decline in spirometry readings.[25] Surrounding alveoli and interstitium are often, but not always, normal. As a pathological entity it is no different from obliterative bronchiolitis caused by non-transplant-related aetiological factors, such as toxic fume inhalation, drug side effects and connective tissue disorders.[26]

In 1990 an ad hoc committee under the auspices of the International Society for Heart and Lung Transplantation proposed a working formulation for the standardisation of nomenclature and for clinical staging of chronic dysfunction in lung allografts.[27]

The formulation described the following staging system:

1. Stage 0: no significant abnormality; FEV_1 80% or more of baseline value.
2. Stage 1: mild bronchiolitis obliterans syndrome; FEV_1 66–88%.
3. Stage 2: moderate bronchiolitis obliterans syndrome; FEV_1 51–65%.
4. Stage 3: severe bronchiolitis obliterans syndrome; FEV_1 50% or less.

Within each stage, an 'a' and 'b' category exist: 'a' denotes no histological evidence of bronchiolitis obliterans or an absence of biopsy material and 'b' denotes a positive diagnosis obtained on biopsy material.

Pancreas

CTD accounts for over half of all pancreas graft losses 5 years post-transplantation.[28] Deterioration in graft function is not easy to detect and is usually manifested by hyperglycaemic episodes with a low C-peptide level following a glucose challenge.[29] There are no serial markers of graft deterioration in pancreas transplantation and, in the absence of concurrent acute rejection, serum amylase is often normal.

Graft biopsy is required to confirm the diagnosis. The typical histological features seen are septal fibrosis with acinar loss and fibrointimal vascular proliferation. Vessels are seldom seen on graft biopsies and therefore vascular changes cannot be relied on for diagnosis.

PATHOPHYSIOLOGY AND IMMUNOLOGY

Overview

Many of the risk factors associated with CTD have been identified, but their respective roles in the pathogenesis remain unclear. This section provides a simplified overview of the pathophysiology of CTD, reviewing the events at cellular level and highlighting the key molecular mediators and their interaction with the cellular components. The use of experimental models is also discussed.

The unifying histopathological lesion indicative of CTD, irrespective of organ type, is graft arteriosclerosis.[30] If graft arteriosclerosis is considered to be the cardinal injury in solid-organ allografts undergoing CTD, then the majority of organ-specific changes can be explained simply on the basis of resulting ischaemia.

Graft arteriosclerosis affects the whole length of the involved vessel, and its distribution within the wall of the vessel is concentric in nature.[30,31] This differs from classical atherosclerosis, where there is a patchy distribution of the disease and eccentric placement of lesions within the vessel wall. Both endothelial inflammation and injury appear to be potent initiating events in the development of graft arteriosclerosis, but a variety of factors can cause or contribute to endothelial cell injury. One of the most important events in the initiation of the endothelial cell response is alloimmune recognition of donor major histocompatibility (MHC) antigens on the endothelial cells.[32–34] Experimental evidence supports this theory, demonstrating that immune recognition of endovascular MHC antigens causes endothelial cell inflammation, which results in a combination of increased permeability of the endothelium, increased exposure of host antigens and a prominent inflammatory response by endothelial cells.[35] The last factor is considered to represent the first stage of tissue repair by endothelial cells.

Although alloimmune mechanisms are paramount in the evolution of the events described above, the injury itself and the endothelial response may be further exacerbated by a variety of other factors such as organ ischaemia, acute rejection episodes, reperfusion injury, hypertension, hyperlipidaemia and cytomegalovirus (CMV) disease.

Endothelial injury results in the release of cytokines and growth factors to mediate cellular repair mechanisms.[30,36–38] These molecular mediators subsequently exert a complex myriad of effects on their targets, including chemotaxis, cell activation, cell division and cell differentiation. Their actions are both paracrine and autocrine in fashion with self-amplifying loops being set up to propagate the process.

Following the endothelial response, smooth muscle cells are seen to migrate from the media into the intima, where they replicate and initiate endothelial repair. There is some debate as to whether these cells are donor or recipient derived.[39] Their migration is facilitated by solubilisation of the intracellular matrix and the occurrence of small breaks within the internal elastic lamina. Their continued migration, replication and attempts to repair lead to intimal fibrosis and luminal obliteration of the affected vessels.[36,37,40] Other predominant cell types identified at this time include T and B lymphocytes and monocytes/macrophages.

The timing of endothelial injury in the development of CTD is not well established. It is thought that the early post-transplant events of ischaemia, alloimmune recognition, reperfusion injury and acute rejection are the cause of graft arteriosclerosis, with their effects only becoming apparent at a later stage. Alternatively, the injury may be considered to be ongoing and more diffuse in nature, with the processes of subclinical rejection, hypertension and

hyperlipidaemia, for example, causing a progressive injury that only becomes apparent when an 'injury threshold' has been exceeded. Clearly, the two different time courses may not be mutually exclusive but may act synergistically in the overall pathogenesis of chronic rejection.

The end result of graft arteriosclerosis, regardless of initiating mechanisms, is the concentric narrowing and eventual obliteration of the vascular lumen that characterises chronic rejection. The fibrotic response and luminal obliteration seen in the hollow structures within each organ (bronchi, bile ducts, renal tubules, etc.) may well be secondary to the resultant ischaemia associated with a disordered response to tissue injury and repair.

Experimental models

The majority of randomised clinical trials have been designed to look at strategies for treating acute rejection. Very few have been designed and powered to look at chronic changes because of the numbers of patients and the timescale required. As an adjunct to clinical studies, experimental models have been developed that are capable of producing similar patterns of 'chronic' injury. Immunosuppressive therapy is not a prerequisite in many animal models where inbred strains are used. Clearly these models have their limitations and caution must be exercised when translating findings back into the clinical field. They have, however, facilitated research into molecular and cellular components involved in the pathogenesis of chronic rejection and have enabled clinical research to be more specifically directed at one area of interest. There is also an increasing amount of work using 'knockout' strains of animals who have had specific genes removed allowing highly directed research to be produced. The commonest models currently used are those involving rodents, predominantly inbred strains of rats and mice.

KIDNEY MODELS

White et al. in 1969 described a rat allograft model between two rat strains – the Fisher and Lewis strains – with a minor histocompatibility difference.[41] This allowed allotransplantation in the absence of immunosuppression, leading to graft changes mirroring the morphological and functional changes of human allografts undergoing chronic rejection. Allograft recipients in this model develop proteinuria, hypertension, declining glomerular filtration rate (GFR) and the histological changes of arteriosclerosis, glomerulosclerosis and interstitial fibrosis. Other models have since been described using various combinations of discordant strains of inbred rats.

The surgical technique in all these models involves either ortho- or heterotopic placement of the kidney by microvascular anastomosis. More recently, mouse models have been developed allowing new possibilities in the study of recipient mice with genetic alterations of macrophage function, MHC expression, T- and B-cell immunity or combined immune deficiencies.[42]

HEART MODELS

Several rodent models have been described employing heterotopic cardiac transplantation.[43–45] Models initially involved discordant rat strains, but, again, mouse models have been developed with the advantage of employing genetically modified strains.

Aortic allograft model

As a simplification of the solid-organ transplant model, the aortic allograft model was developed to allow the study of graft arteriosclerosis alone.[46] The models described employ a transplant between the same animal strains as those for solid-organ models described above. A section of infrarenal aorta is transplanted as an interposition graft in the donor animal and after 1–3 months the aortic allograft demonstrates the typical changes of graft arteriosclerosis. Although it does not provide information on organ-specific changes it is technically less demanding.

Carotid denudation model

This is a mechanical trauma model of endothelial cell damage designed to facilitate the study of the endothelial response to injury in the absence of immune mechanisms. The trauma is usually provided by balloon inflation or chemical injury.

LUNG MODELS

Although less commonly employed, several lung models have been described, including rat single-lung transplant, rat tracheal implants into recipient omentum and porcine subcutaneous implants of lung containing terminal bronchioles.[21]

Cellular effectors

Once endothelial inflammation and disruption have occurred, monocyte and macrophage infiltration appears to be a critical early step in the progression to graft arteriosclerosis in both the clinical and experimental settings.[41,47] Endothelial inflammation leads to increased antigen presentation, thereby attracting T cells. Upregulation of cell adhesion molecules and release of cytokines and growth factors[37] facilitate the process of T-cell attraction and graft infiltration. Antigen presentation and T-cell activation may then aid B lymphocytes in the production of antidonor antibody. A combination of endothelial cell injury and release of cytokines causes the smooth muscle cell activation, replication and migration into the intima described above.

ENDOTHELIAL CELLS

It appears that integrity of the endothelium may be a prerequisite for the prevention of intimal proliferation.[36] The potential causes of endothelial cell injury have been described above. It is now apparent that the endothelial cell is not necessarily a 'passive' victim in this process, but rather the cell becomes activated in response to the injury.

As a result, the endothelial cells are seen to retract, causing breaks in their functional integrity and exposure of adhesion molecules such as inter-cellular adhesion molecule 1 (ICAM-1) and vascular cell adhesion molecule 1 (VCAM-1).[48] Antigenic molecules are also exposed, and this fact, in combination with exposure of adhesion molecules, causes chemotaxis of T lymphocytes and monocytes. There is also marked release of platelet-derived growth factor (PDGF), tumour necrosis factor α (TNF-α), epidermal growth factor (EGF) and thromboxane A (TXA).[36,48] Damaged areas of endothelium cause platelet aggregation, which in turn releases growth factors such as PDGF and eicosanoids – leukotriene B_4 (LTB$_4$) and thromboxane A_2 (TXA$_2$).[48]

Breaches in the endothelium allow inward migration of monocytes, macrophages and lympho-cytes from the luminal surface. Smooth muscle cells migrate in the opposite direction from the media to the intimal surface to begin the process of vascular remodelling.

SMOOTH MUSCLE CELL

Release of growth factors by the activated endothelium causes chemotaxis of smooth muscle cells and, in addition, promotes their replication and differentiation.[30,36,38] There is a phenotypic change in the nature of the smooth muscle cell and it becomes migratory rather than secretory. The migration from the media to the intima is facilitated by altered dynamics of the extracellular matrix and metalloproteinase inhibitor activity. Once in the intima, the smooth muscle cells initiate vascular remodelling but the excessive response results in intimal fibrosis. The disordered control of vascular repair affects all vessels uniformly as evidenced by the concentric and homogeneous distribution of the lesions.

The cytokines, growth factors and eicosanoids acting on smooth muscle cells are summarised in **Fig. 13.4** and further explained in **Box 13.1**.

T LYMPHOCYTES

The role of T lymphocytes in hyperacute and acute rejection is well established, but is less clear in CTD. In acute rejection, the cytotoxic CD8+ population predominates but it is also represented by the CD4+ T-helper population. The latter facilitates B lymphocytes in alloantibody production.[49] When chronic rejection is established within the graft, CD4+ T-helper lymphocytes predominate over CD8+ lymphocytes. Two separate subclasses of CD4+ lymphocytes exist on the basis of their differing cytokine profiles. T-helper type 1 (Th1) cells are associated with the production of interferon γ (IFN-γ), TNF-β and interleukin 2 (IL-2) whilst T-helper type 2 (Th2) cells produce IL-4, IL-5, IL-6, IL-10 and IL-13.[49] Their actions are consequently very different. The Th1 subset is implicated in acute rejection, where their associated cytokines readily activate cytotoxic T lymphocytes and macrophages. In contrast the Th2 population predominantly plays a helper role in enabling B lymphocytes to differentiate into antibody-producing cells.[49] It has been proposed that CTD may result from repeated Th1-mediated cytotoxic lymphocyte attack,[21] whilst Th2 lymphocytes may facilitate the deposition of alloantibody seen in arteriosclerotic vessels and other chronically rejecting tissue components. Each of the subclasses is known to suppress activity in the other subclass and it is interesting that in models of animal tolerance there is a reduction in Th1 activity and a predominance of Th2 lymphocytes.[49] Some authors have reported a reduction in graft arteriosclerosis in recipient mice with defects in MHC class II or CD4 expression, whereas the degree of graft arteriosclerosis remains unchanged in mice with defects in MHC class I or CD8 expression.[50] However, other authors have not reported these findings in studies of a similar nature.[42]

B LYMPHOCYTES AND THE HUMORAL RESPONSE

A role for humoral factors in CTD has been suspected for many years, and as early as 1970 authors were reporting the presence of post-transplant antibodies in patients with a chronically rejecting graft.[51] A high panel-reactive antibody (PRA) level prior to transplantation and the appearance of post-transplant antibodies are associated with the development of CTD. There is good evidence for the presence of immunoglobulins, complement and antibodies to graft components in clinical and experimental studies.[49,52,53] Serum transfer studies in rodent models and studies involving genetically modified mice support the fact that humoral responses are directly implicated. When antidonor antibody is transferred to recipient mice with severe combined immunodeficiency syndrome in a cardiac transplant model, the mice develop graft arteriosclerosis that is otherwise absent or minimal when donor serum is not transferred.[43] Equally, the severity of graft arteriosclerosis in these models is reduced in strain combinations where no detectable antibody is formed compared with those where significant antibody responses occur.

In mice with altered B-cell immune mechanisms, graft arteriosclerosis has been reported to be absent.[44] The role of T lymphocytes is not ruled out by such studies because it is recognised that T- and B-cell interaction is one of the regulatory components of the immune system and that defects in B-cell activity may in effect be altering T-cell-mediated actions.

In addition to antibodies against donor MHC antigens, antibodies have also been detected clinically against a diverse range of organ components,

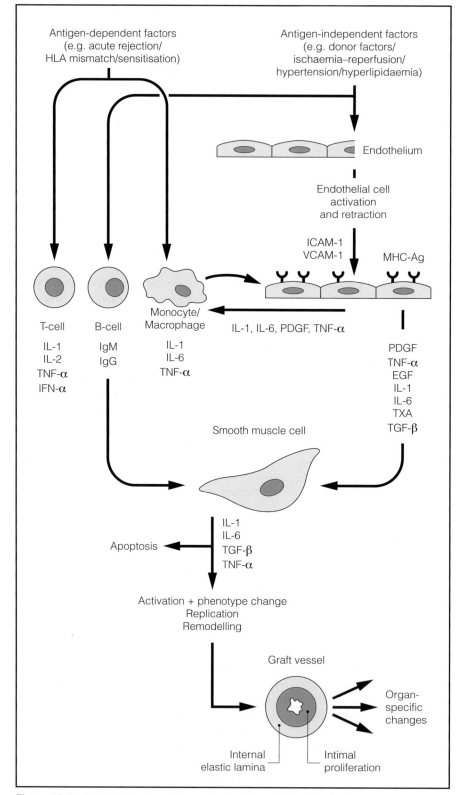

Figure 13.4 • A schematic view of the pathophysiology of chronic rejection.

Box 13.1 • Abbreviations used in Fig. 13.4

IL-1	Interleukin 1
IL-2	Interleukin 2
IL-6	Interleukin 6
TNF-α	Tumour necrosis factor α
TGF-β	Transforming growth factor β
IFN-γ	Interferon γ
TXA	Thromboxane
EGF	Epidermal growth factor
PDGF	Platelet-derived growth factor
BFGF	Basic fibroblast growth factor
ICAM-1	Intracellular adhesion molecule 1
VCAM-1	Vascular cell adhesion molecule 1
MHC-Ag	Major histocompatibility antigen

including the glomerular basement membrane, tubular epithelial cells, mesangial cells and endothelium in renal and cardiac allografts and antitissue antibodies in liver allografts.[45,54,55] Autoantibodies and those antibodies reacting against a broad panel do not appear to be involved in the development of CTD.[56]

The mechanisms by which antibodies cause CTD have yet to be fully explained. It has been demonstrated experimentally that anti-HLA class I antibodies induce the expression of fibroblast growth factor receptor on the surface of endothelial and smooth muscle cells, conferring a theoretical increase in their ability to replicate under the influence of basic fibroblast growth factor.[57] This has not been confirmed in vivo.

MONOCYTES AND MACROPHAGES

Monocyte/macrophage infiltration is a prominent phenomenon in chronically rejecting grafts both experimentally and clinically. Macrophages are seen to undergo transformation to foam cells and these are found deposited in the subendothelial region. Their activity is associated with upregulation of the cytokines IL-1, IL-6 and TNF.[58] Transforming growth factor β (TGF-β) is also upregulated, and together these molecular mediators are likely to promote the fibrotic changes seen within chronically rejecting grafts.[58]

Molecular mediators

CYTOKINES

The cytokines found to be upregulated during CTD in animal models and clinical studies are illustrated in **Fig. 13.4**. The findings in different studies are not always consistent, but upregulation of IL-1, IL-6 and TNF-α have been reported in some clinical studies.[59] These cytokines are predominantly associated with monocyte and macrophage activity. During acute rejection IL-2, IL-4, TNF-α and IFN-γ are seen and these may impinge on the subsequent development of chronic rejection.[60,61]

GROWTH FACTORS

The growth factors associated with the development of CTD are also illustrated in **Fig. 13.4**. The key factors identified include TGF-β, PDGF and basic fibroblast growth factor (bFGF), although many more have been described.[60,61] TGF-β is a powerful profibrotic factor. It is chemotactic for fibroblasts and appears to exert its effects predominantly in the extracellular matrix, where it may be partly responsible for the development of interstitial fibrosis. There is a wide body of experimental and clinical data to support its upregulation during CTD and its putative role in the development of graft fibrosis. PDGF appears to be important in smooth muscle cell chemoattraction and may also have a role to play in monocyte/ macrophage responses.[62] bFGF is released from injured smooth muscle cells in the area adjacent to the damage.[59,63]

Cell senescence

Senescence is a natural phenomenon of cells whereby, after a finite number of divisions, key regulatory processes cease and cell replication no longer occurs. It has been proposed that graft parenchymal cells subjected to repeated damage undergo earlier or accelerated cell senescence with premature termination of these central regulatory processes.[64] One of the processes normally under the control of non-senescent cells is that of fibrosis. In early senescence, cellular control of fibrosis may be lost or disordered, thereby leading to widespread organ fibrosis.

AETIOLOGICAL FACTORS

Although many of the risk factors associated with the development of CTD have been identified, the precise aetiology and the way in which each of these factors interacts remain unknown. As CTD frequently overlaps, both clinically and histologically, with other causes of graft dysfunction, it is essential that a core needle biopsy be taken. There are currently no reliable surrogate markers for the presence of CTD and the use of biopsy-proven diagnosis in clinical studies is mandatory for credible results.

Assessing the impact of risk factor modification on the development and progression of CTD is problematic, as there are no reliable surrogate endpoints aside from graft loss. These studies usually require significant numbers of patients to be followed for long periods of time for differences in outcome to become apparent. However, the Barcelona group have shown that a protocol biopsy at 3 months may allow a reduction in sample size and the time of follow-up in trials aimed at preventing CAN.[65] The quest to unravel the aetiology of the disease is driven by the hope that further information in this area will lead to a breakthrough in the development of primary and secondary treatment strategies for what is currently an irreversible process. Both non-immune (antigen-independent) and immune (antigen-dependent) factors (**Table 13.1**) appear to have a role in the overall development and progression of the disease but the relative roles played by each is unclear.

It is difficult to determine the relative impact of each of these factors on the subsequent development of CTD and this is illustrated in the number of different animal models employed in experimental studies. For example, it is possible to demonstrate the histological changes of CTD in these models not only with varying combinations of immune and non-immune factors but also with wholly immune or wholly non-immune factors independently. It is likely that the aetiology of CTD is multifactorial and that an initial 'injury' is required after which time the graft goes on to develop the insidious and progressive changes of CTD. The major immune-mediated and non-immune-mediated aetiological risk factors will now be considered in greater detail.

Immune factors

ACUTE REJECTION EPISODES

In kidney, heart, lung and liver transplant recipients, acute rejection episodes correlate strongly with the subsequent development of CTD. In one series, recipients of cadaveric renal allografts who had never experienced an acute rejection episode were found to have a 5-year graft survival rate of 92%. In contrast, recipients experiencing one or more acute rejection episodes had an overall graft survival at 5 years of 45%.[66]

Further studies of both living-donor and cadaveric renal allografts showed that it was not simply the presence or absence of an acute rejection episode that predicted the likelihood of subsequent CAN but rather the nature of the rejection episode.[67–70] Early acute rejection episodes that are completely reversed do not appear to confer any greater degree of risk for the later development of CAN.[69]

Table 13.1 • Risk factors for chronic transplant dysfunction

Antigen-dependent	Antigen-independent
Acute rejection	Donor factors
HLA matching	Brainstem death
Host antibody response	Ischaemia/reperfusion
Non-compliance	Hypertension
	Hyperlipidaemia
	Cytomegalovirus
	Drug toxicity
	Functioning renal mass

The greatest risk factors for the development of CAN following an acute rejection episode are:[67–70]

1. Rejection episodes occurring after 3 months.
2. Recurrent rejection episodes.
3. Rejection episodes where the predominant histological changes are vascular rather than interstitial.
4. Incompletely reversed rejection episodes.

In lung allografts, the features of acute rejection associated with the development of bronchiolitis obliterans syndrome are:[71,72]

1. Repeated episodes.

2. Acute cellular rejection.

3. Increasing severity of the episode.

Combinations of these risk factors may prove to be more than additive when determining the relative risk for the development of CTD.

There are several theories to explain the late injury caused by these early immunological events although there is little scientific evidence to favour one explanation over another. In kidneys, the damage caused by the rejection episode may cause a reduction in the functioning nephron mass, subjecting the remaining nephrons to hyperfiltration thereby producing fibrotic changes. Alternatively, the rejection episode may persist in a subclinical form, despite apparent treatment, allowing ongoing immunologically mediated cell damage.[73]

Despite newer improved immunosuppressive agents resulting in less acute rejection there has not been any improvement in long-term graft survival. The main reason for this is that studies used to assess acute rejection rates were never powered to look at long-term graft outcomes. However, it may be that a greater number of marginal recipients are being transplanted with expanded criteria donor organs and therefore improvements caused by reduced acute rejection have been masked. Alternatively, acute rejection may be subclinical in its presentation and therefore not diagnosed and treated.

Despite the current lack of evidence for improved long-term graft survival with a reduction in acute rejection episodes, the association between acute and chronic rejection is so strong that, empirically, it seems justified to continue to aim to minimise the number and severity of acute rejection episodes.

HUMAN LEUCOCYTE ANTIGEN (HLA) MATCHING

Histocompatibility in solid-organ transplantation is of prime importance, as illustrated by data shown in **Fig. 13.5** from the Collaborative Transplant Study. They reveal that the optimal outcome for renal allografts with regard to long-term graft survival occurs in those patients who receive a fully matched organ.

It is also apparent that as the total number of mismatches at the six HLA loci increases, the half-

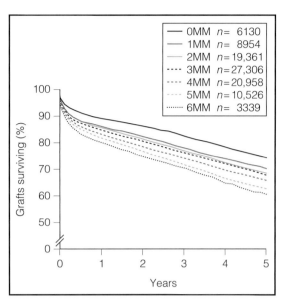

Figure 13.5 • HLA-A+B+DR mismatches for first cadaver kidney transplants 1985–2001. Reproduced with permission of Prof. G. Opelz, Collaborative Transplant Study.

life of the graft decreases. This holds true for all solid-organ transplants.[74,75]

Mismatches at the HLA-DR locus are associated with a poorer outcome than mismatches at the A and B loci. Multivariate analysis in lung transplantation has shown that mismatches at the HLA-A locus are the most predictive of CTD.[71] Transplants performed between monozygotic twins develop only minimal changes of CTD, if any at all.[76]

To confound the issue of HLA matching, the negative effect of a poorly mismatched graft can be overcome in live-donor transplantation. The benefits of a living-donor transplant such as short cold ischaemic time and absence of brainstem death-associated injury appear to negate the effect of a poor HLA mismatch, and excellent long-term graft survival is achieved.

ANTIBODIES

Although the role of the B lymphocyte and antibody response is well defined in hyperacute and, to a lesser extent, acute rejection, its role in CTD is less clear. Patients with raised levels of cytotoxic antibodies prior to transplantation demonstrate shorter graft half-lives than those patients in whom there is minimal sensitisation.[77] Similarly, the appearance of de novo antibodies in the post-transplant period is associated with an increased incidence of CTD.[56,78]

The nature of these antibodies is not well characterised but they are almost certainly directed at both the major and minor histocompatibility antigens. These have classically been described as cytotoxic antibodies. So-called non-cytotoxic antibodies have now also been described, with their exact role in chronic rejection still being unclear: for example, antibodies against cardiac and renal endothelial antigens, kidney tubular antigens and liver cell antigens.[45,55,79]

Clearly, the association between pre- and post-transplant antibody titres and the incidence of CTD does not prove a direct causal link between the two. There is, however, a growing body of experimental and clinical evidence upon which to base this assumption.

IMMUNOSUPPRESSION

Further data from the Collaborative Transplant Study (CTS) demonstrate differences in graft half-life depending on the maintenance immuno-suppression regimen used (**Fig. 13.6**). These data may be confusing, as they do not represent randomised trials of therapy. Previous CTS data of ciclosporin-based immunosuppression, illustrated in the previous edition of this chapter, showed that

although patients on monotherapy appear to have the most impressive graft survival, the group as a whole may be self-selecting and represent a group who require little immunosuppression anyway. Other registry data suggest that corticosteroids exert a negative effect on long-term graft outcome, but, equally, some studies assessing steroid withdrawal have reported the opposite.

Ciclosporin and tacrolimus have had a dramatic impact on reducing the number of acute rejection episodes in the first year post-transplantation but, as yet, have not demonstrated long-term benefit.[80] Similarly, sirolimus and mycophenolate mofetil have reduced acute rejection rates still further, but their use is now being pushed more directly towards the management of CTD as will be discussed later.

It must be remembered that differences in graft survival in relation to immunosuppressive regimens may not be due to purely immunological events. For instance, the calcineurin inhibitors tacrolimus and ciclosporin are well documented as being nephrotoxic. Both cause arteriolar vasoconstriction within the graft leading to chronic ischaemia and also upregulate the production of some growth factors and cytokines already implicated in CTD, such as TGF-β.

Non-immune factors

When long-term graft survival is compared between cadaveric (excluding 000 mismatched grafts) and non-HLA-identical live-donor transplants, the grafts from living donors have significantly better half-lives at all points post-transplantation.[1] By implication, the advantages conferred on these grafts must be related in part to the events involved in brainstem death, organ retrieval and organ preservation. It is now apparent that events occurring prior to transplantation may be as critical as many of the events occurring after it. Equally, organs with comparable pretransplantation characteristics are seen to have differing long-term outcomes where the graft half-lives are associated with differences in recipient characteristics such as blood pressure and lipid abnormalities.

DONOR FACTORS

UNOS (United Network of Organ Sharing) data have been used to identify donor factors predictive

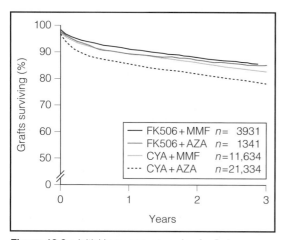

Figure 13.6 • Initial immunosuppression for first cadaver kidney transplants 1995–2001. FK506, tacrolimus; CYA, ciclosporin; MMF, mycophenolate mofetil; AZA, azathioprine. Reproduced with permission of Prof. G. Opelz, Collaborative Transplant Study.

of chronic allograft nephropathy.[81] Organs removed from donors at the extremes of age are associated with poorer long-term graft survival compared with young to middle-aged donors.[82] This may be related to the reduction in the transplanted nephron mass, and this theory is discussed later. Other donor risk factors include death from an acute cerebral haemorrhage, pre-existing hypertension, female gender and Afro-Caribbean ethnic origin.[1]

Brainstem death is significantly associated with a poor long-term graft survival and an increased incidence of delayed graft function and acute rejection.[83] Although the condition of brainstem death is well defined legally and neurologically, the systemic sequelae on the potential donor are very poorly understood. The effects of an irreversible and catastrophic injury to the brainstem include labile blood pressure, alterations in thermal regulation, endocrine and biochemical derangements plus pulmonary changes. Surges in catecholamine release are experienced, with resultant physical and structural changes affecting the vital organs. It may also be the trigger for the systemic release of a range of cytokines, causing a greater exposure of antigenic surface molecules, possibly as a result of endothelial cell retraction. The transplanted organ may prove more immunogenic to the recipient as a result.

ISCHAEMIA–REPERFUSION INJURY

Removal of the graft from the donor includes a short period of warm ischaemia, a more prolonged period of cold ischaemia and a subsequent reperfusion stage. All three events have been shown to produce organ damage, and the degree of ischaemia correlates with the subsequent development of CTD. There is widespread endothelial cell retraction and injury, causing antigen exposure, leucocyte adherence and upregulation of adhesion molecules [ICAM, VCAM and leucocyte functional antigen (LFA-1)] on the surface of the endothelium.[83,84] The antigenicity of the graft may be increased, as shown by an increased incidence of both acute rejection episodes and delayed graft function in grafts undergoing prolonged ischaemia.

HYPERTENSION

Hypertension is a risk factor for the development of CTD and is particularly important in relation to heart and kidney transplantation, and the majority of research has been focused on these two areas. Worsening degrees of post-transplant hypertension[85] have been shown to correlate with both the development of CTD and its rate of progression over time. There are currently no clinical trials to show that treating hypertension has any impact on either of these facts, although experimental animal models suggest that this may be the case.

HYPERLIPIDAEMIA

The post-transplant lipid profile is characterised by an increase in total cholesterol concentration with a predominance of cholesterol carried in low-density lipoproteins (LDL). There is also a significant increase in the percentage of cholesterol and triglycerides carried in very low-density lipoproteins (VLDL).[86] The effects of renal impairment and the hyperlipidaemic nature of immunosuppressive agents (steroids, ciclosporin and sirolimus in particular) cause these abnormalities.

Elevated levels of cholesterol and triglyceride are independent risk factors for CTD.[86] They are associated with adverse morphological changes on the Banff criteria, reduced glomerular filtration rate and proteinuria. There is also a strong correlation between hyperlipidaemia and the other main cause of late graft loss, death with a functioning graft.

Lipid-lowering agents may prove beneficial not only in the prevention of CTD but also in its treatment. Statins have been studied in experimental models and their action in reducing CTD appears to be related to inhibition of smooth muscle cell migration and proliferation in the endothelium.

CYTOMEGALOVIRUS DISEASE AND OTHER VIRAL DISEASE

Cytomegalovirus (CMV) replication can be detected in over 50% of allograft recipients and remains one of the most clinically significant organisms in solid-organ transplantation.[87] Apart from its direct role in causing clinical manifestations of active disease it may also be implicated in the pathogenesis of CTD, a theory proposed as far back as 1971.[88] Experimental evidence supports this theory in animal models of cardiac, renal and lung transplantation.[87] The true relevance of CMV and its involvement in the progression of CAN is still a topic of much deliberation. One large study in renal transplant recipients[89] suggested that CMV infection alone is not a risk factor for CAN. However, if acute rejection and CMV infection were present together then the progression of changes was far more rapid than if there was acute rejection alone. This result is contradicted by several studies in heart transplant recipients where transplant-associated coronary artery disease was much more common in those patients who received grafts from CMV-seropositive donors or who were themselves CMV seropositive either pretransplant or who subsequently acquired CMV seropositivity. Everett et al.[90] found in their cohort of 129 heart transplant recipients that neither primary CMV infection nor previous exposure to CMV antigens were risk factors for the development of graft vasculopathy. However, the presence of ongoing CMV viraemia and its duration was significant in the progression of vascular changes.

Experimentally, treatment of CMV disease and CMV viraemia with ganciclovir reduces the incidence and severity of CTD in experimental allografts but there are still no long-term data in the clinical setting to support this.

Interest is now turning to the role of other viral infections (particularly of the herpes class) and the role that they play in the development of chronic allograft disease. Polyoma virus (also called BK and JC virus) causes no symptoms in healthy individuals. In the presence of immunosuppression it has been documented as causing a tubulo-interstitial nephritis in kidney allografts and usually presents in a way that mimics acute rejection.[91] The true significance of the injury caused by this agent, and its impact on the development of chronic rejection in solid-organ transplants is still not clear.

OBESITY

Recipient obesity is an independent risk factor for the development of chronic rejection[1] and, in particular, when there is donor/recipient body mass index mismatch. The effect is probably related to the hyperfiltration effect of an inadequate nephron mass.[92]

HYPERFILTRATION

Hyperfiltration is a phenomenon seen specifically in kidney transplantation when there is inadequate functioning renal mass to provide for the needs of the transplant recipient. It may result in chronic renal allograft failure with functional and morphological

changes overlapping with those seen in chronic rejection.[93] Brenner et al. pioneered the hypothesis that a limited number of nephrons, regardless of aetiology, resulted in hyperperfusion, increased glomerular pressure and hence hyperfiltration in the remaining nephrons.

A limited functional nephron mass may arise in the following circumstances:[94]

1. Small kidneys from donors aged 4 to 6 years.
2. Transplants into large recipients (over 100 kg).
3. Grafts from females to males compared with males to females.
4. Kidneys that experience severe rejection episodes.
5. Cadaveric grafts compared with living-donor grafts.

Animal models of reduced nephron mass and hyperfiltration have reinforced the correlation between transplanted nephron mass and the subsequent changes of CTD.[95] In addition, augmenting limited nephron mass in these experimental models significantly reduces the incidence and severity of CTD.[96] It has been hypothesised by some groups[94] that late renal allograft loss in the absence of ongoing acute rejection in patients who have had a high serum creatinine from early on may actually occur as a consequence of hyperfiltration. Attributing causality to this phenomenon, however, remains difficult.

THERAPEUTIC OPTIONS

Currently there are no established and effective treatment regimens for the prevention or treatment of chronic rejection although much work has been done in the experimental setting towards looking for such agents. There is an increasing body of evidence that the newer immunosuppressants may aid in reducing the incidence and minimising the progression of CTD. Interpreting data from existing clinical studies is difficult because of low patient numbers in trials or because of the heterogeneity of large cohorts from multiple centres. Few trials are randomised, patients frequently act as their own controls and follow-up is limited. Control groups have been drawn from historical groups of transplant patients but this is of limited value due to the rapid progression that has been made in all aspects of transplantation.

The difficulties encountered in designing studies in this area are well documented, and several publications have provided comprehensive overviews of the individual problems faced.[97,98] The commonest problems are:

1. Establishment of endpoints – at present graft loss is the only reliable endpoint, although there is some evidence to show that findings on protocol biopsy at 3 months may be reliable.[65]
2. Designation of entry criteria – the establishment of diagnostic criteria has enabled uniformity of entry criteria.
3. Identification of a control population.
4. Funding – graft loss is insidious and it is necessary to follow large groups of patients for lengthy periods to show conclusive differences between treatment groups. The cost of such studies is considerable.

To overcome some of these difficulties, it would be beneficial to identify early surrogate markers of chronic rejection. Many units are now moving towards performing surveillance protocol biopsies that will not only aid in providing accurate histological assessment of the clinical problem of CTD but will also allow for treatment modifications to be assessed.

Future study design will need to include suitable endpoints whilst providing adequate patient numbers and follow-up periods to power studies to detect differences in long-term outcomes. One of the reasons that earlier studies of new immunosuppressive agents have not shown improved graft half-life is that these studies were never powered to detect long-term differences. They were designed instead to look primarily at the effect upon acute rejection episodes in the early post-transplant period, this being deemed of greater importance.

The ultimate aim with CTD is to prevent its occurrence (primary prevention). This 'gold standard' will almost certainly prove elusive in the majority and therefore accurate diagnosis and subsequent treatment – secondary treatment – is more attainable. The aim of both of these strategies is to prolong allograft survival. If the diagnosis is missed, eventually there will come a point of no return beyond which, despite intervention, the graft will not be salvageable. At this point graft fibrosis and graft arteriosclerosis are too extensive to be amenable to treatment.

A variety of non-immunological as well as immunological therapeutic treatment options have been explored in recent years, with the former representing the earliest trials of therapy and the latter now assuming precedence.

In addition, risk factor avoidance is likely to play a significant role in reducing the relative risk of an individual developing CTD. The evidence for the efficacy of this approach is so far lacking because, although the risk factors have been well described, authors have seldom gone on to prove a causal relationship between such factors and the development of chronic rejection.

Primary prevention

Prevention of the disease process is likely to remain one of the foremost challenges within the field of transplantation. It is perhaps unrealistic to presume that a single agent or single risk factor modification will achieve this goal. Prevention, therefore, must start empirically with the reduction of known risk factors. The following factors are potentially modifiable:

1. Minimisation of organ ischaemia.
2. Avoidance of HLA mismatches.
3. Avoidance of body mass index discrepancies between donor and recipient.
4. Cautious use of expanded criteria donors.
5. Reduction in the incidence of acute rejection episodes and, in particular, those episodes occurring late with prominent vascular changes.
6. Avoidance of immunosuppressive drug toxicity.
7. Avoidance of suboptimal immunosuppression and non-compliance.
8. Aggressive control of hypertension.
9. Control of conventional risk factors for atherosclerosis, e.g. dyslipidaemia, diabetes, smoking.
10. Prevention and aggressive treatment of CMV/viral disease.

To date, prospective randomised studies of risk factor modification have not been performed and consequently the available results are from registry data. The problems of such data analysis have already been alluded to.

Secondary treatment

NON-IMMUNOLOGICAL AGENTS

Prior to the advent of an expanded armamentarium of immunosuppressive agents, the majority of experimental and clinical studies reported results based on the use of non-immunological agents. Most of the study designs were not robust and therefore results have to be interpreted with caution. The results achieved were generally poor with few of the measures established in clinical practice. An exception to this may be the use of statin therapy in the treatment of hyperlipidaemia. As discussed below, this may be attributable to the fact that the range and mode of action of non-immune agents is more diverse than was first considered. The types of non-immunological agents that have been investigated in recent years are briefly outlined below with an overview of clinical and experimental studies provided in **Table 13.2**.

Prostacyclin analogues and thromboxane antagonists

Patients with CTD have significantly lower levels of prostaglandins and raised levels of thromboxane when compared with matched controls.[99] The normal action of prostaglandins is to inhibit platelet aggregation and smooth muscle cell proliferation. Thromboxanes have the opposite effect and the resultant imbalance promotes a state of increased platelet aggregability and smooth muscle cell proliferation. The use of prostacyclin analogues and thromboxane antagonists is designed to redress the balance.

Antiplatelet drugs

The use of agents such as aspirin, dipyridamole and indomethacin has been tried in an effort to reduce platelet aggregability and adhesion. This is based on the rationale that a reduction in release of growth factors results in downregulatuion of the immune cascade, which plays a role in the development of the arteriosclerotic lesions of CTD.

Polyunsaturated fatty acids

Modulation of dietary polyunsaturated fatty acids is thought to reduce platelet aggregability, reduce hyperlipidaemia, aid restoration of the thromboxane–prostacyclin imbalance and alter the inflammatory response.[100] This approach is reliant on the omega-3 group of polyunsaturated fatty acids.

Statins (hydroxymethylglutaryl-CoA reductase inhibitors)

Statins not only reduce LDL cholesterol levels but are also known to act directly on smooth muscle cells, preventing their migration. They may also cause vasodilatation as a result of nitric oxide synthesis. Their direct action on smooth muscle cells is a promising feature in their potential role in altering the progression of CTD, as a reduction in smooth muscle cell migration may lessen the degree of graft arteriosclerosis.

Angiopeptin

Angiopeptin is a somatostatin analogue and its therapeutic effect is likely to be related to its inhibitory effects on the release of growth factors involved in intimal proliferation. Its inhibitory action affects many growth factors including PDGF, EGF, insulin-like growth factor 1 (IGF-1) and TGF-α.[101]

Heparin and its derivatives

Heparins have been shown to reduce smooth muscle cell proliferation.[102] As previously stated downregulation of smooth muscle cell proliferation may impact on the degree of graft arteriosclerosis.[86]

Nitric oxide synthase upregulation

Nitric oxide synthase (and hence nitric oxide) is upregulated in chronically rejecting allografts and is protective against allograft arteriosclerosis[103,104] and post-transplant obliterative airways disease.[105] This is achieved by inhibiting platelet and leucocyte adhesion on the endothelium and also by suppressing the activity of neointimal smooth muscle cells.

IMMUNOLOGICAL AGENTS

The use of immunological agents in the prevention and treatment of CTD has come to the forefront with the advent of newer immunosuppressive

Table 13.2 • Non-immunological agents in chronic transplant dysfunction

Agent	Ref.	Study type	Results/comments
Antiplatelet drugs	Musket and Burton (1987)[134]	Cardiac transplant (rat)	No effect (aspirin/dipyridamole)
	Hoyt et al. (1984)[135]	Cardiac transplant (rat)	No effect (aspirin/dipyridamole in conjunction with ciclosporin)
	Michielson et al. (1990)[136]	Clinical (renal)	Improvement in graft survival in a percentage of patients (indomethacin)
	Matthew et al. (1974)[137]	Clinical (renal)	Warfarin and dipyridamole – ineffective
	Teraoka et al. (1997)[138]	Clinical (renal)	Satigrel – improvement in stage of CAN and renal function
Polyunsaturated fatty acids	Yun et al. (1991)[139]	Cardiac transplant (rabbit)	Reduced graft arteriosclerosis
	Sweeny et al. (1989)[140]	Clinical (renal)	Reduced rate of decline of graft function
Prostacyclin analogues/ thromboxane antagonists	Fellstrom et al. (1991)[141]	Cardiac transplant (rabbit)	Iloprost infusion – reduced chronic rejection
	Leithner et al. (1981)[142]	Clinical (renal)	Improved short-term graft function
	Teraoka et al. (1987)[99]	Clinical (renal)	Reduced graft loss (prostacyclin analogue + antiplatelet agent + anticomplement)
	Paul and Fellstrom (1992)[143]	Clinical (renal)	Improved graft function (prostacyclin analogue + salicylate + dipyridamole)
	Teraoka et al. (1987)[144]	Clinical (renal)	Reduced rate of decline in renal function (thromboxane antagonist)
Statins	Katznelson et al. (1995)[145]	Clinical (heart)	Reduced intimal hyperplasia
	ALERT study (ongoing)	Clinical (renal)	European multicentre trial – effect of statins on cardiac events and chronic rejection (awaited)
Angiopeptin	Asotra et al. (1989)[146]	Aortic balloon injury (rabbit)	Inhibitor of intimal cell proliferation
	Foegh (1993)[147]	Cardiac transplant (rabbit)	Inhibitor of graft arteriosclerosis
	Meiser et al. (1992)[148]	Cardiac transplant (rat)	Inhibitor of myointimal hyperplasia
	Fellstrom et al. (1991)[141]	Cardiac transplant (rat)	Reduced intimal proliferation
Heparins	Clowes and Clowes (1989)[149]	Balloon injury (rat)	Reduced graft arteriosclerosis
Nitric oxide synthase upregulation	Albrecht et al. (2003)[150]	Aortic transplant (rat)	L-arginine is protective against graft arteriosclerosis
Protein restriction	Feehally et al. (1986)[151]	Clinical (renal)	Reduced rate of graft loss
Oestrogens	Foegh et al. (1989)[152]	Cardiac transplant (rabbit)	Reduced graft arteriosclerosis
	Cheng et al. (1991)[153]	Aortic transplant (rabbit)	Reduced graft arteriosclerosis
Carbon monoxide	Otterbein et al. (2003)[154]	Carotid balloon injury (rats and mice)	Reduced vascular stenosis in response to injury
Perfenidone	Waller et al. (2002)[155]	Carotid balloon injury (rat)	Inhibition of intimal thickening

agents. Immunosuppressive regimens have been developed that are capable of markedly reducing acute rejection rates during the first year post-transplant compared with previous regimens. Despite lower acute rejection rates improvements in long-term graft survival are yet to be seen. This may be because studies have not used this as an objective endpoint. Ciclosporin was the first immuno-suppressant to achieve a dramatic reduction in the incidence of acute rejection episodes in the first year. It demonstrated a 20% improvement in 1-year graft survival rates. Further improvements in the incidence of acute rejection during this first year have been demonstrated with tacrolimus and mycophenolate mofetil, and more recently with sirolimus and the IL-2 receptor antagonists (basiliximab and daclizumab).

Tacrolimus has achieved a reduced rate of acute rejection episodes in liver and kidney transplantation in both US trials and the European Multicentre trials when compared with conventional ciclosporin therapy.[106–108] In addition, there was a trend towards improved renal function and significantly improved lipid profiles in those patients treated with tacrolimus. Significant differences in patient or graft survival have not been shown to date.

Mycophenolate mofetil (MMF) was initially used as a replacement agent for azathioprine in triple drug immunosuppressive regimes in kidney trans-plantation. Three large multicentre trials have demonstrated the efficacy of MMF in reducing acute rejection rates when being used in con-junction with ciclosporin and steroids.[109] There was no demonstrable improvement in graft survival at three years.[110] In cardiac recipients a difference in graft survival in favour of MMF has also been demonstrated on a treated, but not on an intention-to-treat analysis.[111]

With regard to the treatment of established CTD, immunosuppressive agents appear to have a role to play. The early work in this area was performed in kidney transplantation as this provided the largest patient population. The calcineurin inhibitors are known to be nephrotoxic and the hypothesis was that if the dose of these agents could be reduced or withdrawn then this might remove the poten-tially nephrotoxic effect. There was a risk that the resultant reduction in immunosuppression would

lead to acute rejection. Underimmunosuppression is known as one potential risk factor for chronic allograft nephropathy.[112]

Tacrolimus was initially used as a replacement for ciclosporin because of its reduced nephrotoxicity. The early results suggested that a percentage of patients respond to conversion therapy either by a reduction in the rate of decline of renal function or, in some instances, by a partial recovery in renal function.[113] Associated benefits include a reduced requirement for antihypertensives and an improved lipid profile.

MMF has shown much more promise. The initial trials involved combination immunosuppressive therapy where MMF was added to the existing ciclosporin maintenance regimen with good short-term effect in a percentage of patients.[114,115] Following this, several authors have reported a further improvement in short-term outcomes with ciclosporin reduction regimes.[116] The same group has since reported longer-term follow-up on this cohort of patients, again suggesting long-term benefits in renal allograft function.[117] Several groups have now demonstrated the advantages of complete calcineurin inhibitor withdrawal in patients with deteriorating renal allograft function without complications associated with the reduced level of immunosuppression.[118,119] Advantages were also seen in blood pressure control, the number of anti-hypertensive medications required and lipid profiles, thus further modifying aetiological factors important in the slowing of progression in CTD.

The work in kidney transplantation is now being translated into other solid-organ transplants. MMF is increasingly being used to protect native renal function where calcineurin inhibitors have been used for other solid-organ transplants. Barkmann et al.[120] showed that both acute nephrotoxicity and chronic renal failure could be improved in liver transplant recipients on cyclosporin when MMF was substituted. MMF has also been used as the primary agent in liver transplantation thus avoiding the need for calcineurin inhibitors altogether.

Sirolimus and everolimus may be used as alter-natives or an adjunct to MMF in calcineurin inhibitor-sparing regimes. They have been used in combination with calcineurin inhibitors, with a reduction in acute rejection rates, and have been shown in experimental models to reduce the amount of graft arteriosclerosis even when organs have been exposed to long periods of cold ischaemia.[121,122] The latter finding was something of a surprise considering their hyperlipidaemic effect. Their action is to inhibit the intracellular signalling distal to the IL-2 receptor and they are therefore potentially useful even if significant IL-2 release has already occurred. More recently, longer-term follow-up (2 years) has been reported showing improvements or stability in renal function in patients maintained on sirolimus following ciclosporin withdrawal.[123] Everolimus has been shown in cardiac transplantation to reduce graft vasculopathy although data are only available at 1 year.[124] These agents could therefore offer a potential treatment alternative for patients with allograft failure who are unable to tolerate MMF.

FTY720 is a new immunosuppressive agent that is still in the experimental and very early clinical phase of its development. By altering T-cell trafficking, the expression of certain cell adhesion molecules is affected and has improved acute rejection rates. The work in CTD is limited to rat heterotopic cardiac transplantation where it is already showing promise in reducing allograft vasculopathy.[125,126]

FUTURE PROSPECTS

The scope for improving management of patients with CTD is huge. Many treatment modalities could be used in order to achieve this goal. The majority of work is still directed at therapeutic approaches that will prevent or manipulate the process of CTD by modulating the immune response.

As has been described, the role and use of MMF and sirolimus in the treatment of established CTD is fast gaining acceptance.

The current aim of most working groups is to prevent CTD from developing, and therefore many studies are in progress aiming to answer the question how early can calcineurin inhibitors be reduced and/ or withdrawn from immunosuppression protocols? The balance that needs to be achieved is to maintain

adequate immunosuppression and therefore avoid acute rejection episodes whilst still gaining the benefits of reduced nephrotoxicity.

The use of monoclonal antibodies in CTD has not yet been examined in the clinical arena.

As the mechanisms of co-stimulation are investigated further new monoclonal antibodies are being developed. These aim to target specific cell-surface epitopes that play a role in T-cell stimulation, in particular CD4+ T cells. The idea being entertained is that indirect alloantigen recognition plays a vital role in the pathogenesis of true immunologically mediated chronic rejection and that by manipulating this pathway a state of 'tolerance' may be achieved. The main cell-surface targets of monoclonal antibodies at present are CTLA4,[127] CD28,[128] CD40/CD154,[129] CD45[130] and CD52.[131] These are all showing promise in various experimental models of allograft vascular disease but little work has been transferred into clinical trials to date.

Monoclonal antibody work is also being directed at the depletion of specific subsets of T cells, with evidence that both CD4+ and CD8+ cells may play important roles. Modulation of cell apoptosis guided by CD8+ cytotoxic T cells is one target,[132] and CD4 T-cell depletion (thus blocking indirect allorecognition) is another.[133] Only experimental vascular models have been used for these studies.

Solving the problem of CTD remains a key aim for those involved in the field of transplantation. A multidisciplinary team approach will be required with interventions being necessary from the time of organ retrieval throughout the effective life of that graft. The ultimate aim should be to create a scenario where a transplanted organ is for life and where re-transplantation is almost eliminated, or at the very least where organ and patient survival are maximised as far as possible. Now that the clinical problem of acute rejection has been thoroughly addressed more emphasis needs to be placed on designing large well-controlled randomised trials to look specifically at CTD rather than treating it as a secondary issue.

Key points

- Chronic transplant dysfunction is the commonest cause of graft loss after the first post-transplant year.
- It is manifested as a progressive decline in organ function in the absence of any other diagnosed cause for this deterioration, such as an acute rejection episode, drug nephrotoxicity or recurrence of the original disease.
- The histological features common to all organ types are graft vessel arteriosclerosis, perivascular inflammation and organ fibrosis.
- Both non-immune (antigen-independent) and immune (antigen-dependent) factors have a role in the overall development and progression of CTD.
- There are no established and effective regimens for the prevention and treatment of CTD; but primary prevention by minimising known risk factors, and secondary treatment with some of the newer immunosuppressive agents have shown promise.

REFERENCES

1. Cecka J, Terasaki P. In: Terasaki PI, Cecka MJ eds. Clinical Transplants 1994, Los Angeles, California: UCLA Tissue Typing Laboratory 1995; pp. 1–18.

2. Johnson DE, Alderman EL, Schroeder JS et al. Transplant coronary artery disease: histopathological correlation with angiographic morphology. J Am Coll Cardiol 1991; 17(2):449–57.

3. Gao SZ, Alderman EL, Schroeder JS et al. Accelerated coronary vascular disease in the heart transplant patient: coronary arteriographic findings. J Am Coll Cardiol 1988; 12:334.

4. Nissen SE, Yock P. Intravascular ultrasound: novel pathophysiological insights and current clinical applications. Circulation 2001; 14:604–16.

5. Mehra MR, Ventura HO, Stapleton DD et al. Presence of severe intimal thickening by intravascular ultrasonography predicts cardiac events in cardiac allograft vasculopathy. Circulation 1995; 14:632–9.

6. Billingham ME. Graft coronary disease: the lesions and the patients. Transplant Proc 1989; 21(4): 3665–6.

7. Paul LC, Hayry P, Foegh M et al. Diagnostic criteria for chronic rejection/accelerated graft arteriosclerosis in heart and kidney transplant recipients: joint proposal from the Fourth Alexis Carrel Conference on chronic rejection and accelerated graft arteriosclerosis in transplanted organs. Transplant Proc 1993; 25(2):2022–3.

   This paper gives the consensus view of the diagnostic criteria for chronic rejection in kidney and heart transplants that arose out of a multidisciplinary conference to examine the problem. The criteria are listed in the text.

8. Dennis M, Foster MC, Ryan JJ et al. The increasing importance of chronic rejection as a late cause of renal allograft failure. Transplant Int 1989; 2:214–17.

9. Isoniemi HM, Krogerus L, von Willibrand E et al. Histopathological findings in well-functioning, long-term renal allografts. Kidney Int 1992; 41:155–60.

10. Isoniemi H, Taskinen E, Hayry P. Histological chronic allograft damage index accurately predicts chronic renal allograft rejection. Transplantation 1994; 58(11):1195–8.

11. Solez K, Axelson RA, Benediktsson H et al. International standardisation of criteria for the histologic diagnosis of renal allograft rejection: the Banff working classification of kidney transplant pathology. Kidney Int 1993; 44:411–22.

12. Racusen LC, Solez K, Colvin RB et al. The Banff 97 working classification of renal allograft pathology. Kidney Int 1999; 55:713–23.

   The Banff classification of renal allograft pathology is an international consensus that was devised to standardise biopsy interpretation, both to guide therapy and establish objective endpoints for clinical trials. This is the current published working version.

13. Candinas D, Gunson B, Nightingale P et al. Sex mismatch as a risk factor for chronic rejection for liver allografts. Lancet 1995; 346:1117–21.

14. Freese DK, Snover DC, Sharp HL et al. Chronic rejection after liver transplantation: a study of clinical, histopathological and immunological features. Hepatology 1991; 13(5):882–91.

15. Deligeorgi-Politi H, Wight DGD, Calne RY et al. Chronic rejection of liver transplants revisited. Transplant Int 1994; 7:442–7.

16. Pirsch JD, Kalayoglu M, Hafez GR et al. Evidence that the vanishing bile duct syndrome is vanishing. Transplantation 1990; 49:1015–18.

17. Hayry P, Isoniemi H, Yilmaz S et al. Chronic allograft rejection. Immunol Rev 1993; 134:33–80.

18. Demetris AJ, Seaburg EC, Batss KP et al. Chronic liver allograft rejection: a National Institute of Diabetes and Digestive and Kidney Diseases institutional study analyzing the reliability of

current criteria and proposal of an expanded definition. Am J Surg Pathol 1998; 22(1):28–39.

19. Oguma S, Belle S, Starzl TE et al. A histometric analysis of chronically rejected human liver allografts: insights into the mechanisms of bile duct loss: direct immunologic and ischaemic factors. Hepatology 1989; 9:204–9.

20. Reichenspurner H, Girgis RE, Robbins RC et al. Stanford experience with obliterative bronchiolitis after lung and heart-lung transplantation. Ann Thorac Surg 1996; 62(5):1467–72.

21. Garone S, Ross DJ. Bronchiolitis obliterans syndrome. Curr Opin Organ Transplant 1999; 4(3):254–63.

22. Kelly K, Hertz MI. Obliterative bronchiolitis. Clin Chest Med 1997; 18(2):319–38.

23. Yousem SA, Bery GJ, Cagle PT et al. Revision of the 1990 working formulation for the classification of pulmonary allograft rejection: Lung Rejection Study Group. J Heart Lung Transplant 1996; 15:1–15.

24. Ikonen T, Kivisaari L, Harjula AL. Value of high-resolution computed tomography in routine evaluation of lung transplantation recipients during development of bronchiolitis obliterans syndrome. J Heart Lung Transplant 1996; 15(6):587–95.

25. Tazelaar H, Yousem S. Pathologic findings in heart-lung transplantation. Hum Pathol 1988; 208:371–8.

26. Wyatt SE, Nunn P, Hows JM et al. Airways obstruction associated with graft versus host disease after bone marrow transplantation. Thorax 1984; 39:887–94.

27. Cooper JD, Billingham ME, Egan T et al. A working formulation for the standardisation of nomenclature and for clinical staging of chronic dysfunction in lung allografts. J Heart Lung Transplant 1993; 12(5):713–16.

These are the published working formulations of a committee of the ISHLT with regard to staging and standardisation of chronic dysfunction in lung transplants.

28. Sutherland DER, Gruessner A. Long-term function (>5 years) of pancreas grafts from the international transplant registry database. Transplant Proc 1995; 27:2977–80.

29. Allen RDM. Pancreas transplantation. In: Forsythe JLR (ed.) Transplantation surgery, 1st edn. London: WB Saunders, 1997; pp. 167–201.

30. Hayry P, Alatalo S, Myllarniemi M et al. Cellular and molecular biology of chronic rejection. Transplant Proc 1995; 27(1):71–4.

31. Demetris AJ, Zerbe T, Banner B. Morphology of solid organ arteriopathy: identification of proliferating intimal cell populations. Transplant Proc 1989; 21:3667–72.

32. Vella JP, Knoflach A, Waaga AM et al. T-cell mediated immune responses in chronic rejection: role of indirect allorecognition and co-stimulation. Graft 1998; 2(suppl. 2):13–17.

33. Abe M, Kawai T, Tanabe K et al. Post-operative production of anti-donor antibody and chronic rejection in renal transplantation. Transplantation 1997; 64:795–800.

34. Davenport A, Younie M, Parsons J et al. Development of cytotoxic antibodies following renal allograft transplantation is associated with reduced graft survival due to chronic vascular rejection. Nephrol Dial Transplant 1994; 9:1315–19.

35. Cramer DV. The role of humoral responses in chronic rejection. Graft 1998; 1(2):18–20.

36. Foegh ML. Chronic rejection – graft arteriosclerosis. Transplant Proc 1990; 22(1):119–22.

37. Lemstrom K, Koskinen P, Hayry P. Molecular mechanisms of chronic renal allograft damage. Kidney Int 1995; 48(suppl. 52):S2–10.

38. Hayry P, Aavik E, Savolainen H. Mechanisms of chronic rejection. Transplant Proc 1999; 31(suppl. 7A):5S–8S.

39. Hillebrands J-L, Klatter FA, Rozing J. Origin of vascular smooth muscle cells and the role of circulating stem cells in transplant arteriosclerosis. Art Thromb Vasc Biol 2003; 23:380–7.

40. Hayry P. Chronic rejection – an update on the mechanism. Transplant Proc 1998; 30:3993–5.

41. White E, Hildeman WH, Mullen Y. Chronic kidney allograft rejection in rats. Transplantation 1969; 8:602–17.

42. Mannon RB, Kopp JB, Ruiz P et al. Chronic rejection of mouse kidney allografts. Kidney Int 1999; 55:1935–44.

43. Russel PS, Chase CM, Winn HJ. Coronary atherosclerosis in transplanted mouse hearts. J Immunol 1994; 152(10):5135–41.

44. Russel PS, Chase CM, Colvin RB. Contributions of cellular and humoral immunity to arteriopathic lesions in transplanted mouse hearts. Transplant Proc 1997; 29(6):2527–8.

45. Rose EA, Smith CR, Petrossian GR et al. Humoral immune responses after cardiac transplantation: correlation with fatal rejection and graft arteriosclerosis. Surgery 1989; 106:203–7.

46. Hayry P, Renkonen R, Leszczynski D et al. Rat aortic allografts: an experimental model for chronic renal allograft arteriosclerosis. Transplant Proc 1991; 23:611–12.

47. Tullius SG, Heeman UW, Hancock WW. Long-term kidney isografts develop functional and morphologic changes that mimic those of chronic allograft rejection. Ann Surg 1994; 220(4):425–32.

48. Tullius SG, Tilney NL. Both alloantigen-dependent and -indepedent factors influence chronic allograft rejection. Transplantation 1995; 59(3):313–18.

49. Paul LC. Experimental models of chronic rejection. Transplant Proc 1995; 27(3):2126–8.

50. Paul LC. Antibodies and chronic organ graft rejection. Curr Opin Organ Transplant 1999; 4:23–7.

51. Jeanett M, Pinn VW, Flax MH et al. Humoral antibodies in renal allotransplantation in man. N Eng J Med 1970; 282:111–17.

52. Paul LC, Muralidharan J, Muzaffer SA et al. Antibodies against mesangial cells and their secretory products in chronic renal allograft rejection in the rat. Am J Pathol 1998; 152:1209–23.

53. De Heer E, Davidoff A, van der Waal A et al. Chronic renal allograft rejection in the rat: transplant induced antibodies against basement membrane antigens. Lab Invest 1994; 70:494–502.

54. Mohanakumar T, Waldrep JC, Phibbs M et al. Serological characterisation of antibodies eluted from chronically rejected human renal allografts. Transplantation 1981; 32:61–6.

55. Paul LC, Baldwin WM, Van Es LA. Vascular endothelial antigens in renal transplantation. Transplantation 1985; 40:117–23.

56. Sucia-Foca N, Reed E, d'Agati DV et al. Soluble HLA-antigens, anti-HLA-antibodies and anti-idiotypic antibodies in the circulation of renal transplant recipients. Transplantation 1991; 51:593–601.

57. Harris PE, Bian H, Reed EF. Induction of high affinity fibroblast growth factor receptor expression and proliferation in the human endothelial cell by anti-HLA antibodies: a possible mechanism for transplant atherosclerosis. Immunology 1997; 159: 5697–704.

58. Nadeau KC, Azuma H, Tinley NL. Sequential cytokine dynamics in chronic rejection of rat renal allografts: roles for cytokines RANTES and MCP-1. Proc Natl Acad Sci USA 1995; 92(19):8729–33.

59. Lindner V, Reidy MA. Proliferation of smooth muscle cells after vascular injury is inhibited by an antibody against basic fibroblast growth factor. Proc Natl Acad Sci USA 1991; 88:3739–43.

60. Norohna IL, Weis H, Hartley B et al. Expression of cytokines, growth factors and their receptors in renal allograft biopsies. Transplant Proc 1993; 25: 917–18.

61. Hancock WW, Whitley WD, Baldwin WM et al. Cells, cytokines, adhesion molecules and humoral responses in a rat model of chronic renal allograft rejection. Transplant Proc 1992; 24:2315–16.

62. Ross R, Raines EW, Bowen-Poe DF. The biology of platelet derived growth factor. Cell 1986; 46:155–69.

63. Lindner V, Lappi DA, Baird A et al. Role of basic fibroblast growth factor in vascular lesion formation. Circ Res 1991; 68:106–13.

64. Paul LC. Current knowledge of the pathogenesis of chronic allograft dysfunction. Transplant Proc 1999; 31:1793–5.

65. Seron D, Moreso F, Ramon J et al. Protocol renal allograft biopsies and the design of clinical trials aimed to prevent or treat chronic allograft nephropathy. Transplantation 2000; 69(9):1849–55.

66. Kahan BD. Towards a rational design of clinical trials of immunosuppressive agents in transplantation. Immunol Rev 1993; 136:29–49.

67. Basadonna GP, Matas AJ, Gillingham KJ et al. Early versus late renal allograft rejection: the impact on chronic rejection. Transplantation 1993; 55(5):993–5.

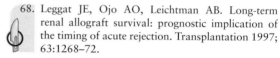

68. Leggat JE, Ojo AO, Leichtman AB. Long-term renal allograft survival: prognostic implication of the timing of acute rejection. Transplantation 1997; 63:1268–72.

A group of 31 600 first cadaveric renal transplants in USA were studied. It was shown that a late episode of rejection either alone or in combination with previous episodes of acute rejection led to inferior graft outcome.

69. Opelz G. Critical evaluation of the association of acute with chronic graft rejection in kidney and heart transplant recipients. Transplant Proc 1997; 29:73–6.

70. Humar A, Kerr S, Hassoun A et al. The association between acute rejection and chronic rejection in kidney transplantation. Transplant Proc 1999; 31:1302–3.

71. Kroshus TJ, Kshetty VR, Savik K et al. Risk factors for the development of bronchiolitis obliterans syndrome after lung transplantation. J Thorac Cardiovasc Surg 1997; 114:195–202.

72. Heng D, Phil M, Sharples LD et al. Bronchiolitis obliterans syndrome: incidence, natural history, prognosis and risk factors. J Heart Lung Transplant 1998; 17(12):1255–63.

A single-centre study of 230 lung transplant patients followed 109 patients who developed BOS. BOS adversely affected outcome and acute rejection was a major prognostic factor.

73. Rush DN, Karpinski ME, Nickerson P et al. Does subclinical rejection contribute to chronic rejection in renal transplant patients? Clin Transplant 1999; 13(6):441–6.

74. Opelz G. Strength of HLA-A, HLA-B and HLA-DR mismatches in relation to short and long-term kidney graft survival. Transplant Int 1991; 5(suppl. 1):S621.

75. O'Grady JG, Alexander G, Sutherland S et al. Cytomegalovirus and donor/recipient HLA antigens: interdependent co-factors in the pathogenesis of vanishing bile duct syndrome after liver transplantation. Lancet 1988; 2(8606):302–5.

76. Tilney NL. Renal transplantation between identical twins: a review. World J Surg 1986; 10:381–8.

77. Cecka JM. Outcome statistics of renal transplants with an emphasis on long-term survival. Clin Transplant 1994; 8(3 Pt 2):324–7.

78. Thomas JM, Thomas FT, Kaplan AM et al. Antibody-dependent cellular cytotoxicity and chronic renal allograft rejection. Transplantation 1976; 62:201–5.

79. Wheeler CH, Collins A, Dunn MJ et al. Characterisation of endothelial antigens associated with transplant associated coronary artery disease. J Heart Lung Transplant 1995; 14:S188–97.

80. European Multicentre Study. Tacrolimus vs. cyclosporin in renal transplantation: five-year follow-up of the European Multicentre study. Am J Transplantation 2002; 2(suppl. 3):238.

81. Chertow GM, Brenner BM, Mackenzie HS et al. Non-immunological predictors of chronic renal allograft failure: data from the United Network of Organ Sharing. Kidney Int 1995; 48(suppl. 52):S48–51.

82. Alexander JW, Bennett LE, Breen TJ. Effect of donor age on outcome of kidney transplantation: a two-year analysis of transplants reported to the United Network of Organ Sharing Registry. Transplantation 1994; 57:871–6.

83. Pratschke J, Kusaka M, Wilhelm MJ et al. Chronic rejection: effect of brain death and ischaemia/reperfusion. Graft 1998; 1(2):34–6.

84. Tilney NL. Chronic rejection and its risk factors. Transplant Proc 1999; 31(suppl. 1/2A):S41–4.

85. Cheigh JS, Haschemaeyer RH, Wang JC et al. Hypertension in kidney transplant recipients: effect of long-term renal allograft survival. Am J Hypertens 1989; 2:341–9.

86. Arnadottir M, Berg A-L. Treatment of hyperlipidaemia in renal transplant recipients. Transplantation 1997; 63(3):339–45.

87. Tolkoff-Rubin NE, Rubin RH. The impact of cytomegalovirus infection on graft function and patient outcome. Graft 1999; 2(2):S101–3.

88. Simmons RL, Fallon RJ, Schulenberg WE. Do mild infections trigger the rejection of renal allografts. Transplant Proc 1970; 1:419–23.

89. Humar A, Gillingham KJ, Payne WD et al. Association between cytomegalovirus disease and chronic rejection in kidney transplant recipients. Transplantation 1999; 68(12):1879–83.

90. Everett JP, Hershberger RE, Norman DJ et al. Prolonged cytomegalovirus infection with viraemia is associated with development of cardiac allograft vasculopathy. J Heart Lung Transplant 1992; 11(3 Pt 2):S133–7.

91. Randhawa PS, Finkelstein S, Scantlebury V et al. Human polyoma virus associated interstitial nephritis in the allograft kidney. Transplantation 1999; 67(1):103–9.

92. Nicholson ML, Windmill DC, Horsburgh T et al. Influence of allograft size to recipient body-weight ratio on the long-term outcome of renal transplantation. Br J Surg 2000; 87(3):314–19.

93. Brenner BM, Cohen RA, Milford EL. In renal transplantation, one size may not fit all. J Am Soc Nephrol 1992; 3:162–9.

94. Terasaki PI, Koyama H, Cecka JM et al. The hyperfiltration hypothesis in human renal transplantation. Transplantation 1994; 57:1450–4.

> The authors conclude that the five conditions, listed in the text, under which hyperfiltration damage might be suspected all had increased failure rates. Such failures are almost never reported as 'due to hyperfiltration' and are probably recorded as rejections.

95. Heeman UW, Tullius SG, Azuma H et al. The association between reduced functioning kidney mass and chronic rejection in rats. Transplant Int 1994; 7(suppl. 1):S328–30.

96. Heeman UW, Azuma H, Tullius SG et al. Influence of renal mass on chronic kidney allograft rejection in rats. Transplant Proc 1995; 27:549.

97. Kasiske BL, Massy ZA, Guijarro C et al. Chronic renal allograft rejection and clinical trial design. Kidney Int 1995; 48(suppl. 52):S116–19.

98. Paul LC, Sijpkens YWJ. Surrogate endpoints in chronic kidney graft rejection studies. Transplantation 1999; 31:1293–4.

99. Teraoka S, Takahashi Y, Toma H. New approach to management of chronic vascular rejection with prostacyclin analogue after kidney transplantation. Transplant Proc 1987; 19:2115–18.

100. Harris WS. Fish oils, plasma lipid and lipoprotein metabolism in humans: a clinical review. J Lipid Res 1989; 30:785.

101. Wanders A, Akyurek ML, Waltenburger J et al. Impact of ischaemia on chronic vascular rejection in the rat – effect of angiopeptin. Transplant Proc 1993; 25(2):2098–9.

102. Castellot JJ, Favreau LV, Karnovsky MJ et al. Inhibition of vascular smooth muscle cell growth by endothelial cell-derived heparin: possible role of platelet endoglycosidase. J Biol Chem 1982; 257:1256–8.

103. Lee PC, Wang ZL, Qian S et al. Endothelial nitric oxide synthase protects aortic allografts from the development of transplant arteriosclerosis. Transplantation 2000; 69(6):1186–92.

104. Romagnani P, Pupilli C, Lasagni L et al. Inducible nitric oxide synthase expression in vascular and glomerular structures of human chronic allograft nephropathy. J Pathol 1999; 187(3):345–50.

105. Romanska HM, Ikonen TS, Bishop AE et al. Up-regulation of inducible nitric oxide synthase in fibroblasts parallels the onset and progression of fibrosis in an experimental model of post-transplant obliterative airway disease. J Pathol 2000; 191(1):71–7.

106. European FK Multicentre Study Group. Randomised trial comparing Tacrolimus (FK506) and cyclosporin in prevention of liver allograft rejection. Lancet 1994; 344:423–8.

107. Pirsch J, Miller J, Deierhoi M et al. A comparison of Tacrolimus (FK506) and cyclosporin for immuno-suppression after cadaveric renal transplantation. Transplantation 1997; 63:977–83.

108. Mayer D, Dmittrewski J, Squifflet J. Multicentre randomised trial comparing Tacrolimus (FK506) and cyclosporin in the prevention of renal allograft rejection: a report of the European Tacrolimus Multicentre Study Group. Transplantation 1997; 64:436–43.

109. Halloran P, Matthew T, Tomlanovitch S et al. Mycophenolate mofetil in renal allograft recipients. Transplantation 1997; 63:39–47.

110. Matthew T. A blinded, long-term, randomised, multicentre trial of Mycophenolate Mofetil in cadaveric renal transplantation: results at three years: tri-continental Mycophenolate Mofetil study group. Transplantation 1998; 65:1450–4.

111. Kobishigawa J, Miller L, Renlund D. A randomised active-controlled trial of Mycophenolate Mofetil in heart transplant recipients: Mycophenolate Mofetil investigators. Transplantation 1998; 66:507–15.

112. Kuo P, Manaco AP. Chronic rejection and sub-optimal immunosuppression. Transplant Proc 1993; 25(2):2082–4.

113. Morris-Stiff G, Baboolal K, Singh J et al. Conversion from cyclosporin to Tacrolimus in renal allograft recipients with chronic allograft neph-ropathy. Transplant Proc 1998; 30:1245–6.

114. Jirasiritham S, Sumethkul V, Mavichak S et al. Treatment of chronic rejection in renal trans-plantation by Mycophenolate Mofetil (MMF): a preliminary report of six-month experience. Transplant Proc 1998; 30:3576–7.

115. Kliem V, Boeck A, Eisenberger U et al. Treatment of chronic renal allograft failure by addition of Mycophenolate Mofetil: single centre experience in 40 patients. Transplant Proc 1999; 31:1312–13.

116. Weir MR, Anderson L, Fink JC et al. A novel approach to the treatment of chronic allograft neph-ropathy. Transplantation 1997; 64(12):1706–10.

117. Weir MR, Ward MT, Lahut SA et al. Long-term impact of discontinued or reduced calcineurin inhibitor in patients with chronic allograft neph-ropathy. Kidney Int 2001; 59(4):1567–73.

118. Francois H, Durrbach A, Amor M et al. The long-term effect of switching from Cyclosporin A to Mycophenolate Mofetil in chronic renal graft dys-function compared with conventional management. Nephrol Dial Transplant 2003; 18(9):1909–16.

119. Graetz K, O'Dair J, Boswell A et al. Does conversion to Mycophenolate Mofetil in chronic allograft nephropathy prolong graft survival? Presented at American Congress of Transplantation, Washington 2003. Am J Transplantation 2003; 3(suppl. 5):555.

120. Barkmann A, Nashan B, Schmidt HH et al. Improvement of acute and chronic renal dysfunction in liver transplant patients after substitution of calcineurin inhibitors by Mycophenolate Mofetil. Transplantation 2000; 69(9):1886–90.

121. Schmid C, Heeman U, Azuma H et al. Rapamycin inhibits transplant vasculopathy in long-surviving rat heart allografts. Transplantation 1995; 60:729–33.

122. Cole OJ, Shehata M, Rigg KM. Effects of SDZ-RAD on transplant arteriosclerosis in the rat aortic model. Transplant Proc 1998; 30(5):2200–3.

123. Oberbauer R, Kreis H, Johnson RW et al. Long-term improvement in renal function with Sirolimus after early Cyclosporin withdrawal in renal trans-plant recipients: 2-year results of the Rapamune Maintenance Regimen Study. Transplantation 2003; 76(2):364–70.

124. RAD B253 Study Group. Everolimus for the prevention of allograft rejection and vasculopathy in cardiac transplant recipients. N Engl J Med 2003; 349(9):847–58.

125. Koshiba T, Van Damme B, Rutgeerts O et al. FTY720, an immunosuppressant that alters lympho-cyte trafficking, abrogates chronic rejection in combination with Cyclosporine A. Transplantation 2003; 75(7):945–52.

126. Cheuh SC, Chen JR, Chen J et al. FTY720 prevents chronic rejection of rat heterotopic cardiac allo-grafts. Transplant Proc 2001; 33(1-2):542–3.

127. Sayegh M, Zheng X, Magee C et al. Donor antigen is necessary for the prevention of chronic rejection in CTLA4-Ig treated murine cardiac allografts. Transplantation 1997; 64: 1646–50.

128. Laskowski IA, Pratscke J, Wilhelm MJ et al. Anti-CD28 monoclonal antibody therapy prevents chronic rejection of renal allografts in rats. J Am Soc Nephrol 2002; 13(2):519–27.

129. Yuan X, Dong VM, Coito AJ et al. A novel CD154 monoclonal antibody in acute and chronic rat vascularized cardiac allograft rejection. Transplantation 2002; 73(11):1736–42.

130. Sho M, Harada H, Rothstein DM et al. CD45RB targeting strategies for promoting long-term allograft survival and preventing chronic allograft vasculopathy. Transplantation 2003; 75(8):1142–6.

131. Knechtle SJ, Pirsch JD, Fechner J et al. Campath-1H induction plus Rapamycin monotherapy for renal transplantation: results of a pilot study. Am J Transplant 2003; 3(6):722–30.

132. Legare J, Issekutz T, Lee T et al. CD8+ T-lymphocytes mediate destruction of the vascular media in a model of chronic rejection. Am J Pathol 2000; 157:859–65.

133. Szeto WY, Krasinskas AM, Kriesal D et al. Depletion of recipient CD4+ but not CD8+ T-lymphocytes prevents the development of cardiac allograft vasculopathy. Transplantation 2002; 73(7):1116–22.

134. Muskett A, Burton NA. The effect of antiplatelet drugs on graft arteriosclerosis in rat heterotopic cardiac allografts. Transplant Proc 1987; 19(4):74–6.

135. Hoyt G, Collin G, Billingham M et al. Effect of antiplatelet regimes in combination with cyclosporin on heart allograft vessel disease. J Heart Transplant 1984; 4:54–7.

136. Michielson P, Vanrenterghem Y, Roels L et al. Is there a treatment for chronic rejection? In: Proceedings of the 21st CITIC. Transplantation Immunology 1990:209.

137. Matthew TH, Kincaid-Smith P, Saker BM et al. A controlled trial of oral anticoagulants and dipyridamole in cadaveric renal allografts. Lancet 1974; 1(7870):1307–10.

138. Teraoka S, Ota K, Tanabe K et al. Multi centre trial of the therapeutic effect of a newly developed anti-platelet agent, Satigrel, on biopsy-proven chronic rejection after kidney transplantaiton. Transplant Proc 1997; 29: 266–71.

139. Yun KL, Fann JI, Sokoloff MH et al. Dose response of fish oil versus sunflower oil on graft arterio-sclerosis in rabbit heterotopic cardiac allografts. Ann Surg 1991; 214:155–67.

140. Sweeney P, Wheeler DC, Lui SF et al. Dietary fish oil supplements preserve renal function in renal transplant recipients with chronic vascular rejection. Nephrol Dial Transplant 1989; 4: 1070–5.

141. Fellstrom B, Dimeny E, Foegh ML et al. Accelerated atherosclerosis in heart transplants in the rat simulating chronic vascular rejection: effects of prostacyclin and angiopeptin. Transplant Proc 1991; 23: 525–8.

142. Leithner C, Sinzinger H, Schwartz M. Treatment of chronic kidney transplant rejection with prostacyclin. Prostaglandins 1981; 22(5):783–8.

143. Paul LC, Fellstrom B. Chronic vascular rejection of the heart and the kidney – have rational treatment options emerged? Transplantation 1992; 53:1169–79.

144. Teraoka S, Oba A, Takahashi K et al. Therapeutic effect of antiplatelet agents on obstructive vascular lesions after kidney transplantation with cyclosporin. Transplant Proc 1987; 19:77–81.

145. Katznelson S, Kobashigawa JA. Dual roles of HMG-CoA reductase inhibitors in solid organ trans-plantation: lipid lowering and immunosuppression. Kidney Int 1995; 52:S112–15.

146. Asotra NS, Foegh ML, Vargas R. Inhibition of thymidine incorporation by angiopeptin in the aortas of rabbits after balloon angioplasty. Transplant Proc 1989; 21(4):3695–6.

147. Foegh ML. Accelerated cardiac transplant athero-sclerosis/chronic rejection in rabbits: inhibition by angiopeptin. Transplant Proc 1993; 25(2)2095–7.

148. Meiser BM, Wolf S, Devens C et al. Continuous infusion of angiopeptin significantly reduces accelerated graft vessel disease induced by FK506 in rat allograft model. Transplant Proc 1992; 24(5):1671–2.

149. Clowes AW, Clowes MM. Inhibition of smooth muscle cell proliferation by heparin molecules. Transplant Proc 1989; 21(4):3700–1.

150. Albrecht EW, van Goor H, Smit-van Oosten A et al. Long-term dietary L-arginine supplementation attenuates proteinuria and focal glomerulosclerosis in experimental chronic renal transplant failure. Nitric Oxide 2003; 8(1):53–8.

151. Feehally J, Harris KPG, Bennett SE et al. Is chronic renal transplant rejection a non-immunological phenomenon? Lancet 1986; 2:486–9.

152. Foegh ML, Khiribadi BS, Chambers E. Peptide inhibition of accelerated transplant atherosclerosis. Transplant Proc 1989; 21(4):3674–6.

153. Cheng LP, Kuwahara M, Jacobsson J et al. Inhibition of myointimal hyperplasia and macro-phage infiltration by estradiol in aorta allografts. Transplantation 1991; 52(6):967–72.

154. Otterbein LE, Zuckerbraun BS, Haga M et al. Carbon monoxide suppresses arteriosclerotic lesions associated with chronic graft rejection and with balloon injury. Nature Med 2003; 9(2):183–90.

155. Waller JR, Toomey D, Metcalfe MS et al. Pirfenidone inhibits early neointimal proliferation following arterial injury. Transplant Proc 2002; 34(5):1486–8.

Index